NPLEX Homeopathic Materia Medica Study Guide

Steve Olsen ND, DHANP

ISBN-13: 978-1494871413

ISBN-10: 1494871416

All rights reserved, including translation. No part of this book may be used, reproduced, or transmitted in any form electronic or mechanical, including print, photocopying, recording or any retrieval or storage system, or by any other means whatsoever without the prior written permission of the copyright holder.

Self-published by Author, Steve Olsen ND

Snohomish, Washington USA

Copyright August, 2014

Printed in the USA

All rights reserved

steveolsen@iinet.com

REFERENCES

There are many quotes and references in this text taken from current and past authors. I have tried to integrate this information with what is most useful and pertinent to each remedy combined with my own experience. Every author and homeopath has had to do the same, that is build on information from provings made by Hahnemann and others; then built on provings with cured cases and therefore each remedy can gradually become known in all of its aspects. Lippe for example in his materia medica listed below makes reference to 72 other authors! They all deserve our deep felt acknowledgment and appreciation.

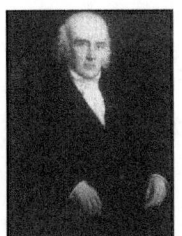
Hahnemann

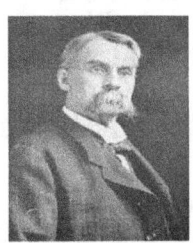
Kent

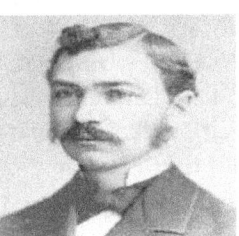
Boericke

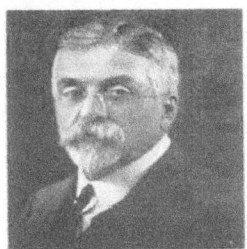
Clark

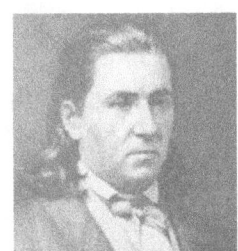
Hering

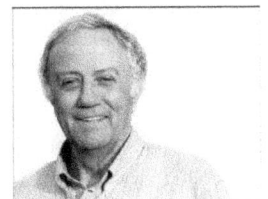
Vithoulkas

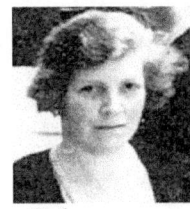
Tyler

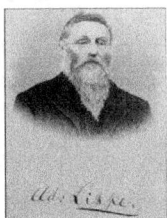
Lippe

These remedies have been used over and over for the symptoms and conditions that I have listed. This Study Guide I have written is useful as a starting point for many remedies but it is only the beginning as there is always more to learn. One can best begin to learn a remedy within a framework that can later be filled in with more details. At the beginning it is not the totality of symptoms for each remedy one is expected to learn but rather a summary of symptoms put into order from most to least important.

Recommended Reading

Lectured on Homeopathic Materia Medica J.T. Kent
Keynotes & Red Line Symptoms   by Lippe
Keynotes and Characteristics of the Materia Medica by Allen, H. C.
Leaders in Homeopathic Therapeutics by Nash, E. B.
Pocket Manual of Homeopathic Materia Medica with Repertory by William Boericke, W.
Materia Medica Viva by George Vithoulkas.
Books by C.M.Boger.
Farrington: Clinical Lectures
Books by Edwin Moses Hale.
Materia Medica by Carol Dunham.
New, Old and Forgotten Remedies: Dr. E. P. Anshutz.
Materia Medica by Massimo Mangialavori.

Table of Contents

Acknowledgements   i

Forward   i

Chapter 1 First Aid Remedies   5

Chapter 2 Remedies for Chronic Ailments   39

Appendix One, Case Studies   355

Appendix Two, The Periodic Table   369

Appendix Three, Wound Healing, Systemic Infections   389

Appendix Four, Snake Remedies   407

Appendix Five, On Line Resources   422

Alphabetical Index

ACONITUM NAPELLUS...6
AESCULUS HIPPOCASTANUM 40
AGARICUS MUSCARIUS..41
AILANTHUS GLANDULOSA..43
ALLIUM CEPA..46
ALOE...44
AMBRA GRESIA...48
AMBROSIA 50
ANACARDIUM ORIENTALE..50
ANDROCTONUS..52
ANTIMONIUM TARTARICUM.......................................56
ANTIMONIUM CRUDUM...53
APIS MELLIFICA..8
APOCYNUM CANNABINUM..58
ARGENTUM NITRICUM...59
ARNICA MONTANA...12
Arnica Montana Case Study.......................................355
ARSENICUM ALBUM...65
ARSENICUM IODATUM...64
ARUM TRIPHYLLUM...74
ARUNDO DONAX..74
AURUM METALLICUM..75
AURUM SULPH...80
AURUM MURIATICUM..79
BAMBUSA...81
BAPTISIA...85
BAPTISIA TINCTORIA 399
BARYTA CARBONICA...81
BELLADONNA...87
BELLIS PERENNIS...17
BOTHROPS LANCEOLATUS..94
BRYONIA ALBA...97
Bufo rana..391

CALCAREA PHOSPHORICA..119
CALCAREA CARBONICA..115
CALCAREA IODATUM..118
CALCAREA SULPHURICUM..129
CALENDULA..18
CAMPHORA...131
CANTHARIS..20
CARBO ANIMALIS..21
CARBO-VEG...133
Carcinosin..138
CARCINOSIN..138
CARDUUS MARIANUM...142
Case Studies..355
CAUSTICUM...144
Cenchris...407
CHAMOMILLA..146
CHELIDONIUM MAJUS...149
CHOCOLATE..150
CINA MARITIMA...151
CINCHONA...156
COCA..160
COCCULUS INDICUS 163
COCCUS CACTI..164
COFFEA CRUDA 165
COLOCYNTHIS 168
CONIUM MACULATUM 169
CONVALARIA MAJALIS 197
CRATAEGUS 199
Crotalus cascavella 414
Crotalus horridus...414
CUBEBA 200
CUPRUM METALLICUM..201
CYCLAMEN 204
CYPRIPEDIUM 205
DROSERA..206

DULCAMARA	206
ECHINACEA	390
ELAPS CORALLINUS	208
EUPATORIUM PERFOLIATUM	222
EUPHRASIA	223
FERRUM METALLICUM (Iron)	223
FERRUM PHOSPHORICUM	224
GELSEMIUM	226
GINSENG	229
GLONOIN	230
HEPAR SULPHUR CALCAREUM	233
HYDRASTIS	238
HYOSCYAMUS	239
HYPERICUM PERFORATUM	23
Ignatia	26
IGNATIA AMARA	25
IODUM	242
IPECACUANHA	244
KALI BICHROMICUM	253
KALI CARBONICA	255
KALI MURIATICUM	257
KALI NITRICUM	257
KALI SULPHURICUM	261
KALI-PHOHORICUM	258
LAC-CANINUM	262
LAC-HUMANUM	264
LACHESIS	267
LECITHINUM	270
LEDUM PULUSTRE	29
LYCOPODIUM	272
MAGNESIA CARBONICA	276
MAGNESIA PHOSPHORICUM	281
MAGNESIA SULPHURICA	282
MAGNESIUM MURIATICUM	281

MEDORRHINUM..286
MERCURIUS..282
MYRISTICA..406
Naja..417
NATRUM SULPHURICUM..296
NATRUM CARBONICUM..292
NATRUM MURIATICUM...293
NATRUM PHOSPHORICA...295
NICCOLUM..296
NUX MOSCHATA..297
NUX VOMICA..297
On-Line Resources..422
OPIUM...300
PETROLEUM...301
PHOSPHORUS..301
PHYTOLACCA...309
PLATINA...311
PODOPHYLUM..312
PSORINUM...313
PULSATILLA...314
PYROGENIUM..405
RHUS TOXICODENDRON...32
Ruta..34
RUTA GRAVEOLENS 34
SANICULA AQUA...318
SEPIA..319
SILICA...322
Snake Remedies...407
SPONGIA..327
STAPHASAGRIA..330
STRAMONIUM..335
Strychninum..300
SULPHUR...337
SULPHUR IODATUM...340
SULPHUROSUM ACID..340

SYMPHYTUM	36
Systemic Infections	390
TABACUM	340
TARENTULA	341
TAXUS BREVIFOLIA	343
The periodic table	369
THUJA	343
URTICA URENS	348
VERATRUM ALBUM	348
VIOLA ODORATA	353
Vipera berus	419
Wound Healing – Systemic Infections	389

ACKNOWLEDGMENTS

To my students, patients and teachers.

Foreword

The information provided here is the beginning point for any student of homeopathy and it will help you to pass your board exam. I have been teaching this same material since 1988, at various Naturopathic schools. I have found this information to be the most reliable for my daily practice.

It has often been asked, how can one study and learn the materia medica? There are so many remedies and each remedy has so many symptoms. Far too many symptoms to remember. Many remedies also have the same symptoms as other remedies, therefore how can one be distinguished from the other? Here are six ways to think about this problem.

1. **Unusual symptoms**: Always look for what are the most unusual symptoms for each remedy. As Hahnemann said, always look for: *the more striking, exceptional, unusual, and odd (characteristic) sign and symptoms <in the patient>*. (Aphorism 153). It is the same when we learn each remedy, we need to find out and remember what is striking and unusual about it but also seen in most patients that need that remedy. If these peculiar symptoms of the remedy correspond with the peculiar symptoms of the patient then most likely you have found the correct remedy or are very close to finding it. For lack of a better word we call these 'keynote' symptoms.

2. **Modalities:** Hahnemann goes on to say: *The more common and intermediate symptoms (lack of appetite, headaches, lassitude, restless sleep, discomfort, etc) are to be seen with almost every disease and medicine and thus deserve little attention ...* (Aphorism 153). In other words it is not helpful to try and remember common symptoms such as pain, or nausea or fatigue but rather what is special about the pain or nausea or fatigue; such as the type of pain, when it comes on, what makes it better or worse etc. Common symptoms such as pain, paint a blurry unfocused picture, the picture of the remedy needs to be sharpened and brought into focus by modalities; such as what makes the symptom better or worse.

3. **Themes and Mental Emotional Symptoms**: Discover and remember the main theme or themes of the remedy, a main idea that makes that remedy come to life in some way, a theme that is usually present for all who need that remedy. For example: Chamomilla has great *irritability*, Aconite has a marked *fear of death*, Pulsatilla is very *mild and yielding*. This helps us because as soon as you meet your patient this theme will usually be evident even without asking one question. For chronic and most acute cases the remedy will have to match the main themes of the

patient.

4. **General Symptoms and Sensations**: Learn the strong general symptoms and strong sensations for each remedy. For Hepar sulphur we have: *great sensitivity to cold*, for Pulsatilla we have: *desire for fresh air,* for Euphorbium we have *very strong burning pains* etc. These symptoms are present for almost every patient that needs that remedy.

5. **Causation:** Some remedies are best known for the strong exciting causes such as never well since an injury (Arnica) or never well since grief (Ignatia).

6. **Pathology:** The pathology of what the remedy can treat is also important; Magnesia remedies treat the liver, Lachesis treats headaches, Ceanothus treats the spleen etc, but it comes in last place in what you need to know, as many remedies will treat almost any pathology and you can use a remedy for a pathology that it is not listed for when all or many of the symptoms in the four other categories above are present. Some remedies we only know according to what pathology and common symptoms they treat but this makes it very difficult to decide when to use that remedy. We need modalities, general symptoms, the emotional state and themes to help us.

Following these six criteria is the most sure method to learn materia medica. If you can learn all the keynotes, themes of the mental state, modalities, sensations, general symptoms and pathology then you have learned a meaningful totality of symptoms for each remedy. Each remedy will also become unique and not like any other.

One can think if this totality of symptoms as a story or a picture. Imagine a child locked out of their house on a dark night. They are all alone, wild animals are snarling nearby with huge sharp teeth. The child runs but is chased down and devoured. The elements of this story or image are: Fear of dark, fear of being attacked, the attempt to defend themselves out of fear of death, feeling of terror, fear to be alone at night, feeling abandoned. This is the story or image of Stramonium and many patients who need this remedy will tell you that emotionally they have this same story *as if* they were alone at night etc but it may be a veteran with PTSD or an abused child or for some other reason such as being bullied at school. The remedy treats the reaction to the stress and this is the image we need to learn for each remedy.

Each remedy is like this. It is a picture that we can add to as we learn more about it. When the patient tells their symptoms it is a story full of images, colors, textures, emotions and facts you are painting, the image of which you then try to match to a remedy with the same image.

Example of learning a remedy and bringing it into focus. Each remedy can be broken down into separate characteristics and symptoms. If we can see enough of these unique symptoms we can recognize that person or remedy as unique. By analogy we can look at the nose (special characteristics), ears (special characteristics), forehead (special characteristics), hair (special characteristics), chin (special characteristics), etc but finally we want to see a meaningful totality. For each of us these parts are unique and we have an amazing ability to see how all the parts fit together so we can all be recognized as individuals. Here is an example:

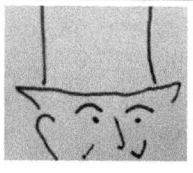
Who is this? This is often the image one can get after studying the main pathology of a remedy such as it treats ear infections and severe pain. It is the information one can get in the first 15 minutes of case taking. It is not in focus as we need a theme, modalities, keynotes and the strong general symptoms.

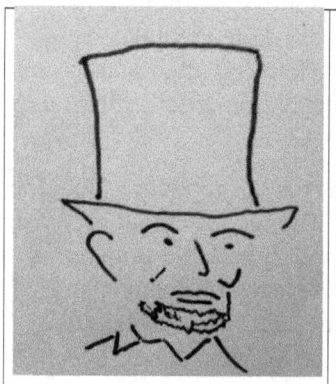
Finally we see the clear image of Abraham Lincoln. After one hour plus of case taking or after learning the characteristic symptoms of a remedy we can draw the images to the left. The characteristic traits will fit together in a recognizable way.

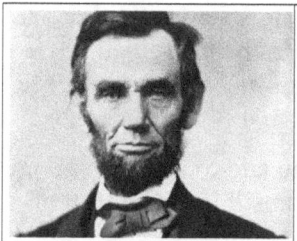
We can learn a remedy as well we can see to the right if and when one gets to use it successfully a few times. Only a few times a year will the image be this clear in a patient.

After you give the correct remedy and the patient is better it always looks very clear in retrospect as you know what is important to look at :-)

Another way to look at how to collect symptoms in the problem of naming birds correctly. It is not helpful to determine the name of a bird because the bird has feathers, wings, eyes as as all birds have these characteristics; just as most sick people have pain, fatigue and loss of sleep. But there are many people who can tell one bird from the other very easily. 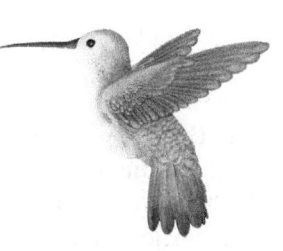 They learn what is characteristic and special about each one such as the song, its coloration, what it eats, how it flies and many other special criteria. It is the same with our remedies; there are special things about each one.

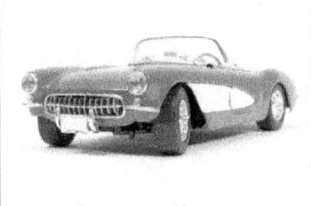 For those who love cars there is a final analogy. When you build a car one piece has to fit with the next piece till you recognize what you have. It is the same with learning a remedy. Add one characteristic symptoms to the next till you see the whole unique subject. What is the name of this car? We could find out because it has very distinguishing (unique) characteristics.

CHAPTER 1

FIRST AID

These are the twelve remedies which are used most often for first aid situations. But they are also useful for acute illnesses and even many chronic complaints are treated with them; but primarily they are used for first aid. One way to learn these remedies is to know that each one is able to heal a specific tissues.

Arnica: Muscle tissue. Tendons and ligaments. *Soreness as if beaten.*

Bellis perennis: Muscle, tendons, connective tissue. *Overuse.*

Calendula: Epithelial (skin) tissue. *Cuts and scrapes.*

Aconite: Neurological tissue. *Fear of death.*

Hypericum: Nerve tissue. *Shooting pains.*

Ledum: All soft tissues such as muscles, blood vessels, tendons, immune system.

Rhus tox: Muscles and tendons leading to stiffness.

Ruta: Connective tissue, white fibrous tissues. Overuse injuries.

Cantharis: Burns to epithelial tissue.

Ignatia: Neurological tissue, grief.

Apis: Immune system, allergic reactions.

Carbo animalis: Muscle and connective tissue, *weakness.*

Remedies for Accidents and Injuries
These remedies also treat many chronic ailments

ACONITUM NAPELLUS
(Monkshood)

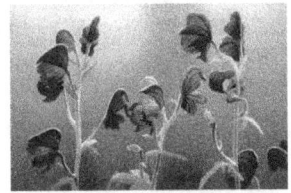

Rapid onset of acute symptoms attended with <u>sudden</u> ANXIETY and FEAR OF DEATH.

Examples: Anxiety after a car accident. Fear and panic after a natural disaster such as an earthquake. Panic feeling after being attacked or chased.

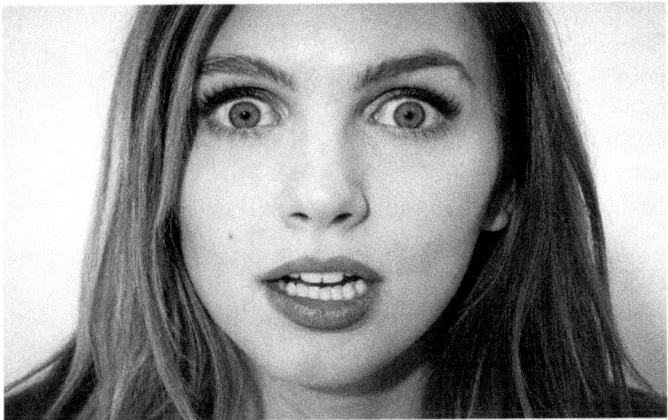

Sudden severe complaints attended with ***an agonizing fear of imminent death.*** A fright arising from a shock - such as a car accident, heart attack injury that threatens ones life.

Case: 1. A 35 year old women driving on ice, her car spun out and hit the guard rail, then when she was out looking at her car another car hit the same ice sheet and amost crashed into her!! After this she went into shock with papitations, anxiety and trembling. A year later when she came to see me she was still having sudden anxiety episodes when she would drive her car, get on an airplane or go through a tunnel or over a bridge. After a few doses of Aconite 30c these fears went a way.

2. I received a call late at night from a distraught parent. Their 4 year old child has a sudden onset of a fever of 104 deg F. (40d Cel.) The child was very anxious as she was having trouble breathing and was restless. A dose of Aconite 30c calmed the child, the fever went down and the parents called me the next day to say she had slept well, with no symptoms to report.

3. A 55 year old women with anxiety. Her father would yell at her so violently as a child she would shake and almost faint. After Aconite 30c she is much calmer and no longer has panic attacks.

Physical symptoms include:
- skin dry, swollen and hot with fever
- violent pains that are intolerable accompanied by acute inflammations
- intense thirst
- rapid heartbeat with anxiety
- restless
- hyperventilating
- trembling
- heart palpitations
- tossing about with anguish and restlessness

Mental symptoms include:
- anxiety of the mind
- panic
- fear of open spaces
- fear of crowds
- fear of narrow places
- distressed
- agitated
- inconsolable
- in severe acute inflammatory conditions the fear may be intense

An illness which comes on suddenly (often only minutes or hours):
- after exposure to dry cold wind, fright, or shock.
- such as colds, influenza, fever, pneumonia, or inflammation of almost any organ system.

Aconite is helpful during labor or before surgery, if the person is terrified of dying.

Some remedies, including Aconite, are especially effective when the cause of fright is known. Aconite is very helpful, for example, when the cause of the fright is from a sudden and intense specific stress; such as a car accident, earthquake, upcoming surgery, or labor. When the stress is accompanied with the possibility of losing one's life.

Many times, people who have experienced a shock like this become fearful of crowds, narrow places, further earthquakes, tunnels, being on airplanes, etc. If these symptoms become chronic Aconite can still be the correct remedy.

Chronic phobic or anxiety states are often helped by Aconite. The anxiety being an overwhelming, SUDDEN, intense fear accompanied with palpitations of the heart that is out of proportion to the situation at hand. This may last for hours or suddenly stop. After calming down, the anxiety is easily triggered again, thus becoming a chronic cycle. A phobia is an intense, specific fear of something, such as an intense fear of death, which they feel all the time for no apparent reason.

Children needing Aconite typically experience:
- night terrors 10 minutes after falling asleep
- trouble breathing
- the feeling of suffocation
- the feeling they are dying
- stuttering following a fright (Stram)
- vision, hearing, or the sense of smell become distorted after a fright
- numbness and tingling in the extremities

APIS MELLIFICA
(Honey-Bee)

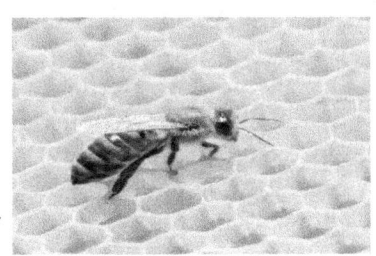

SWELLING WORSE FROM HEAT.
Bee **stings. Allergic reactions. Hives.**

Apis is a wonderful remedy. We all know

the symptoms of a bee sting and these are also the symptoms it will cure such as edematous *swelling* (swelling of the skin as if it were filled with water), stinging pains, redness, *itching*, a sensation of heat and *allergic* reactions.

It will also with great success treat urticaria which is <u>worse from heat,</u> and infections with swelling, pain and redness. Generally the person feels <u>worse in a warm room</u> and is thirstless.

For example, Apis is the first remedy to treat the effects of a bee sting. One dose will prevent all the usual symptoms of a sting from developing and save the patient from much suffering, especially if they happen to be allergic to stings.

This remedy is a perfect example of the law of similars. A large dose of bee venom injected into the body by an angry bee will produce edematous swelling, stinging pains, redness and itching, or perhaps even a more severe allergic reaction, such as swelling of the air passages leading to anaphylaxis or an acute asthma attack.

With diluted homeopathic doses of Apis venom, the body will have a very strong reaction against the remedy and, as a result, it will build up its defense forces to protect itself from the remedy. These same healing responses also work to cure any swelling or allergic reactions which occur in the body as a result of the bee sting.

It is interesting that there is a type of arthritis which responds positively to bee stings. These people purposefully expose themselves to live bees with the hope of being stung. The arthritis subsequently improves for some time after this therapy. This is an example of the same law of similars at work; the joints are also red, inflamed and swollen and therefore respond to small doses of bee venom. It would be much easier and less painful to take a few doses of homeopathic Apis instead! For first aid, use Apis for the following reasons:

☼. Sun allergy with swelling of the skin, itching and burning or stinging pain. May have dermatographia (light scraping of the skin produces a red raised histamine/allergic rash).
☼ Bee, wasp, ant and any other insect bite or sting. Look for the typical swelling, redness, itching, stinging inflammatory process.

ⴰ Allergic reactions from any cause, such as nettles, poison oak, pollen, dust, animal dander, animal or insect bites or foods such as shellfish etc. which lead to swollen eyes, runny itchy eyes, swelling of the sinuses, painful sinuses, mucous from the sinuses, swelling or itching of the throat, swelling of the uvula (a soft grape like sack that hangs from the roof of the mouth), swelling of the bronchi leading to a difficulty in breathing, rashes, swelling of the skin, *hives* on the skin, welts, red raised itchy patches of swollen skin and burning or stinging pain in any of these tissues.

ⴰ *Anaphylactic shock* (an allergic hypersensitivity reaction), resulting in difficult breathing, blueness of body parts, sometime convulsions, unconsciousness and possible death due to any cause, such as a bee sting, blood transfusion, eating shellfish, peanuts, injection of a medical agent, i.e., vaccination, antibiotic, etc.

During my third year at the Bastyr clinic, a severely asthmatic person collapsed and stop breathing. She turned blue and looked as if she were about to die. The attending naturopathic physician opened her mouth and put a dose of homeopathic Apis 30c under her tongue. Within seconds she coughed and started to suck in air again. I believe Apis saved this woman's life.

In a situation needing Apis, the observation of some type of allergic or histamine type of reaction, which leads to swelling, inflammation and a heat induced aggravation is clear. In many cases, there will be a rash and a sensation as if the organ is about to burst from pressure.

Various types of kidney inflammation, glomerulonephritis, nephritic syndrome, renal failure etc.

Mental state: Apis works well for people who have a tendency to anger and jealousy. They are often very energetic people, quick to respond, loyal with family, assertive and confident. Like Belladonna, Nux vomica and Ferrum metallicum they can get angry from contradiction.

Kent says of this remedy: *This remedy has so many symptoms on the surface of the body we will study the outer aspect first. All over the body is found a thick rash, sometimes of a rose color. It is rough and can be felt as a rough rash under the fingers. The patient at this time is greatly distressed by heat and the skin is sensitive to touch with the rash or without it. Nodular swellings here and there come and go. Then conies an erysipelatous inflammatory condition, in patches, here and there, about the head, with great tumefaction about the face, eyes and eyelids. Erysipelas may occur anywhere, but it more commonly belongs to the face and runs to a high degree of inflammatory action, with stinging, burning and oedema. In the extremities we have a marked dropsy, swelling with pitting upon pressure. A general anasarca may appear. The face is greatly swollen at times, the eyelids look like water bags, the uvula hangs down like a water bag, the abdominal walls are of great thickness and pit upon pressure, and the mucous membranes in any part look as if they would discharge water if they were punctured. Puffing or oedema, with pitting upon pressure, is a general condition that may be present in any inflammatory state.*

There is a general amelioration from cold and aggravation from heat. The skin symptoms and the patient are aggravated from heat. This prevails also in the mental state, in inflammatory conditions; in cardiac conditions, in dropsy, in sore throat, etc. Sometimes this aggravation amounts to aggravation from warm drinks, warm room, warm clothing, warmth of the fire, etc.; if it is heat the patient is greatly disturbed. In brain troubles, if you put an Apis patient with congestion of the brain into a warm bath he will go into convulsions, and consequently warm bathing is not always "good for fits." It is taught in old school text-books so much that the old women and nurses know that a hot bath is good for fits, and before you get there just as like as not you will have a dead baby.

This congestion of the brain, with little twitchings and threatening convulsions, makes them put the baby in a hot bath, and it is in an awful state when you get there. If the baby needs OPIUM or Apis in congestion of the brain the fits become worse by bathing in hot water. If the nurse has been doing that kind of business you have learned the remedy as soon as you enter the house, for she will say the child has been worse ever since the warm bath, has become pale as a ghost and she was afraid he was going to die. There you have convulsions worse from heat, pointing especially to OPIUM and Apis. That is the way with Apis all through. It is not laid down in the books that Apis is worse in the throat symptoms from warm drinks and wants altogether cold things, and will not take warm things which aggravate, but one of our graduates wrote me that by making use simply of the generals, as he had been instructed, Apis conforming to all the rest of the case, he made a beautiful cure of a case of diphtheria which had the relief from cold, which shows how generals are continued into particulars and how they can be made use

Study Guide

of. *The generals continue to build and enlarge our Materia Medica.* (J.T. Kent <u>Lectures on Materia Medica</u>)

Pharmacology:
Apis, used in homeopathic doses, corrects dysfunctions of that part of the body's healing system which treats hyper-allergic responses. The result is a stabilizing of white blood cells such as lymphocytes, mast cells and basophils, so that they do not react so violently and cause an allergic response.

For example after Apis, mast cells will not break open so easily and release histamine. Histamine and similar substances are what usually cause edema and allergic reactions. Antihistamine type drugs also act to chemically stabilize white blood cells but do nothing to strengthen the body's healing system to control the entire allergic response. Therefore, in chronic conditions, when the antihistamine drug is withdrawn, the original complaint will return because the root cause was never treated. If Apis is the correct medicine for the chronic condition, the correction to the body's defense mechanism allows the illness to go into remission and remain alleviated.

Summary: Think of what a bee sting can do and you will know when to give Apis. Used only for the occasional bee sting, it will have fulfilled its purpose but it can do a lot more. Allergic reactions from any cause which lead to tissues being filled with fluid, stinging pains and inflammation will very often respond to a few doses of Apis.

ARNICA MONTANA
(Leopard's Bane)

The first remedy to give for PAIN or shock **from** *PHYSICAL TRAUMA.*

<u>It is best to use this remedy as soon as possible after any physical trauma.</u>

Sprains, strains

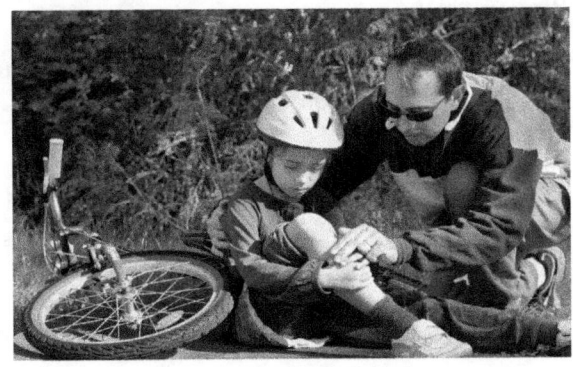

Contusions, falls, sports injuries, head trauma and concussion.

Sudden extreme exertion resulting in pain. Heart strain; such as trying to run a marathon when one has not trained for it. Arnica will usually work for all of these but it will work 99.9% of the time for injuries **from blunt trauma** where the injury is very sensitive to touch.

<u>Bruises</u>, car accidents, surgery, childbirth - for baby and mother.
Main symptoms: PAIN, as if hit with a stick, BRUISED, black and blue all over, swelling. Worse from touch.

With the flu – the muscles are sore and *very sensitive to touch and pressure;* so the patient has to keep turning over.

Emotions: Delusions well, sends the doctor home. Fear of touch. Stupor from a head injury.

Chronic picture: depression, feels good for nothing but keeps trying. Feels beaten down. Chronic physical conditions: Arthritis, back pains, herniated disc, bladder infections.

Case: 1. A child falls down the stairs, HITS THEIR HEAD and looses consciousness. A few seconds after Arnica he opens his eyes and goes on to feeling well within the same day.

2. Playing tennis he twists his ankle and falls to the ground in extreme pain. After one dose of Arnica 200c he plays again less than ten minutes later. The next day he still can't believe Arnica could have healed him in such a short time.

3. A boy slams his hand in a door. After Arnica 30c there is no bruising the next day.

4. After a car accident he feels in shock and time seems to move too slowly. Dazed and confused. Ten minutes after Arnica 30c he feels normal again.

5. I ran into a concrete park bench one time trying to catch a Frisbee. After Arnica 30c the pain, within thirty seconds, left my body and the next day there was no bruise on my leg.

6. A women with Lupus in her uterus. The bleeding is continuous, she feels insignificant and of little consequence. After a few doses of Arnica 30c the hemorrhage stops and she is able to stop taking prednizone.

7. After playing football his disc was ruptured, with sciatica, pain on any flexion of the spine in the lumbar area. After Arnica 200c he was able to go back playing sports within a week.

8. In this case a woman lost everything in the stock market – her house was taken from her. She was in a type of stupor, dazed and mentally bruised by the shock. Arnica set her right, along with all her old sports injuries.

9. In another case a 66 year old woman came to me for depression. She had been taking Hydrobromide as an antidepressant for many years. She had a type of lethargy and very low vitality. "I feel inadequate" she said. "I am not good for anything, I have never been smart. My father used to spank me with a razor strap. He broke my heart (trauma). My father adored me but he died when I was eleven years old (trauma). From this death I felt he did not want me (feels low and of no consequence). At work I feel less than others. I could never do public speaking I was terrified of it – I had a fear to make a fool of myself and of being rejected. I am embarrassed easily. Arthritis worse from cold. Arms are sore to touch. Painful stiffness. I am hard on myself and very sensitive to criticism. Painful coition so avoids it for many years. Does not bruise easily." After Arnica 30c one dose a week for a month: Energy is much better i.e. used to be five out of ten now it is eight out of ten. Confidence is much improved and she is not so hard on herself. "I feel more equal to others" she says. Back and arthritis is much better. Memory improved for words.

10. This next Arnica case is of a 70 year old women who is a real workaholic. She suffers from depression. She won't clean her house, she won't cook for herself and won't exercise. She is self critical. She is isolated from people and from her family. "I am full of self doubt; I can't recover from my financial losses. I easily feel devastated and rejected, it is as if I am not respected. I feel that I have no value then I start to cry. I never felt that my parents loved me. My parents never complimented me so I always felt inferior. I feel ugly and gray." Pain in her knee joint and back pain after eating wheat. Also has some chest and heart pain. Two weeks after Arnica 200c she says she feels a lot better in general. "I felt so much better that I cleaned up my house. I am eating better and crave wholesome food now where as before I was eating a gallon of ice cream for dinner. I have had some days that I really enjoyed – this has not happened for years. I feel that I look better now and that I am reclaiming my life. I used to feel rage when other people did not do things right, now this is also a lot improved. I like to be in my house now." Aurum metallicum is very similar: – i.e. depression, self reproach, isolation and unable to recover from financial loss.

11. Painful acne. See appendix case study.

12. Female age 35; chronic bladder infections. It feels bruised and sore in the pelvic area worse from touch. Arnica 30c one dose cleared it up in about a day. These infections did not appear again.

13. 26 year old female. Acute influenza, sore all over worse from touch and lying on her side. Lethargic and self critical person. Arnica 30c one dose; all better the next day with lots of vitality.

14. Ten years previous had a car accident. Arms and legs are weak, no vitality to speak of, muscles feel sore all over and sensitive to touch and pressure. After Arnica 30c she could not sleep as she had too much vitality, she cleaned her whole house, lifted and moved all the furniture, muscle pain and weakness all better.

This is the most used remedy in homeopathy. It should be carried where-ever one goes as injuries can happen at any time.

Kent has this to say about Arnica: *All over the body there is a lameness, and soreness, and a feeling as if bruised; a rheumatic lameness; the joints are swollen, sore and lame.*

If an acute disease becomes more severe, we shall find the mental symptoms as described, and there will be an increasing soreness in the muscles. Arnica is very suitable for that sore, bruised condition of the body, therefore Arnica is a very important remedy in injuries, bruises and shocks, injuries of joints, injury of the back with lameness and soreness. In such conditions Arnica becomes one of the first remedies, and unless there are general decided symptoms calling for other remedies it should be the first remedy.

Arnica will very often take all the soreness out of a sprained ankle and permit him in a few days to go walking about, to the surprise of everybody. The black and blue appearance of sprained joints will go away in a surprisingly short time, the soreness will disappear, and he will be able to manipulate that joint with surprising ease.

I have seen a sprained ankle when it was black and blue, so swollen that the shoe could not be put on, but after a dose of Arnica, the swelling disappeared in an astonishing way, the discoloration faded out and the patient was able to stand on the foot. No such result can be obtained with the use of Arnica lotion externally.

A high potency of Arnica is most satisfactory in bruises, and when no decided contra-indication is present Arnica is the first remedy; but for the weakness of tendons that follows such a condition Arnica is not always sufficient, and then RHUS TOX. is its natural follower.

If the weakness and tenderness remain in the joints, follow the RHUS with CALCAREA. One will not, of course, give these remedies all on the same day, and not in the same glass, but will wait until all the good has been gotten out of the Arnica before following with RHUS. It is quite a common thing for aching and restlessness and weakness to come into a part that has been injured, and RHUS is then a suitable remedy; and it is quite common for a joint that has been badly treated to remain sore and weak, and then CALCAREA comes in as a natural follower of the RHUS.

In inflammation of the kidneys and bladder, of the liver, and even in pneumonia, the mental state and the sore, bruised feeling all over the body would enable you to do astonishing work in such cases, even though Arnica has never produced pneumonia.

It has ... rusty expectoration, with all the soreness of the chest and catarrhal state, the coughing and gagging, and sore, bruised feeling all over the body, and then add to this the condition of stupor and the mental state that belongs to the inflammatory condition of any organ and is especially strong in this medicine.

A general feature also of the remedy is that the body is cold and the head hot; the whole body and the extremities are cold, but the head feels hot. This is a marked condition in sudden congestive attacks, in congestive chill and congestive intermittent fevers. (Kent)

BELLIS PERENNIS
(Daisy)

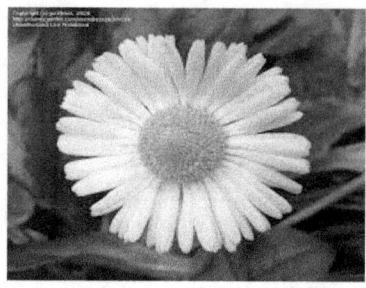

Muscle soreness after injury or after excessive physical exercise or a strenuous work out.
The muscles become very sore, painful and somewhat stiff after a day of heavy physical labor. Arnica can help this situation but Bellis is even more effective. (Will Taylor)

For people of older age who love to work for hours in the garden. When they are *stiff and sore all over the next day* then this remedy is called for.

Worse from touch like Arnica. Joints lame as if sprained. Back is sore from sitting for too long. This is the first remedy that can be used after surgery to deeper organs. Septic wounds from surgery. After a car accident when the internal organs are bruised or bleeding. After surgery to the internal organs to stimulate healing and vitality.

Varicose veins; they feel sore and bruised. Engorged breasts and uterus. The uterus feels as if squeezed. Enlarged spleen, boils. Tumors develop after an injury. Waking too early then can't get back to sleep. Worse from heat better from cold.

Boericke says: *It acts upon the muscular fibers of the blood-vessels. Much muscular soreness. Lameness, as if sprained. Venous congestion, due to mechanical causes. First remedy in injuries to the deeper tissues, after major surgical work. Results of injuries to nerves with intense soreness and intolerance of cold bathing.*

Skin.--Boils. Ecchymosis, swelling, very sensitive to touch. Venous congestion due to mechanical causes. Varicose veins with bruised sore feeling. Exudations and swellings. Acne. (Boericke)

Case 1: Pain in the adductors worse after heavy work (lifting) and after tennis. Pain has become chronic. He does work and exercise to excess. He has so much vitality but it takes its toll on his body. Bellis 30c and then 200c relieved this ailment. He is now also able to sleep past 5 am. In the past felt he could not wait to get up and go back to work.

CALENDULA
(Marigold)

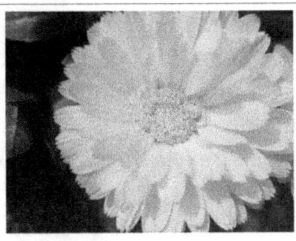

Cuts and scraps to prevent wounds from becoming infected.

Lacerations, physical wounds. Use this remedy before and after surgery.

Pain or INFECTIONS from cuts, surgery or scrapes.

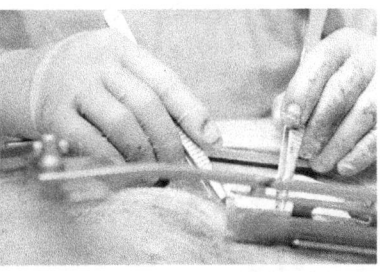

Over 140,000 people die every year from post surgical infections in Canada and the US combined – It is therefore best to give this remedy the day before surgery, right after surgery and then at least once a day for three days, then every other day for a week.

The chronic picture of this remedy can have the following: Never well since a wound such as surgery. After surgery the tissues heal very slowly, become infected – the patient could die if this remedy is not taken. After surgery the pain continues such as fibromyalgia pain, cutting pains, referred pains to other parts of the body. Anxiety: the patient wakes at night with the pain and thinks that *something terrible is happening and they will die*. Such as they have chest pain and think they are having a heart attack – they rush themselves to the hospital but nothing is wrong (except they need Calendula). In the repertory it is listed under: *Mind, fear happen, something bad*. This is often a valuable symptom to confirm Calendula.

Use topically for minor cuts and scrapes. Use 30c for infected wounds and for the chronic conditions.

Case 1: A few years after back surgery she feels extreme pain in her ankle as if it had been cut off. Since this pain started soon after the back surgery I used the rubric: Ailments from surgery and gave Calendula 30c.

After this the pain in the ankle is all better.

2. A 38 year old women presented with fibromyalgia in the upper half of her body. It started after breast reduction surgery eight years previously. The surgery scars did not heal, kept opening up and became infected. She also wakes often at night with chest oppression and a feeling as if she is having a heart attack with anxiety. After Calendula 30c once a week for a month she is much better in all ways. Then scars itched for about a week.

What we can learn from this case is that this women was a Calendula case even before the surgery as she had always had a tendency to feel anxiety and that something bad was going to happen. This also explains why her wounds would not heal and she became chronically sick after the surgery. Look in the rubric: Mind, fear happen, something will: There we find Calendula.

3. After he cut his hand on an ax blade the wound became infected. Calendula cured this case in a few days.

4. A sixty year old man put two of his fingers through a table saw. The flesh was badly torn and abraded. Calendula 30c then 200c and finally 1m over a period of months led to a total recovery. He never took any antibiotics and his surgeon said: "What-ever you are doing is working, so keep doing it."

5. Fifty year old male with an infected knee since knee surgery. Swelling, redness and pain in the knee. After many courses of antibiotics the whole leg was gray and the blood supply was shutting down. An amputation was recommended. He came in with this situation and after a few doses of Calendula 30c a day he showed signs of recovery within 24 hours. He did not need an amputation as with Calendula he made a full recovery.

6. There was such a feeling as if some overwhelming calamity was hovering over me as to be almost unbearable. I have been plagued by back pain which has spoiled my love for walking. This dreadful feeling became very much exaggerated, especially when exposed to a chill. I've always, since a child, been afraid of such things, as if I were going to fall forever when I fell asleep, or if I heard music or noises and I would start easily. Calendula was given with a good result.

CANTHARIS
(Spanish fly)

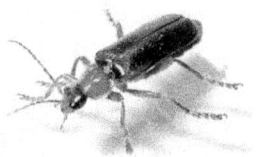

For BURNS from fire, heat or hot water.

PAIN and BLISTERING from a burn.

This remedy can relieve burn pain often within a few minutes.

Case 1: The child touched the hot wood stove and the skin burned and blistered. After a dose of Cantharis 30c, she then put her gloves on and went to play in the snow. After that as she pulled her gloves off, the blister also tore off. She looked at her hand but there was no pain and so had no reaction. This shows how well Cantharis can be used effectively to treat burn pain.

2: The boiling water from the kettle blistered his fingers. After taking Cantharis 30c the pain was relieved in thirty seconds.

3: After mowing the lawn my neighbor put his hand on the red hot muffler and scorched his whole hand. The pain was so intense he put a bag of ice on his palm and could not take it off. The 30c Cantharis relieved the pain for minute but he had to keep taking it. A dose of Cantharis 200c took all the pain away and so there was no more need of the ice. He slept well that night and the next day reported to me that still there was no pain.

4: The fire scorched his back, it was red, blistered and crusted. Cantharis 30c, then 200c and finally 1m took away all the pain.

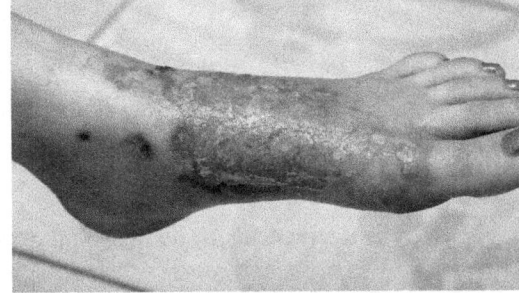

If after three doses of the 30c the pain continues to relapse then try the 200c potency. If this is used three times then use the

1m potency or even a dose of the 10m potency if the 1m does not hold after three doses.

Enough evidence is available to allow Cantharis to be used as a routine medicine in hospital emergency and burn wards.

Acute Situations
Cantharis can also be used for acute situations such as infections. The most common situation is in the treatment of acute bladder infection. It can be used for irritation or infection of mucous membranes with **burning pains during urination**.

Internal mucous membranes include urinary passages, lungs, esophagus, stomach, small intestine, and colon.

For a person who needs Cantharis, these mucous membranes will become highly irritated with sensations of intense burning pain. The nerves around these passages also become irritated and cause violent spasms and constrictions. The irritation then leads to a violent rapid inflammation and infection. Finally these tissue decay.

On the emotional and mental level, irritation, restlessness, anger, and excitability are experienced. In the beginning stages of these infections all that is noticed by the patient is burning with urination, and a frequent desire to urinate.

Boericke: *Intolerable urging and tenesmus. Nephritis with bloody urine. Violent paroxysms of cutting and burning in whole renal region, with painful urging to urinate and bloody urine, by drops. Intolerable tenesmus, cutting before, during, and after urine. Urine scalds him, and is passed drop by drop. Constant desire to urinate. Membranous scales looking like bran in water. Urine jelly-like, shreddy.* (BOERICKE)

CARBO ANIMALIS
(Animal Charcoal Leather)

WEAKNESS after an injury – weakness *worse from lifting*.

This remedy is derived from the charcoal of burnt leather. Its main indications of use are: *weakness* of *muscles* after an injury and/or severe and painful muscular spasms after an injury.

There is also a characteristic *aggravation from lifting or carrying anything* or doing any strenuous exercise.

This triad of symptoms is often found after a severe injury such as a major car accident, ski accident or similar incident where the whole body is severely shaken.

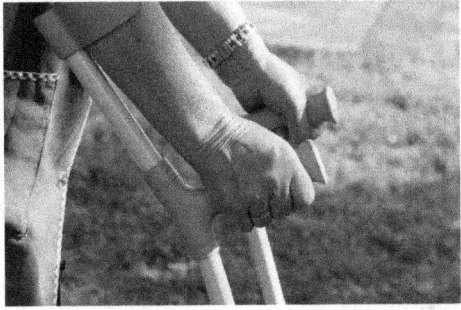

Case 1: In one patient I treated, the back muscles had become tight, swollen, stiff, extremely weak and painful after a car accident. In this case the back pains caused interrupted sleep and the patient felt worse in general after lifting things. Two weeks after taking Carbo Animalis, the muscle spasms were significantly improved as did her overall strength.

2: In another case, the right shoulder of a middle-aged woman had become stiff and frozen ever since she injured it during a fall from a chair. She could not tolerate any lifting tasks. Carbo animalis 30c given once a week brought her back to health.

In some of the cases I have treated, there were, in addition to the joint symptoms: chills and coldness while sleeping and/or night sweats. Some of them had sinus headaches with a sense of dullness in the head.

Consider using Carbo animalis after Arnica has done its work to treat the initial bruising. That is to say, when Arnica has been used and subsequent doses of Arnica produce no further improvement, then consider this remedy, if the symptoms agree.

For chronic conditions this remedy is useful for a variety of other ailments including cancer. With many of these ailments the weakness is present and characteristic chills during the night in bed.

Kent: *It is not surprising that this remedy has been one of the most suitable for old, stubborn cancerous affections; for cancerous ulcers. They all burn, they are all surrounded by infiltrated, hardened, dark-colored tissue, and they all ooze an acrid ichorous fluid.*

It has cured these troubles in old feeble constitutions with night-sweats and much bleeding. It has relieved in incurable cases, and has apparently removed the cancerous condition for years, even though it comes back afterward and kills. This remedy is often a great palliative for the pains that occur in cancer, the indurations and the stinging, burning pains.

Of course we do not want to teach, nor do we wish to have you infer, that a patient with a well-advanced cancerous affection, such as scirrhus, may be restored to perfect health and the cancerous affection removed. We may comfort that patient, and restore order at least temporarily, so that there is freedom from suffering in these malignant affections.

Summary:
Falls and injuries can lead to a weakness of the whole body or of a specific joint. If this weakness is aggravated after lifting or carrying heavy things, then this remedy will most likely be of benefit. Repeat it when the healing of the previous dose has exhausted its action or when there is a relapse for two days in a row.

HYPERICUM PERFORATUM
(St John's Wort)

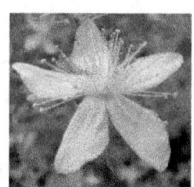

NERVE INJURIES. shooting pains, tingling, numbness. Puncture wounds. Examples: after dental work, after a car accident, after a sports injury.

Case: 1. I once had to have a dental filling replaced. Instead of taking a shot of Novocaine I insisted on taking a dose of Hypericum 30c instead. The dentist drilled away and cleaned out the deep filling. He could not believe that I did not have any pain.

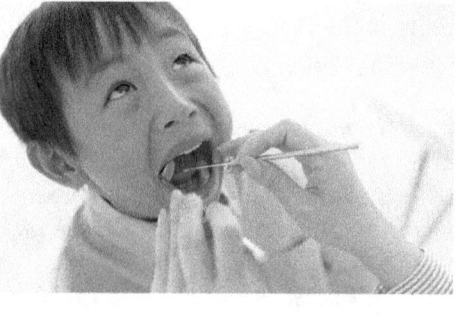

2. A patient of mine was in a car accident. Her arm was severely stretched backward. Two weeks later it was still numb, tingling and felt swollen. Hypericum 30c a few doses healed these parasthesias.

3. This was a case of depression, she was nervous and overly sensitive to pain.

4. A 70 year old gentleman came to see me for emphysema. He could not walk down his driveway any longer to get his mail as he was too out of breath. He smoked for many years. His <u>breathing</u> was much <u>worse in foggy weather</u>. *Generalities: weather, foggy weather agg.* (Synthesis) After Hypericum 30c his respiratory doctor could not believe it as he went on to recover and renovated his house and regained the vitality and health he had in his 30's and 40's.

Pains – shooting and sharp or severe, shooting upward along the nerves.

- Injuries – contusions, lacerations, punctures to parts rich in nerves – fingers, toes, eyes, lips, teeth, nails, genitalia
- Spinal injuries esp. to the coccyx after a fall, blow
- Pain in lower back and coccyx during labor, delivery, difficult childbirth
- Spinal wounds, after spinal injections
- Head injuries, wounds, concussions, after forceps birth if child becomes nervous
- Puncture wounds, deep gaping wounds where nerves have been injured
- After surgery if nerves have been cut
- After dental surgery involving nerves – i.e. root canals
- Nerve pain after injury – neuralgia, neuritis, sciatica
- Alternate with Arnica (for shock, and to reduce bruising, swelling)
- Helps with shock after injury
- Treats depression after injury, surgery, amputation
- For pain of amputation and phantom pains
- Carpal tunnel syndrome with pains shooting upwards
- It could be used for a certain type of depression (St. John's wort)
- Crushing, severing of fingers, toes (i.e. caught in car door)
- Tearing off a fingernail, torn-off skin
- Splinters
- Second and third degree burns (Cantharis, Caust, Urtica urens)

- Helps prevent tetanus, lockjaw
- After animal bites, inflamed insect bites

Pain in coccyx during, after or since delivery. Injury to coccyx from falls, blows, birth trauma.

Asthma from foggy weather.

When lying in bed a sensation as if being lifted up high into the air, **floating;** with great anxiety lest he fall from this height (Allen, Boericke.)

Nervous; **hurried feeling** as if there was something that must be done at once.

Lachrymose mood; melancholy and feels like crying.

Hall wrote: *Hypericum people are quick to do everything. Quick to grow, quick to mature, quick to dive headlong into life. Their coordination may sometimes suffer with the speed of their nervous energy, and occasional clumsiness may mark them out.*

Fear of physical pain such as dental work and injections. Sharp pains are experienced vividly and remembered for a long time. More than most people, they take decisive and speedy action to settle problems with others. These people are speedy. They gallop through the day, their agile minds often leaping ahead of them and causing the above uncoordination.

Often intellectually bright, they enjoy their education only if the teacher is not boring or slow. The Hypericum child can be precocious and later in life they seek out new experiences and intellectual challenges. They have hyper acute senses such as hearing, taste and most of all touch.
(Hall)

IGNATIA AMARA
(St. Ignatius Bean)

Disappointment from high expectations.

Silent GRIEF, sighing. *Strong idealism.*
Changeable moods. Lump in the throat.   GRIEF SHOCK

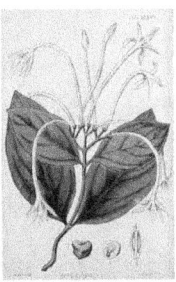

This is a first aid remedy for the symptoms of *grief* or *sudden disappointment*. This remedy is most commonly indicated when the loss of a friend, loved one or relative was unexpected, producing emotional shock and often a tremendous amount of emotional pain.

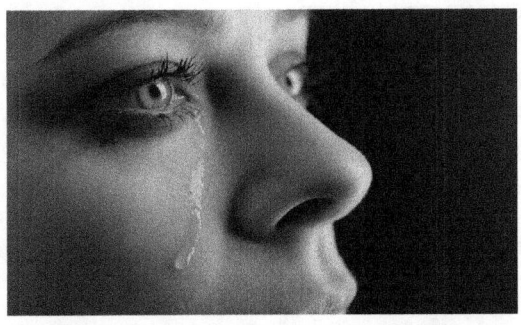

Boericke: *.. quick to perceive, rapid in execution. Rapid change of mental and physical condition, opposite to each other. Great contradictions. Alert, nervous, apprehensive, rigid, trembling patients who suffer acutely in mind or body, at the same time made worse by drinking coffee. The superficial and erratic character of its symptoms is most characteristic. Effects of grief and worry. Cannot bear tobacco.*

Changeable mood; introspective; silently brooding. Melancholic, sad, tearful. Not communicative. Sighing and sobbing. After shocks, grief, disappointment.

Some common symptoms revealing the need for Ignatia are:

※ *Changeable moods, such as crying, then silent grief, then episodes of irritability will often occur.*

※ Grief followed by sighing, i.e. slow deep breaths with rapid expiration, are common symptoms of a need for Ignatia.

※ <u>Romantic disappointments,</u> which lead to silent brooding and feelings of despondency. Who has not felt this type of emotion but only some of us will need Ignatia.

Ailments following grief such as *sleeplessness, loss of appetite*, stomach pains, sore throats, coughs, muscle spasms in the neck and back, headaches, constipation, numbness and tingling in the extremities will also benefit from this remedy.

In general, people who need Ignatia will be emotionally oversensitive, depressed, weighed down with sadness.

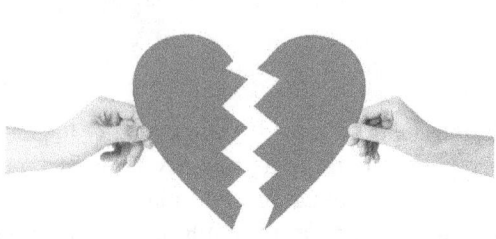

They often find it difficult to accept the truth of what has occurred. It is as if they are determined to change the past. Often, there is a <u>sensation of a lump in the throat</u>. The smell of tobacco smoke can aggravate them as well. They can be very artistic people, refined and or overly sophisticated.

Cold in general bothers them and they are easily chilled. Consolation from a friend can create more irritability. Therefore they feel better when alone.

Case 1: I have seen Ignatia cure a type of neurological paralysis (weak arms and legs with numbness) in a woman who acquired these symptoms after finding out that her husband was being unfaithful to her. She would stagger down the hallway of my office bumping into both walls as she tried to not fall over. After Ignatia this neurological ailment was reversed and all her coordination and strength returned.

2: A woman experienced crying fits whenever she thought about her mother, who had died. She had a lump in her throat and was sighing frequently.

3: A teenager who had fallen in love for the first time was rudely rejected. He displayed a sullen irritability with very sad eyes. Subsequently he could not sleep, eat and he refused to go to school. Ignatia brought him out of it.

4: A man in his 40's had hiccoughs ever since he found out his teenage daughter was pregnant. After a dose of Ignatia the hiccoughs stopped the next day.

5: A 30 year old man became obsessed with his x-girlfriend. She had rejected him for someone else but he could not let go. He followed her from place to place, confronted her etc (also think of Naja for obsession). After Ignatia 30c, then 200c, then 1m then 10m then 50m he was able to sleep again, eat again, stopped his obsession and was able to move on. Each potency helped the grief but only the 50m could finally take away all remnants.

6: This is case I heard about at a seminar. An elderly women went into a coma after she was treated very rudely by her granddaughter (Mind, ailments from disappointment). The grandmother had held this child in such high esteem, idealized her, and then to have her speak in such a way was a shock she could not process and became unconscious. After Ignatia all health was restored.

7: This was another one that I saw by video at a seminar. It was of a boy with encephalitis from chicken pox. He was paralyzed and his prognosis was poor. His parents had split up (Mind, forsaken feeling: Ign) and then as they both had to work he felt extreme grief and sadness over the whole situation. Within a few days of taking Ignatia he started to rally and within a week was up and about, walking, eating well again and made a full recovery. Quite a few us were in tears from this case as it was so dramatic.

In all these examples, Ignatia was the remedy to heal the emotional wounds such as grief, emotional shock and disappointment.

There are more than forty remedies that can be used to alleviate grief. Ignatia is one of the most common of these remedies and it will help many people in the acute first aid stages of grief. Recommendation: If this remedy is indicated, use the 30c potency once and then repeat when a relapse occurs, and repeat when the healing reaction stops showing improvements until the grief and physical symptoms are all resolved.

If your the case is showing good improvement with about four doses of the remedy and then with the 5th dose there is no more improvement it is best to give the 200c of the same remedy before trying to find a better remedy. This is good advice and one can try the other way, that being if the symptoms have really changed in many respects to try a new remedy, but most often, all one needs to do is give a higher potency of the same remedy that was working before. This one can keep doing all the way to 50m if one needs to.

Kent: *"Weakness of the body coming on suddenly. Hysterical debility and fainting fits. Fainting in a crowd." It is especially useful in the tearful, nervous, sad, yielding, sensitive minds. "Jerking and twitching. Convulsive twitchings."*

Children are convulsed in sleep after punishment. "Convulsions in children in the first period of dentition. Spasms in children from fright." The child is cold and pale, and has a fixed staring look, like Cina.

"Convulsions with loss of consciousness. Violent convulsions. Tetanic convulsions. Tetanus after fright. Emotional chorea. After fright, or grief." Choreic girls. Emotional epilepsy, or epileptiform manifestations. Paralytic weakness. (Kent)

Summary
Ignatia is the best remedy to give for the shock of grief or sudden disappointment. To confirm this prescription there will often be a sensation of a lump in the throat, sighing and a changeable moods.

LEDUM PULUSTRE
(Marsh Tea)

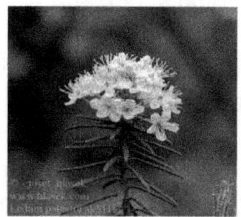

PUNCTURE wounds. Better from COLD applications. Mosquito bites.

Ledum is indicated for a variety of ailments. Its main use is in the treatment of all types of *puncture wounds*. Examples: stepping on a nail, animal bites, and the effects of insect bites. Wounds which could lead to tetanus. It can prevent mosquito bites from itching or swelling.

Case 1: I have used this remedy mostly for patients that were affected for days and weeks after mosquito bites. The bites would not stop itching and were better from the application of ice.

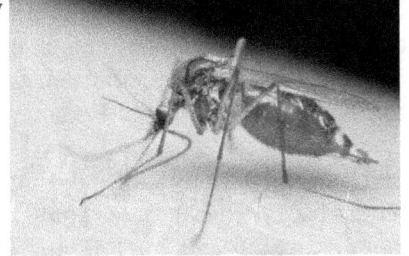

2. This case is from a lecture by James Tyler Kent: *The only relief that patient gets is by sitting, with the feet in a tub of ice cold water. I remember the first time I ever saw this in a patient. He was an old syphilitic, whose nasal bones had been eaten out by syphilis, and his nose was a flabby piece of skin; it had no stiffening in it. He was a drunkard, and was extremely abusive to his family when drunk.*

He had been for several years unwilling to work, having lost his ambition, and he would sit in the house and allow his wife to wait upon him. He had practically become a tramp, only he could not tramp, for this dropsical condition had come on and his feet were so badly swollen and sensitive that he sat in the house day after day. When I first saw him he had before him a good-sized old-fashioned wash-tub, and there he sat with the ice water two-thirds up to his knees and pieces of ice floating around on the top of the water, which he liked to have coming in contact with the skin. When that ice was out he would put in more. The wife described his sufferings by saying he "suffered agonies something dreadful." Ledum took his feet out of the ice water so that he never used it afterwards. It caused the purpleness to disappear, the bloating went out of his feet, and he quit drinking. Ledum cured him of his syphilitic trouble, and he never had a return of that original state.(Kent)

Ledum is also highly useful if the wound becomes swollen, mottled purple, and with a red or blue streak extending up the limb away from the injury. Ledum is especially indicated for sprained ankles and bruises to soft tissues even when the wound has become infected, and has an aching pain associated with it, Ledum is still highly effective. Take Hypericum if there are any shooting pains from a puncture wound. Ledum has some healing properties, which are similar to those of Arnica. After an injury to a muscle or joint, Arnica is the best first remedy to use.

If Arnica does not completely heal the pain, bruising and swelling then stop using the Arnica. Instead use one dose of Ledum 30c to speed up the re-absorption of fluids. In this way, Ledum complements the action of Arnica and takes the healing process a step further. If soaking the injury in cold water helps relieve the pain, Ledum is a sure remedy to help. This could be a sprained wrist, black eye, or crushed finger. In these injuries, the skin is puffy, blue, mottled, and painful. Often, Hypericum is given for puncture wounds but Ledum may be the better remedy.

Stepping on a rusty nail, jabbing the finger with a thumb-tack, or being bitten by an insect or animal are all considered as types of puncture wounds which call for Ledum. There have been some cases where it is thought that taking Ledum prevented tetanus, but this is so far anecdotal evidence. If tetanus is suspected then clean the wound, take Ledum and obtain a tetanus shot.

The puncture wounds in which Ledum is indicated are those producing a strong *ache*. In cases where Hypericum is indicated, the infection of a damaged nerve leads to a *shooting pain* rather than to an aching pain.

Ledum wounds can feel cold, but they are relieved with cold applications and are often aggravated by heat, such as a hot compress or a hot bath. Ledum is needed for very painful wounds that become swollen and blue. For insect bites, such as a wasp or bee sting, Apis is the first remedy to use, but if no benefit is noticed then take Ledum. Pain, itching and swelling are the indicating symptoms. Ledum is recommended as the first remedy for mosquito bites, flea-bites and spider bites, especially if a person has an allergic reaction to them.

Summary: Ledum covers a variety of injuries, including puncture wounds, contusions, bruises, sprains, infected wounds, animal and insect bites. It can be used to complement the effects of Arnica, Apis, and Hypericum, or used when these remedies fail to have any benefit.

The strong symptoms to indicate the use of Ledum are: wounds which are slow to heal, wounds that are aggravated by heat and improve with cold applications. The affected parts become blue, mottled and/or purple and there is often swelling, infection, pain, aching pains, and sometimes numbness of the affected area. Ledum is a valuable remedy to consider.

Chronic: Alcoholism effects from – joint pains better from cold applications. Mean and abusive temperament.

RHUS TOXICODENDRON
(Poison Ivy)

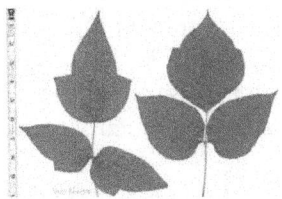

STIFFNESS of JOINTS – worse from rest – worse beginning motion; better from CONTINUED MOTION. Worse from cold and damp weather. The joints are acting like a rusty gate.

Rhus Tox is another remedy like Ledum, Ruta, and Bryonia, which can be used after Arnica has healed the initial stages of trauma to a joint.

After trauma to a joint, such as a sports injury, the joint can become very *stiff at rest*, then painful at the onset of motion and *less painful with continued motion and heat.* If these are the main symptoms a dose of Rhus tox is needed.

For example, the joint will be very stiff and difficult to move upon waking. *If heat and continued motion are applied to the joint for some time, it will become more flexible and feel better.*

Rhust tox is like a rusty hinge joint. They feel stiff and there is pain when they start to move but limber up with continued motion.

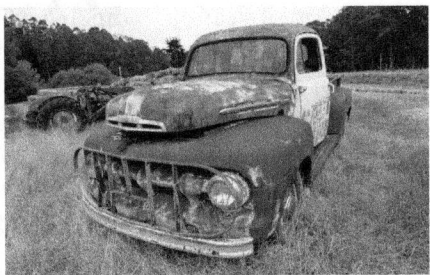

After the person rests, then once again, the stiffness will set in. At night, there is often restlessness of that joint because it becomes more painful if it is not moved to keep it flexible; the next morning the stiffness is there again and the whole cycle is repeated.

WORSE FROM COLD DAMP WEATHER. In order for Rhus Tox to work for a chronic joint condition such as arthritis the patient needs to have this symptom. If weather is rainy and cold they definitely feel worse.

The cold and damp weather will aggravate the pain and stiffness in a person who needs Rhus Tox. In fact, if the stiffness is improved with a cold application, then Rhus Tox will not bring any benefit. Often there has been a sports injury, a work related injury or a car accident. Rhus tox is used for general trauma to the body or specifically to one or more joints. It can be used when this condition is recent or when it has continued for many years and the ailment is now defined as arthritis.

The main symptom of the arthritis is pain and stiffness. It is worse when beginning to move but better from continued motion. If this joint improves under a hot shower and is worse from cold, damp weather, then usually Rhus tox will be of great benefit. Recommendation: In these chronic cases, repeat the 30c potency about once per week for a month. Repeat it for two days in a row if the pain returns.

Summary: Rhus tox is a deep-acting medicine for joint injuries when stiffness is the main symptom. Remember that the pain needs to improve from continued motion and to become worse from rest and cold applications or cold damp weather.

Rhus tox does not seem to affect the mind to any great extent. The people who need this remedy seem to be for the most part well balanced. It is listed for mental restlessness and physically they are also restlessness when they have a fever or an infection.

Case 1: An 80 year old women came to see me for general arthritis which she had suffered from for over 40 years. The joints of her hands were all swollen, with bony nodules and very limited range of motion. The pain she said was quite severe most of the time but better when she was in the hot dry climate of Arizona.

On these trips she was always getting into trouble on the airplane as the only way to stop the pains in her back, hips and legs was to walk up and down the aisle of the plane. The flight attendant would tell her to stay in her seat but she could not and had to walk to feel better. I had only been working as a homeopath for a few weeks at this time back in 1979 and looking at her I thought to myself, 'well she has many symptoms for Rhus tox but this case is too far gone and she is too old to get better'.

After taking Rhus tox 30c every three days she came back a few weeks later to tell me she had no pain at all, she could move her fingers again, the stiffness was mostly better and she was completely satisfied with the effectiveness of the remedy. She sat there looking at her hands and said over and over, *"where has all the pain gone?"*.

I could not believe how her body could make so many changes in such a short amount of time in tissues that had been damaged for so many years.

There are many other cases of arthritis in which I have used Rhus tox according to the guiding symptoms listed above, too many to mention.

RUTA GRAVEOLENS
(Herb of Grace)

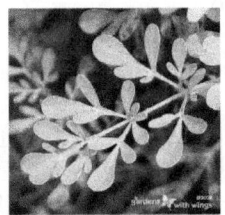

Old STRAINS of connective tissues. Pains at night. GUILT over trifles. Tendinitis. OVER-USE INJURIES (Bellis).

Ruta is one of the remedies, which is called for to take care of the symptoms which are left over after giving Arnica. In the case of Ruta, its greatest affinity is for the healing of fibrous tissue such as *tendons* and *ligaments*.

It is especially indicated for injuries from *over-use*, such as chronic sprains and strains. Inflammation of these tissues, typically causing tendinitis and myositis (muscle inflammation), will usually require Ruta. Eye strain from overuse.

The pains continue during rest. An injury that would respond favorably to Ruta will have a sensation as if 'there is nothing that will ameliorate the constant pain'.

Often there is a sore, bruised sensation and weakness of the joint, or a deep wrenching pain. Cold wet weather will often aggravate the ailments which Ruta treats. Shin splints from running, tennis elbow, a lame feeling in the joint, aching pains, and shooting pains up the spine from an injury, all call for Ruta.

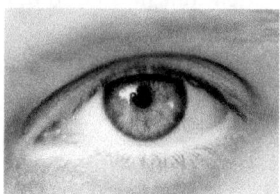

Eye strain, headaches from reading or working in front of a computer screen, a detached retina from a blow to the head and a black eye are also ailments needing this remedy.

Case 1: I used Ruta with good results in the case of a construction worker who repeatedly sprained his back. In order to receive compensation from his employer he had to fill out a lot of forms in a room that was small. In this space he would get panic attacks so he told me he would walk round and round the building trying to get enough courage to go in and fill out these forms. Ruta not only cured his back pains but also the anxiety and claustrophobia.

2: In another case a police officer came to me for chronic tendinitis of the shoulder joints so much so he could no longer drive his patrol car. After Ruta he was able to go back to work with no more pain and also was wondering why he felt no more guilt from writing speeding tickets? But this is not a coincidence as we know Ruta cures guilt. Ruta cures chronic wear-and-tear chronic painful injuries. Each repeat of the sprain is slower to heal; such as often seen in dancers and athletes. With Ruta the back becomes stronger, and the tendency for sprains is greatly decreased.

3: She is a competitive swimmer. Tendonitis is both shoulders. Can no longer train for the Senior Olympics. She collects antiques but has too many of them. Her husband has told her to sell them but she can't as she is afraid she will sell them for too much and thus her conscience bothers her too much. After Ruta 30c her shoulders are all better, able to swim again and feels less pangs of conscience to sell her collectibles.

When Ruta is needed for the root cause of a chronic constitutional imbalance such as the above mentioned cases; the patient will often feel *morbidly conscientious* and extremely guilty over small insignificant details. The guilt is not justified and which acts to paralyze these people. Ruta will reduce this morbid conscientiousness (guilt feelings) and remove the chronic inflammation in the tendons.

The other mental symptom of this remedy is that it can be used for a person who suffers from chronic sprains and who also has a fear of imminent death or experiences panic attacks in a warm, closed-in room (claustrophobia).

In these chronic cases, the ailment will be a chronic tendinitis; the pain will be so severe that it will prevent the use of the arms and prevent sleep. The key symptom is that the pain continues during rest and through the night it seems to get worse (Syph).

SYMPHYTUM
(Comfrey)

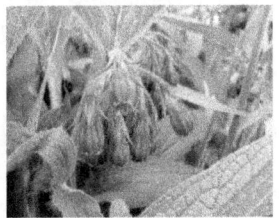

This is the best healer for broken bones. It can also be used for pain from INJURIES to BONES and the periosteum (periosteum: connective tissue, trauma sensing nerve fibers, blood vessels).

Pain from kicking a concrete bench with the shin – lingering deep aching pain in the bone. Many times after an injury many tissues are traumatized. Always give Arnica first to to stop the bleeding and start the overall healing process. Later on try to determine which specific tissues are injured and then give the appropriate remedy such as: Calendula, Symphytum, Hypericum,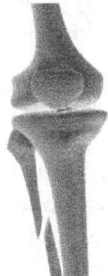
Bryonia, Rhus toxicodendron or Ruta also on that same day as the injury.

Repeat the remedy which is helping the most when those same

symptoms return. Start with 30c; when this stops working start using 200c, then 1m if needed.

Symphytum can also be used to speed up the healing of fractures after the bone is set in its correct alignment. Tendon and ligament injuries often respond to this remedy. Old knee injuries., knees with loose tendons and ligaments. It can be used as a salve for this condition.

Osteomalacia – soft bones. (on x-ray the bone is not white but rather shows a dark shadow; i.e. demineralization of the bone tissue. Patients with this bone condition can complain of bone pain at night or bone pain worse from exercise.

The salve can also be used to treat oseopenia and osteoporosis (Calc-phos, Syph). Rub the Comfrey salve over the spine and hips about three times a week. This salve is also one of the best restorative agents for the skin. It will treat dry cracking skin; bringing moisture back.

Symphytum: 30c, 200c and 1m for pain from bone cancer. Give as needed so that the patient does not have to take as much morphine or none at all.

Cases: 1. A 65 year old man came to see me with intractable hip pain from osteosarcoma. He took Symphytum 30c as needed – about three times a day and so never needed any morphine.

2. An 8 year old was hit in the eye by a baseball. Arnica helped but Symphytum took away the pain and bruising of the bone.

3. At work he hit his finger with a hammer resulting in severe pain. Arnica and Hypericum were tried first with no effect. Then Symphytum was tried and helped right away.

4. Teenager with pain in the knee at night with weakness on walking up a hill. X-ray shows irregular and oval shadows in the femur and the condyles are almost broken off. Symphytum 30c cured and in a month the patches of bone softening are filling in with dense bone and a return of strength to the knee.

5. Dog with bone cancer and given no more than a few months to live. Given the advise to put her down because of the pain. After Symphytum 30c weekly dose; this dog lives pain free for another three years.

Study Guide

6. Patient with chronically dry lips. After Symphytum salve this ailment resolved.

Quiz: Fill in the blank with the name of the remedy.

      1. Stiffness and pain better from motion: _____
      2. Bruises worse from touch: _____
      3. Weakness from over-lifting: _____
      4. Mosquito bites: _____
      5. Bee stings, edema: _____
      6. Sharp shooting pains: _____
      7. Burns and bladder infections: _____
      8. Muscle pain from overexertion: _____
      9. Tendonitis worse from overexertion: _____
      10. Shock with fear of death: _____
      11. Grief with a lump in the throat: _____
      12. Cuts and scrapes: _____

Answers: 1. Rhus-t, 2. Arnica 3. Carb-an, 4. Ledum, 5. Apis, 6. Hypericum, 7. Cantharis, 8. Bellis, 9. Ruta, 10. Aconite, 11. Ignatia, 12. Calendula.

CHAPTER 2

REMEDIES
FOR CHRONIC AILMENTS

Below is the materia medica of some of our best known remedies which mostly treat acute and chronic ailments. The highlighted area shows how for example a remedy can affect a wide range of symptoms both for certain first aid, acute ailments and for certain chronic ailments.

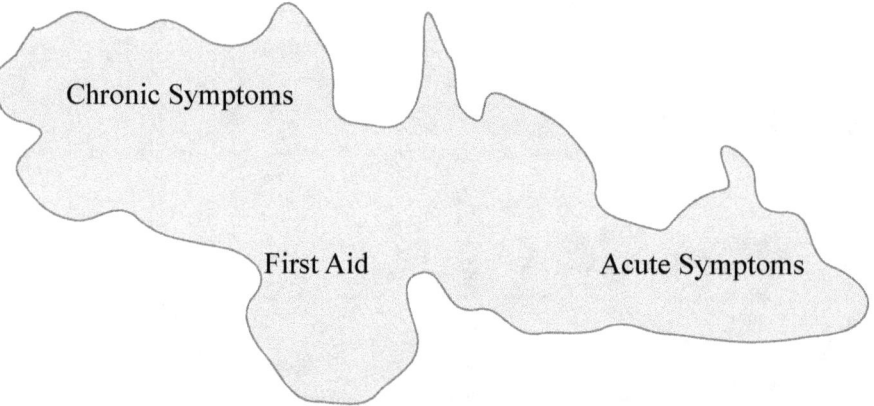

Each remedy rebuilds a certain area of the body's healing system but this could affect many systems and different tissue types in the body. For example if a patient has food poisoning – an acute symptoms such as nausea and vomiting can occur. Arsenicum can treat this in about an hour in most situations but this patient may also need Arsenicum to threat his acute bronchitis, chronic asthma or chronic anxiety attacks. It is best therefor to learn each remedy its for first aid situations, acute situations and for chronic situation.

Study Guide

AESCULUS HIPPOCASTANUM
(Horse Chestnut)

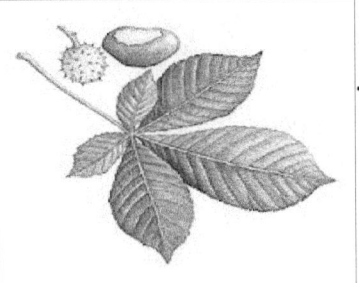

Hemorrhoids – *the rectum feels full of sticks.* Stasis of venous system; *general congestion.*

Plethora – fullness and congestion. Dull and sluggish in the mind. Varicose veins are purple.

Pain in the sacroiliac joint worse from rising from sitting or stooping. Sharp shooting pains in the back.

Worse in the morning on waking, better in cool open air.

Here is what James Kent has to say about this remedy: *A peculiar kind of plethora is found running through this remedy, a vascular fullness which affects the extremities and the whole body, and there are symptoms showing that the brain is similarly affected.*

Modalities: The conditions of Aesculus are worse during sleep, hence symptoms are observed on waking. He wakes up with confusion of mind, looks all around the room in confusion, bewildered, does not know the people, wonders where he is and what is the meaning of the things he sees.

It is especially useful in children that rouse up in sleep frightened and in confusion, like Lycopodium. The remedy produces great sadness, irritability, loss of memory and aversion

Materia Medica

to work. There are times when there is a sense of bodily congestion, fullness of the veins, and then these symptoms are most marked.

It is a general venous stasis, and is sometimes worse in sleep, worse from lying, better from bodily exertion. The symptoms pass away after considerable exertion; moving about, doing something, keeping busy relieves. (Kent, Lectures on Materia Medica).

AGARICUS MUSCARIUS
(Aminita Mushroom)

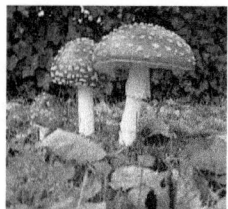

Fearless – daredevil, takes unbelievable chances.

Face is rigid or ***twitching*** of the facial muscles.

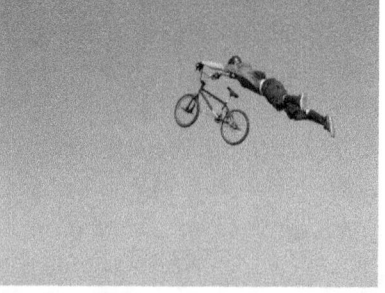

Case 1: For example an 11 year old boy who was a real dare-devil with his bicycle. He had no fear to ride down a sleep hill and then go over a jump across a stream. His mother brought him in because his face had become rigid and paralyzed especially around his mouth with twitching around the eye lids. This remedy in a 30c potency taken once a week resolved this problem and he became more cautious.

Study Guide

2: This was a case of mania. Staying up all night, can't stop talking. *No fear of anything or anyone.* He was driving his car as if he was on a race track. Very angry from contradiction, he almost got into some fights. He was brash, could not see what a turmoil his life was in. Spending money on useless things. After Agaricus he calmed down became rational again.

3: 53 years old male. He had lived a life with no fear. Taking bets on the stock market winning huge amounts and living a lavish lifestyle then loosing it all and living in financial ruin, then winning again. For a time he was addicted to gambling, he was a very colorful character. He liked to take a risk on relationships that others would have run away from. He made friends with known criminals. Spent some time in jail. Now suffers from terrible anxiety with jerking of the arms. After Agar 30c he is much better; he pulled back from living life on the edge. He is more sensible and careful. Able to enjoy life without anxiety.

This remedy is used for lack of fear or the opposite; that being extreme fear; panic attacks with *muscle twitchings*.

Kent: *The most striking things running through this medicine are twitchings and tremblings, jerkings of the muscles and trembling of the limbs; quivering and tremors, everywhere these two features are present in all parts of the body and limbs.*

The twitching of the muscles becomes so extensive that it is a well-developed case of chorea. It has in its nature all that is found in chorea and has cured many cases. This is a general belonging to all parts to all muscles. Throughout the body there is a sensation of creeping and crawling. It is hardly confined to the skin, it is felt as if in the flesh, a sensation as if of ants. (Kent, Lectures on Materia Medica).

AILANTHUS GLANDULOSA
(Chinese Sumach)

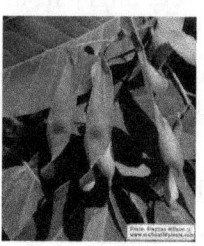

Enlarged glands, puffy skin. Low continued fever. Blue or dark red face. Frightened expression. Swollen throat internally and externally. Strep throat. Throat dark, purple and red (Hell). The neck feels tender. Enlarged tonsils with white puss with an inflamed throat. Offensive discharges (Pyrogen). The throat is very painful worse on swallowing. Can lead to sepsis. The tongue and throat feel dry. Dry hacking cough.

There is often pain in the back of the head and neck. Burning heat in the palms and soles. Dilated pupils.

Mental stupor, the mind is benumbed, stupid and dreamy. There is a constant loss of memory. She may become completely unconscious.

The face may be purple and bloated. The may be bleeding from the gums or nose. Chill during hunger. Tremendous body weakness.

This remedy can treat malignant scarlet fever. The most used remedy for scarlet fever is Belladonna but in that remedy the rash is bright red. Baptisia, Phytolacca and Helleborus like Ailanthus also have the purple dark eruptions with scarlatina.

Kent: *This medicine is especially suitable in the low zymotic forms of sickness, such as we find in diphtheria and scarlet fever, in blood poisoning and in symptomatic typhoids, especially those cases that are characterized by capillary congestion in spots, red mottled spots.*

Scarlet Fever: *Perhaps the most striking manifestation of such a low type of sickness is malignant scarlet fever. The regular rash does not come out, but in its place red spots, roseola-like, make their appearance; the usual uniform spread of the eruption has failed, or has been suppressed, and there is bleeding from the gums and nose, and dreadful tumefaction in the throat.*

The countenance is purple and besotted, the eyes are congested and there is even bleeding from the eyes. There is an appearance of great prostration, but it is really stupefaction; he seems stupid and benumbed.

If you look at the throat you see it is covered with little purple patches, intermingled with an oedematous appearance similar to that found in Baptisia. It is a low depressed type of sickness. (Kent, Lectures on Materia Medica).

ALOE
(Socritine Aloe)

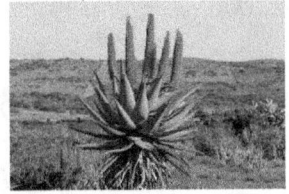

Insecurity of rectum; rectum feels full of heavy fluid, which will fall out, and does, if he does not go to stool immediately.

Diarrhea. *The rectum feels hot and burning so has to put cold applications on it.*

Nash one of the famous Homeopaths from the last century had this to say about Aloe: *Solid stool, passing (in large balls) involuntarily and unnoticed.*

Great fullness and weight in whole abdomen, with feeling of weight in rectum and hemorrhoids protruding like a bunch of grapes; > by cold water applied.

This remedy should be considered alongside of PODOPHYLLUM, because it is one of the so-called cathartics. Although one is as decided a cathartic as the other the characteristics which guide to their choice are very different.

Materia Medica

Both are apt to be worse during hot weather. Both are apt to be worse in the morning. Both are often well supplemented with SULPHUR.

But now let us look at some of the more marked and peculiar symptoms of ALOE. Stools yellow, fecal, bloody or transparent jelly-like mucus. Sometimes this jelly-like mucus (KALI BICH.) comes in great masses, or "gobs," and drops out of the rectum almost unnoticed. Again the stools are often passed involuntarily when expelling flatus or passing urine. There seems to be not only an actual weakness in the sphincter ani, but a distressing SENSE of weakness. The rectum feels as if full of heavy fluid which will fall out or escape from the patient, and in fact does so if he doesn't "git there, Eli." This escape of stool with flatus in ALOE finds its counterpart in OLEANDER. No two remedies are more alike in this respect, though MURIATIC ACID is also similar.

Again a very characteristic symptom in the ALOE diarrhea is "Great rumbling in the abdomen just before stool," and the feeling of weight in the rectum already mentioned is not always confined to the rectum, but is also felt through the whole pelvis and abdomen. Again, the rectum protrudes in ALOE like a bunch of grapes, and is relieved by the application of COLD WATER. MURIATIC ACID is relieved by hot applications. Both of these remedies have blue hemorrhoids; the ALOE itching intensely, while those of MURIATIC ACID are very sore and sensitive to touch, even of the bed clothes. In addition to the aggravations already mentioned, the diarrhea of ALOE is aggravated by walking or standing, after eating or drinking. In dysentery there is violent tenesmus, heat in the rectum, prostration even to fainting and profuse clammy sweats. The weakness of the sphincter ani is also found in constipation. It is a curious symptom, and I would not believe it until I had seen it with my own eyes. "Solid stool passing involuntarily, passing away unnoticed." I was called to treat a child five years of age suffering from birth with a most obstinate form of constipation.

He had to be forced and held to the stool crying and screaming all the while being totally unable to pass any feces even after an

Study Guide

enema. After trying several remedies in vain, I asked the mother to turn the child over (he was in bed) to let me examine the anus and rectum. As she turned down the bed clothes to do so, a large chunk of solid feces appeared in the bed. "There," she said, "that is the way it is. Notwithstanding his inability to pass stool when he tries, we often find these things in the bed, and he does not know when they pass, nor do we."

I then gave a few doses of ALOE 200th and cured the whole trouble quickly and permanently. ALOE like PODOPHYLLUM has also prolapsus uteri, and the feeling of heat, heaviness and fullness in the abdomen, pelvis and rectum guides to its selection. Like PODOPHYLLUM, also, its range of action is not wide, but positive, reliable and satisfactory. (<u>Leaders</u> In Homeopathic Therapeutics by E. B. *NASH)*

ALLIUM CEPA
(Red Onion)

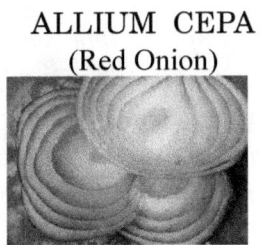

Hay fever or common cold symptoms with watery eyes and burning of the upper lip. <u>Sleepiness.</u> WORSE FROM HEAT.

Allium Cepa is made from a tincture of the red onion. Imagine the symptoms one gets from cutting up an onion: burning irritation of the eyes and this is often one of the symptoms that is present in a person who needs this remedy.

It is an excellent remedy for colds, ear aches and hay fever. The following symptoms when present, indicate its use:
- *hay fever*
- WATERY DISCHARGE from the nose that can BURN THE UPPER LIP
- *watery discharge from the eyes or red burning irritation of the eyes*
- *sleepiness with the cold symptoms or hay fever*

Materia Medica

- *worse in a warm room*
- feel groggy, dull and sleepy in the daytime
- lack motivation
- sneezing, especially when entering a warm room
- scratchy throat, hoarseness
- tickling or burning in the throat
- headache, worse from closing the eyes and worse from a warm room

Sleeping sickness, (Op, Nux-m) wants to sleep all the time, it may be a psychiatric case and when awake will do bizarre things.

All symptoms are worse from a warm room or from becoming overheated, and better in the fresh air. Pains in general described as being threadlike.

Kent: *Further, as to the eye-symptoms that accompany the Allium cepa colds, remember that the discharge from the eye is bland. Although there is burning in the eyes the tears do not excoriate as they flow down over the cheek. Profuse, bland lachrymation. Lachrymation in the evening in a warm room.*

"*Hoarse, harsh, ringing, spasmodic cough, excited by constant tickling in the larynx; cough produces a raw, splitting pain in the larynx, so acute and so severe as to compel the patient to crouch from suffering and to make every effort to suppress the cough.*"

"*Severe, laryngeal cough, which compels the patient to grasp the larynx; feels as if cough would tear it.*"

The child will reach up to the larynx and clutch it. This is wholly different from the Aconite condition, when the child, after exposure to a dry, cold wind, wakes before midnight with a hoarse, barking cough, and clutches the larynx. So Aconite cannot be substituted for Allium cepa.

Study Guide

Traumatic neuritis: Another affection over which this remedy has marvellous power is traumatic neuritis, often met with in a stump after amputation. The pains are almost unbearable, rapidly exhausting the strength of the patient. (Kent, Lectures on Materia Medica).

AMBRA GRESIA
(Half digested Crustacean Shells)

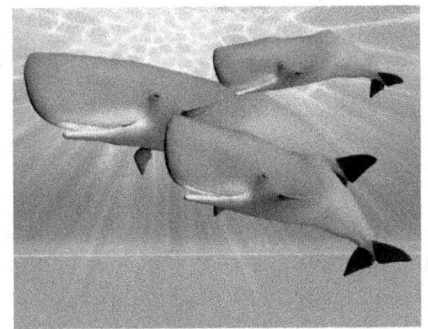

Feels embarrassed very easily; When ever they speak, they start to blush and want to escape. Social anxiety. Blushing from mortification. Feels stupid and inadequate. Feels too inhibited. Anticipation anxiety. Desire to hide away from people (Bar-carb). Lack of self confidence. Numbness of the arms.

More timid than Gelsemium, Silica or Lycopodium. Cramps in legs, twitching and spasms.

The most obvious symptom is that during the interview the patient will blush with embarrassment just from talking about ordinary things.

Kent: *We recognize trembling and a peculiar kind of feebleness that cannot be described by any expression but senility; it is not the confusion of mind belonging to sickness, but the peculiar state we recognize in old people, in declining life; trembling and tottering and a dreamy state of mind with forgetfulness.*

Materia Medica

He goes on from one subject to another, asking a question, and, without waiting for it to be answered, asking another.

So dizzy that they cannot go out on the street; so dizzy upon getting up in the morning that they must wait a while until they can get a-round on their feet. It is the dizziness belonging to senility and to premature old age.

This is a paroxysmal cough, much like whooping cough. Asthmatic dyspnoea from any little exertion, from music, from excitement. Cough with congestion of blood to the head. Cough from thinking and from anxiety. (Kent, Lectures on Materia Medica).

Case 1: Male 22 years old. Many different physical symptoms such as vertigo, heart racing, nausea, numbness of face arms and hands, legs jerk, diarrhea in the mornings and sleep problems. He achieved good grades in hight school but now afraid to go to college. Fear to be around so many people. Fear people will find out he was molested by his uncle. "I feel so much shame; no one knew". He is blushing many times in the interview.

After Ambra 30c he made a total recovery. All his physical symptoms get better and he went off to college. A couple of years later he is still doing well and enjoying his work in computer technology.

Vithoulkas describes these people as socially inhibited. It is for "the person, he says, who come face to face with the idea of 'failure' … they feel put down … or from the loss of their business they feel embarrassment. They seem to loose all their self-confidence instantly …."

Study Guide

AMBROSIA
(Rag Weed)

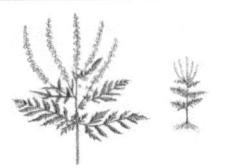

Hay-fever when there is intolerable itching of the eye-lids.

ANACARDIUM ORIENTALE
Marking Nut

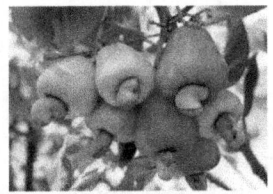

Pathological inferiority and cruelty. The more inferior he feels the more cruel he becomes.

Case 1. A 12 year old girl is neglected by her parents. She feels worthless, teased at school. She becomes aggressive and tries to stab another child at school. After getting in trouble for this she tries to burn the school down. This is typical behavior for Anacardium, the more inferior they feel the more cruel and aggressive they become. During the interview she was quiet and timid. After Anacardium her violent tendencies resolved.

With the inferiority these people often have fear of examinations and loss of memory. Depression from being neglected, then they become hard and aggressive. Desire to curse and swear. Feels a devil on one shoulder and an angel on the other shoulder. Sensation of a band around parts of body. She can feel very easily offended. Malicious and vicious acts of revenge. History of being put down and told they are no good. Tenacious, keeps trying to prove herself. Becomes frustrated leading to mischievous and delinquent behavior. Not doing well in school then slashing tires and violent acts. Sensation of a plug in various parts. Better from eating.

Vesicles are painful. Itchy eczema.

Kent: *The mind appears to be feeble; almost, if not complete imbecility; seems as if in a dream; everything is strange; slow to comprehend. Marked irritability; disturbed by everything; cursing. Weak memory. Forgetful of things in his mind but a moment ago. All his senses seem to vanish and he gropes around as if in a dream.*

Change of states; after states. Dullness and sluggishness of the mind prevail. He is in a continuous controversy with himself. Irresolution marks his character. He cannot settle between doing this and that, he hesitates and often does nothing. He cannot decide, especially in an action of good or evil.

He hears voices commanding him to do this or that, and seems to be between a good and an evil will. He is persuaded by his evil will to do acts of violence and injustice, but is withheld and restrained by a good will. So there is a controversy between two wills, between two impulses.

Unsocial; complains of weak memory. Slight causes make him excessively angry. A strong feature is that all moral feeling is taken out of him. He feels cruel. Can do bodily injury without feeling. Cruel, malicious, wicked.

Bad effects of mental excitement. Weak-minded. Consequences of fright and mortification. Suitable in religious mania when the conflict between the external and internal will is kept up. It is analogous to Hyos.

Study Guide

Many complaints are ameliorated by eating. Sensation here and there of pressure, described as if a plug, all through the body, in the head, eyes, in the navel and down the spine. (Kent, Lectures on Materia Medica)

ANDROCTONUS
(Scorpion)

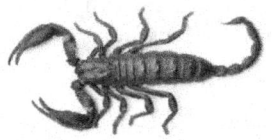

Takes offense very easily leading to acts of cruelty and violence. Cold violence. Feels everyone is the enemy (Merc-sol).

Here are some cases that I treated successfully with this remedy:

Case 1. A women is training her dogs. She beats them unmercifully when they do something wrong. After taking Scorpion the violence stops and she stops hitting her children as well.

2. A women is suddenly angry from being cut off in traffic. She follows them home, then chases them down and beats on them. She is very thankful of this remedy as her temper is so much better and no longer has to go to court.

3. A worker is fired from his job; later on he burns down the building and luckily there were no people in it. After taking this remedy he feels a lot of remorse for what he has done and finds he is no longer loosing his temper.

4. A teen is selling drugs, he feels invincible. He likes to beat on people, take their drugs or get money from them by almost killing them. He tells me he would like to kill someone one day.

After taking this remedy he quits this occupation and enrolls in in the army with the goal of learning how to rescue hostages.

5. The mother says it takes a lot of willpower to not kill her child when he won't stop crying (Alum). After Androc she can more easily moderate her temper and no longer feels cruel.

These people are often overly confident even charismatic. They are single minded in their ambitions. There is great cunning and no hesitation. Paranoid and suspicious. They often have a desire to control others and feel a total indifference toward others welfare.

Aversion to company, feels separate from the world. Selfish and self-centered. Detached. Chilly with lack of vital heat. Better from warm applications. Desire for open air. Lots of headaches. It is too late usually to be giving this remedy after the age of twelve as the harm these individuals can bring to others, their family, community and work place can be irreparable, such as gun violence.

One can only imagine the consequences these people bring to their own or other countries if they happen to be a military leader or hold other positions of power. For all of the violence in this world much of it could be prevented with these remedies such as Androc, Anac, Bell, Hep-sulph, Lach, Hyos and many others.
(Proved by Sher in 1985 – 31 provers)

ANTIMONIUM CRUDUM
(Black Sulphide of Antimony)

Very sentimental. Overwhelmed by emotions so has to isolate. For example he or she sits at home for hours thinking about an intense romantic situation. "She was beautiful, she had the eyes like moon light....I can't meet up with her it would be too intense" He met her on the bus so he keeps the bus ticket so he will always remember her and writes a poem about this infatuation. Much too sentimental but then angry if others try to talk to them about these intense emotions.

Typical for Antimonium crudum are romantic moods that are overwhelming. He or she will collect greeting cards and mementos in order to sustain and enhance the *romantic memories*. They feel things too strongly, and then are too sensitive so they can't cope with real people. In one case I saw he locked himself in his room and wold not communicate with his parents; *if they tried to talk with him he would become angry and the anger was worse if they looked at him.* After taking this remedy he would talk and have dinner with his parents again. He was now about 21 years old and had spent most of his life in his room alone.

She cries over lost love. Writes poetry looking at the moon.

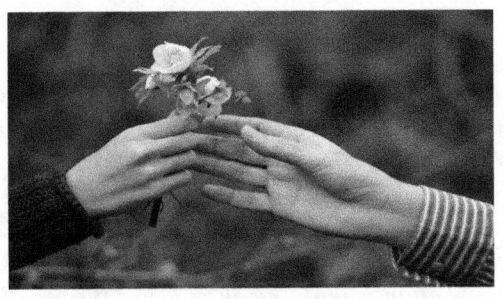

Over-eating tendency. She feels misunderstood, sulky and angry at everything.

Craving for acids and pickles. Ignatia is also very romantic but Ignatia can go out and meet real people and get into a real relationship and then get disappointed while Antimonium crudum is thirty to fifty percent more sensitive so that after a brief meeting with their object of affection they retreat into fantasy and can't meet that person again. In fact it is better not to meet them again as that would spoil it.

Kent: *The pains disturb his stomach and bring, on nausea. With his headache he is sick at the stomach; with all complaints his stomach is out of order, and, on the other hand, whenever he disorders his stomach he is sick all over. Complaints that manifest themselves through the stomach very frequently need this medicine.* (Kent)

Like Ipecac these people can't digest the real world, it makes them feel nausea.

First in importance are the mental symptoms showing the type of constitution likely to need this remedy. It produces a very serious state in the mind, an absence of the desire to live. It is well known to physicians that the case is a serious one if the patient has no desire to live; life is a burden. When I hear a patient say: "Oh, doctor, if I could only die." I do not like such a case; there is some deep-seated trouble in the economy that is hard to remove. Something is threatening, and when it comes it is a common thing to see the patient actually die. (kent)

"Loathing of life. Sentimental mood in the moonlight."

It is a hysterical state, a disorderly outburst of the affections, such affections as can be aroused only in one who is sick, or one who is unbalanced in the general nervous system.

We have running through this remedy a general state that you should keep in mind, that is, a gouty or rheumatic state, in which the symptoms change with the changes of the weather; worse in cold, damp weather, worse from cold bathing, better from the heat of a hot bath, worse from taking sour wine, and worse from stimulants of any kind.

The skin is ulcerated and has a tendency to grow warts, callosities, bad nails and bad hair.

Hard, horny excrescences grow under the nail and are extremely painful. From the ends of the fingers little horn-like excrescences appear.

Study Guide

The slightest pressure will produce a callosity, or a sore place, and in working men you will find an unusual tendency to thickening of the skin on the soles of the feet.

They are very sore to walk upon, because these callous places are sensitive and have numerous centers of little corns. The tendency to build up and indurate belongs to the remedy.

Warts grow upon the hands. The hair is unhealthy. Pustules form upon the skin with red areola.

Pustular eruptions have an inflamed base that is red, and sensitive. (Kent, Lectures on Materia Medica).

ANTIMONIUM TARTARICUM
(Tartar Emetic)

$$2K^+ \left[\begin{array}{c} O \\ O\!-\!Sb\!-\!O \\ O \end{array} \begin{array}{c} O \\ O\!-\!Sb\!-\!O \\ O \end{array} \right]^{2-} \cdot \; 3H_2O$$

This is a remedy that can be used for colds that have progressed toward bronchitis. The keynote symptom to look for is a **RATTLING OF MUCOUS IN THE CHEST** with difficult expectoration.

The bronchioles are full of tough mucous. As the person breaths, there is rattling of this mucous, which feels suffocating at times. Better to sit erect and generally feels worse when lying down.

Burning pains in the chest, a weak feeling in the chest. Hacking cough which has relief when lying on the right side. Dizziness. Cough made worse from eating. Coldness, trembling with chilliness. Cold clammy sweat. *Very sleepy* or wants to sleep many extra hours when has a cold or bronchitis.

The eyes often portray contempt and disdain for others. This can also be true for Antimonium crudum.

Case 1: A ten year old boy. He has a chronic cough; it goes on for months at a time. Sleepy and drowsy all day. He is discontented, whining and uncomfortable. When he looks at me I feel his hatred and disdain. I think to myself: "how can he hate me that much he has only just met me?" I make a mental note of it. Rattling cough. Has to sit up in bed or he can't breath. After Antimonium tart 30c he is completely better and even with a two year follow up he has not relapsed.

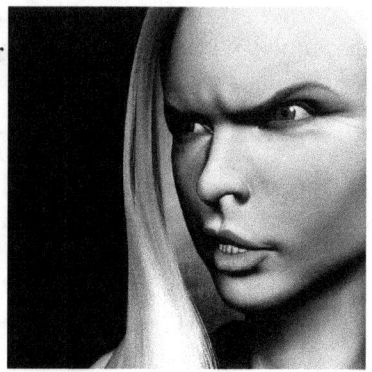

Kent: *The face is pale and sickly; the nose is drawn and shrunken; the eyes are sunken and there are dark rings around the eyes.*

The lips are pale and shriveled. The nostrils are dilated and flapping, and there is a dark, sooty appearance inside of the nostrils.

The face is covered with a cold sweat and is cold and pale. The expression is that of suffering. The atmosphere of the room is pungent, more pungent than foetid or putrid, and makes you feel that death is in it.

Catarrhal conditions of the trachea and the bronchial tubes. Our ears being open we hear coarse rattling and bubblings in the chest.

If you have ever been in the room of the dying you have heard what is called the death rattle. It is coarse like that.

Now and then there is expectoration of a mouthful of light-colored, whitish mucus. The condition is one in which the chest is steadily filling up with mucus, and at first he may be

Study Guide

able to throw it out; but finally he is suffocating from the filling up of mucus and the inability of the chest and lungs to throw it out.

In cases of bronchitis with pneumonia, inflammation of the trachea, inflammation of the air passages in general, the inflammation is likely to be attended with dryness or a scanty flow of mucus.

The child when sick doesn't want to be touched or talked to or looked at. Wants to be let alone. The infant is always keeping up a pitiful whining and moaning. Many times the respiration is a moaning respiration. Rattling and moaning. Always in bad humor, that is, extremely irritable when disturbed.

Antimonium is a common cause of the "fever sore," the lingering indolent ulcer that forms upon the legs following old fevers in broken down constitutions. (Kent, Lectures on Materia Medica).

APOCYNUM CANNABINUM
(Hemp Dogbane)

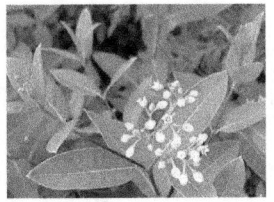

Edema in any part of the body. Slow pulse. *Dropsy, ascites, anasarca and hydrothorax.* Kidney diseases leading to edema. Excessive vomiting, water is immediately ejected with cramps. In rectum feeling as if the sphincter were open and stools ran right out. Low blood pressure. Retention of urine. Heart attack. Weakness, cold extremities, bradycardia, and arrhythmias. The skin is usually dry. *Deeply suppressed emotions.*

Kidney pain with shrieking. Acute nephritis with a high BUN. Hydrocephalus with stupor. Protracted hemorrhages.
Comparison with Apis. Apis is worse from heat and thirst-less while Apocynum is **WORSE FROM COLD and thirsty.** (Digitalis – also has a very slow pulse). Near death from alcoholism when the kidney and liver are severely damaged.

Kent: *This remedy comes in as a good one to contrast with Apis. You will find it analogous in its symptoms and much like the complaints cured by Apis.*

You will be astonished in going over the dropsical condition, the rheumatic condition, the tumefaction of the cellular tissues, the dropsy of the sacs, the scanty urine resulting in dropsy; the inflammatory swellings with oedema, at the great resemblances; and if you were to start in with two cases and work them out from their particulars, and if one feature were left out, the aggravation and the amelioration, the cold and the heat, in many cases you would not be able to distinguish between Apis and Apocynum, so near alike are their swellings, their bleedings, their distensions, and their disturbances. (Kent, Lectures on Materia Medica)

ARGENTUM NITRICUM
Silver Nitrate – AgNO3

Impulses to do dangerous things, but then feels afraid. Such as standing on a cliff, feels the impulse to jump but then experiences anxiety.

Likes to be on stage but then has anticipation anxiety. The mind is too weak and the emotions are too strong. For example he knows in his mind he should not laugh, but he can't help it. May appear as if being too silly or full of quirky jokes. *He looks at an electric outlet and knows not to put a wire in there but then almost does it anyway and gets a shock.* When he is on a height his mind says: *"don't jump"* but the emotions say: *"what would it be like to try and fly?"*. This frightens him as if he had jumped a serious accident or death would have resulted.

She wants to sing on the stage but when up there she feels afraid or *gets diarrhea before her recital from fear*. Stage fright in talented people. May have an uncontrollable temper. Feels hurried for no reason. *Crave sugar but it makes them sick. Fear of bridges or of driving over a bridge. Fear of closed in spaces.*

Anxiety about health. Warty growths, papilomas. Stomach ulcers. Loud belching. Generally worse from heat. Feels better in the cold wind. Violent palpitations. Paralysis; i.e. burned out nervous system.

Case 1: I had a patient who could not cross a bridge in her car. She was generally nervous, talkative and engaging. She also had lots of burning stomach pains. Arg-nit took care of both symptoms.

Kent: *He has all sorts of imaginations, illusions, hallucinations. He is tormented in his mind by the inflowing of troublesome thoughts, and especially at night his thoughts torment him to the extent that he is extremely anxious and this puts him in a hurry and in a fidget and he goes out and walks and walks, and the faster he walks the faster he thinks he must walk, and he walks till fatigued.*

Strange notions and ideas and fears come into his mind. He has an impulse that he is going to have a fit or that he is going to have a sickness.

A strange thought comes into his mind that if be goes past a certain corner of the street he will create a sensation, will fall down and have a fit, and to avoid that he will go around the block.

He avoids going past that corner for fear he will do something strange, He is so reduced in his mental state that he admits into the mind all sorts of impulses.

There is inflowing of strange thoughts into his mind, and when crossing a bridge or high place the thought that he might kill himself, or perhaps he might jump off, or what if he should jump off, and sometimes the actual impulse comes to jump off the bridge into the water.

When looking out of a window the thought comes to his mind what an awful thing it would be to jump out of the window, and sometimes the impulse comes to actually jump out of the window.

There is fear of death, the over-anxious state, that death is near, and often at times like Aconite he predicts the moment he is going to die.

Looking forward to times he is anxious. When looking forward to some thing that he is about to do, or in the expectation of things, he is anxious.

When about to meet an engagement he is anxious until the time comes.

If he is about to take a railroad journey he is anxious, full of fear and anxiety and tremulous nervousness until he is on the car going and then it passes away. If he is about to meet a certain person on the street corner he is anxious and breaks out often in a sweat from anxiety until it is over with.

Everywhere we find ulceration, but particularly upon the mucous membrane. The throat has ulcers in it, the eyelids, and of the cornea; ulceration of the bladder.

Ulcers of the uterus, of the vagina and of the external soft parts. This tendency of ulcerate seems rather strange, peculiar that it should have in its pathogenesis such a tendency, when the old school has been using it to cauterize ulcers, and yet it heals them up.

We know that Phosphorus will burn and it intensifies the tendency to ulcerate, makes the ulcer go deeper, while Argentum nitricum sets it healing. (Most snake remedies also treat ulcers).

There is a tendency to favor the growth of warts and in the throat there are little wart-like growths polypoid growths in the throat and about the genitals and anus; hence its great use in sycotic constitutions.

In Argentum nitricum he wants to be in a cold room, wants cold air, and to swallow cold things. In Hepar he wants warm things to drink, warm clothing, warm room, and cannot put even his hand out of bed or his throat will begin paining him.

Things, you see, just exactly opposite, but they both have "sticks" in the throat. In dry chronic catarrh Alumina and Natrum muriaticum have "sticks" in the throat; but in red throat with tumefaction and pain these two remedies give no relief, the former two are better. "Sticks" in the throat like fish-bones.

Nitric acid, Hepar, and Argentum nitricum, are the most striking remedies for the fish-bone sensation. Many remedies have sticking in the throat, but these are the most prominent.

We know how Argentum nitricum has been used for ulceration in the throat, and here it comes in as one of the most useful remedies in congestion of the throat of long standing. Catarrhs with loss of voice. Warty growths, condylomata, etc.

Loss of voice, tumefaction of the mucous membrane round about the vocal cords and paresis of the vocal cords. Condylomata on the vocal cords.

When it is said that "I cannot eat a teaspoonful of anything with starch, egg or sugar in it without being sick," it is always strange and peculiar, because it is not something that comes in only as a craving and affecting the stomach, but it affects the whole patient.

The patient says: "I become sick" and hence it becomes a general. When the patient gets a diarrhea from eating sugar it is not merely a local and particular symptom, because the whole patient is sick before the diarrhea begins; the diarrhea is the outcome. Hence as it is a general it i necessary that it should be examined into.

"Most gastric ailments arc accompanied by belching. Belching difficult; finally air rushes out with great violence."

"Nausea after every meal; nausea with troublesome efforts to vomit."

I have seen these Argentum nitricum patients vomiting and purging in the same moment, not vomiting one second and purging the next, but gushing out both ways with great exhaustion like cholera morbus, so relaxed, prostrated and weak.

"Anxiety with palpitation and throbbing through the whole body. Violent palpitation from the slightest mental emotion or sudden muscular exertion. Palpitation obliges her to press hand hard against heart for relief. Heart's action irregular, intermittent," etc.

Pain in the lumbar region comes on while sitting, but is better when standing a walking. Pain in the back from flatulence. Sore pain in the spine. Pain in back at night. Great weight in the lumbar region. It is a very useful remedy in locomotor ataxia.

Great restlessness. The nervous symptoms are very numerous. Periodical trembling of the body. Chorea, with tearing in the legs. Convulsions preceded by great restlessness. Nervous faintness, tremulous sensation, etc.

The sleep symptoms are quite general. Distressing nightmares.

Study Guide

The dreams are horrible. Wakens in excitement and with starting. All sorts of strange, horrible things in sleep. Dreams of vicious and violent things, and that everything is going to happen to him. Dreams of departed friends, etc.

On waking in the morning limbs feel bruised aching in the chest. Cannot sleep at night because he is so nervous.

Erysipelatous bed sores.

While riding <in a car>, palpitation and anxiety compelling him to get out of the wagon and walk, and that <being> real fast <walking>.

Purplish rash, such as appears in the most serious forms of scarlet and zymotic diseases.

Its most natural antidote is Natrum muriaticum. When you have the ulceration where the throat has been cauterized or the cervix uteri or eyelids have been cauterized by Nitrate of Silver, study Natrum mur. and see if the symptoms of the case would not justify its administration. It is the most common natural antidote for these vicious practices. (Kent, Lectures on Materia Medica).

ARSENICUM IODATUM
(Arsenic triiodide)

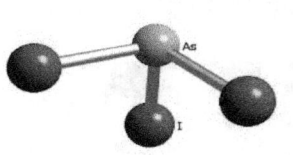

Very hyperactive - (ADD) *restless* and *worse from heat.* **Hypoglycemia. Wants to eat all the time.**

Can be <u>worse from heat and cold.</u> The Arsencium part of this remedy makes the patient or parts of the patient or at certain times very sensitive to cold but the Iodum part makes the patient in certain areas or at certain times very sensitive to heat.

Case 1: Ten year old with hypoglycemia and restlessness. Given no affection as a child so he feels empty and tries to get and demand attention from others to feel secure and wanted. Teacher says he won't sit still in class. Worse from heat and cold. Always getting up from his desk. After Arsen-iod he is much improved in his behavior at school., puts on weight and is no longer hypoglycemic.

Boericke: *Thin, watery, irritating, excoriating discharge from anterior and posterior nares; sneezing. Hay-fever. Irritation and tingling of nose constant desire to sneeze (Pollanin). Chronic nasal catarrh; swollen nose; profuse, thick, yellow discharge; ulcers; membrane sore and excoriated. Aggravation by sneezing.*

Dry, scaly, itching. Marked exfoliation of skin in large scales, leaving a raw exuding surface beneath. Ichthyosis. Enlarged scrofulous glands. Venereal bubo. Debilitating night-sweats. Eczema of the beard; watery, oozing, itching; worse, washing. Emaciation. Psoriasis. Acne hard, indurated base with pustule at apex. (Boericke)

ARSENICUM ALBUM
(White Arsenic - As2O3)

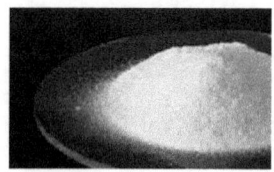

RESTLESS ANXIETY – *he moves from place to place, paces but can't find peace or rest.*

Study Guide

Fear of death – *she thinks every symptom is the sign of a chronic illness, he can't listen to stories about illness as he thinks he will be next. Fear of cancer because cancer is so strongly associated with death.*

FASTIDIOUS – *everything is in order, wants to clean up the house every day, it all has to be perfect. Anxiety and worry if things are not in their right place. Critical of others if they don't have the same standards.* ***Chilly*** – *always feel the room is too cold, wants to stay warm. May like fresh air for head complaints.*

Desire for security – *wants money in the bank. Stingy to spend money* (Bryonia- proporous people who have a fear to spend money, Melaleuca – fear there will be an economic catrastrophe so hoards food and money, Psor – fear of poverty with depression and despair)
First Aid:

It is the first medicine that can be given for FOOD POISONING I have verified it's effectiveness for these complaints many times. Within two or three hours after a dose of this remedy the vomiting and diarrhea will stop and the person will be able to go about their normal routine once more. For this reason it should always be taken when travelling to a country where the water is known to contain organisms that produce <u>diarrhea and vomiting</u>. If a person is prone to food poisoning then this may be a sign they are in need of this remedy for their chronic state.

Acute illness:
For respiratory illness, one will often find the following symptoms: A general feeling of *anxiety, restlessness,* a fear the illness is severe and a *fear to be left alone.* <u>A fear of death.</u> This is the same as the emotional state of Aconite and so they need to be compared. Although, with Arsenicum album, the person is *fastidious;* they want to have everything in order, clean and neat while in the Aconite patient this is not such a priority.

If pneumonia is present:
- Difficulty in breathing
- A worsening from lying down
- Burning in the chest
- Suffocative or dry cough
- Cough being worse from 1:00 – 2:00 am

- Darting pains in the lungs
- Burning heat all over, but a desire to be kept warm but a desire for fresh air
- Cough *worse* from cold drinks, and *better* from warm drinks

Asthma that leaves the person in a panic and full of restlessness.
Cold sweats, always wanting to be kept warm. Very sensitive to the cold and cold drafts.

Fevers with high temperatures, delirium, septic fevers, periodic fevers and exhausting fevers.

Headaches are made better with cold applications. Sore burning or ulcerated throat.

<u>Desire for frequent small sips of water.</u> Aversion to eating.
Can't sleep from midnight until two am. Anxious and restless sleep.
Typical influenza with anxiety and a desire for small sips of water.
Thin watery discharge from the nose. Sneezing without relief.

Always changing position, RESTLESS, <u>wants company</u>, full of worry, lacks courage, despair of recovery, selfish, FASTIDIOUS (sensitive to disorder) and confusion. Wants everything its place, chilly, collapses with exhaustion and burning pains.

In the old literature these people are described as carrying around a gold cane (a symbol of wealth, security and stratification). They walk about the house polishing their precious things and straightening the paintings on the walls. They are alone, they call someone to come over and keep them company. "I feel less anxiety when so and so is over here." They pace the floor wondering if the pains in their lungs or stomach are about to kill them, looking at their cell phone every minute; "when will my friend be here I just called her!" Anyway they are sure it is cancer even though the specialist said it was not cancer from all the tests that were taken. "Best to call the doctor at 6 a.m. tomorrow morning as he did not do such and such a test and then see him again for more questioning and get a second and third opinion. I must insist on that"

So it goes until they happen to come and see you the homeopath; who they will also torment.

Study Guide

In the movie: <u>What About Bob</u> -he drives his psychiatrist crazy. Nitric Acid also has this same anxiety and determination to hound their doctor for many tests.

These are the symptoms to look for. If they are present, the acute ailment no matter what its name, will be helped if not outright cured by Arsenicum. The main symptom to look for are restless anxiety, sensitivity to cold, desire for small sips of water, a need for things to be clean and orderly and feels better with company.

The character 'House' played by the talented Hugh Laurie is a good example of this remedy. He is obsessed about medical obscurities but he can't cure his own ailments which leads to taking all types of medications (Mind, anxiety about health). He is unapologetically selfish, he pretends to not need anyone but desperately stays at work all hours so as not to be alone.

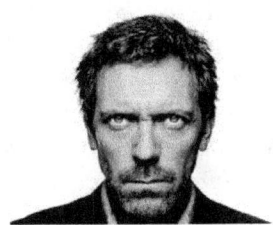

The Arsenicum patient is always busy and cannot rest. When he is alone, he can't find peace, suffers from anxiety which needs to be medicated. He is critical, selfish, alienated from life, (no religious feeling), wants certainty and is severely cynical.

He fights against chaos and death but there is no real answer or guarantee of security or salvation which he can't find in his work or from friends. What happens after death? he has no answer. The Arsenicum patient feels there is no guarantee in life, no real spiritual answer or anything to save us from death, give comfort, no secure purpose or proven God to give us meaning, comfort and security. It is a modern dilema curable with Arsenicum.

If a person has this type of character in real life they may need Arsenicum if the other guiding symptoms listed here are also present.

Money represents security from suffering and chaos; therefore these people can be stingy with it. In one case I treated the patient begged me to not charge her anything for her stomach ulcer. Then after she received Arsenicum which cured her ulcer I found out she was one of the most wealthy people in town.

In another case I saw treated by George Vithoulkas the young women had stopped eating. She was severely anorexic, fear to eat, anxious to look beautiful as if she was not beautiful she would be rejected and alone from her family. She was very beautiful but no one could touch her as it could spoil her. It was a polished elegance not to be spoiled by real affection from others. After Arsenicum she started to eat, let people love her for who she was and no longer needed to maintain the delusional projection of something that was not realy real.

Nash in his book <u>Leaders</u> says: *No remedy is more restless than this one. The ACONITE restlessness comes in the earlier stages of inflammatory diseases, with fever of a high grade. ARSENICUM in the later stages, after the patient has become greatly reduced in strength, or in low grades of fever like typhoids. The ACONITE patient tosses to and fro in agony and fear. The ARSENIC patient is too weak to toss as the anguish and restlessness would incline him to. He cannot move himself around as he desires, but wants to be moved from place to place, or bed to bed, while the least exertion on his own part exhausts terribly. He has fear of death, but not like the ACONITE fear, but rather an anxiety and a feeling that it is useless to take medicine for he is going to die; he is incurable.*

The mental restlessness is as great as the bodily. He has attacks of anxiety that drive him out of bed at night. Even when there is no pain at all he wants to be continually changing place, walking about if strong enough, without any other reason than that he can't keep still. Often the first beneficial effect to be observed in cases calling for this remedy is that the anxiety grows less, the patient lies still, his pain is not so much less, but it does not make him so restless; he can bear it better. This is a good sign and is generally followed by amelioration of all the symptoms. It makes little difference what the disease, if this persistent restlessness and especially if great weakness is also present, don't forget ARSENIC.

ARSENICUM leads all the remedies for burning sensation, especially in acute diseases. It is not by any means confined to acute diseases, but is often found in chronic affections, especially of a malignant character or tending to malignancy. I think perhaps SULPHUR outranks it generally for burnings in chronic affections. There is hardly an organ or tissue in the human system where these burnings of ARSENIC are not found. This burning, strange as it may seem, is greatly ameliorated by heat. Hot applications if they can be gotten in contact with the part, also heat of a warm stove or warm room.

This is the exact opposite of SECALE CORNUTUM, for while the part is objectively cold, it still BURNS, but hot applications are intolerable; they cannot even bear to have it covered; with ARSENICUM, in throat complaints, in connection with acute catarrh, the burnings in throat and from the excoriating nasal discharge are ameliorated by hot application. The burning in throat is better from eating or drinking hot things. This is the chief modality which enables us to choose between this remedy and CEPA and MERCURIUS, for all three have fluent coryza. I once had a case of very severe gastralgia caused by suppression of eczema on the hands. I knew nothing of the suppression, but prescribed ARSENICUM because the pains came on at midnight, lasting until 3 a.m., during which time the patient had to walk the floor in agony, and there was GREAT BURNING in the stomach. She had but one slight attack after taking ARSENICUM, but, said she, when I visited her, "Doctor, would that remedy send out salt rheum?" Then I found out about the suppression which had been caused by the application of an ointment, and told her that she could have back the pain in the stomach any time she wanted it, by suppressing the eruption again. She did not want it.

ARSENICUM is not the only remedy capable of curing these malignant cases, and how do we know after all that it may not be MURIATIC ACID or CARBO VEGETABILIS that will be the remedy after the case is developed. There is no safe or scientific rule but to treat the case with the INDICATED remedy at any and all stages of the disease, without trying to treat expected conditions or future possibilities.

It would be out of place here to give all the indications for ARSENIC in typhoids, as it would take too much space, and they can be found in Raue, Lilienthal or any good work on practice. ARSENIC is also one of our best remedies in intermittents, especially after the abuse of QUININE. Close individualization is necessary here as elsewhere.

ARSENIC profoundly affects the alimentary canal from lips to anus. The lips are so dry and parched and cracked that the patient often licks them to moisten them. The tongue is affected in various ways. It may be dry and red, with raised papillae; or red, with indented edges; or white as chalk or white paint; or lead colored; or dry, brown or black, especially in typhoids. The mouth is dry or aphthous, ulcerated or gangrenous.

The throat the same. The thirst is indescribably intense and peculiar, in that notwithstanding its intensity the patient can TAKE ONLY A LITTLE WATER AT A TIME. The stomach is so irritable that the least food or drink causes distress and pain, or immediately excites vomiting, or stool, or both together. Cold drinks, ice-water, or ice-cream particularly, disagree and create distress. Vomits all kinds and grades of substances from water or mucus to bile, blood, and coffee ground substances.

The pains in stomach are terrible and aggravated by the least food or drink, especially, if COLD. The abdominal pains also are intense, causing the patient to turn and twist in all possible shapes and directions.

Diarrhoea of all kinds of stools, from simple watery to black, bloody and horribly offensive, and finally the end of the tract is reached and we have haemorrhoids. Now in every one of these affections, ranging along the whole length of the canal, and from the lightest grade of irritation to the most intense inflammatory and malignant forms of disease, we will be apt to find everywhere present the characteristic BURNING of this remedy, in greater or lesser degree; and the not less characteristic AMELIORATION FROM HEAT, and also, though not quite so invariably, the MIDNIGHT AGGRAVATION.

ARSENICUM also has its sphere of usefulness in diseases of the respiratory organs. First, for acute coryza it stands in the front rank, the choice often having to be made between this remedy, CEPA and MERCURIUS. ARSENICUM has the fluent discharge which corrodes the lips and wings of the nose and more BURNING than the other two remedies. It often follows well after MERCURIUS, if that remedy only partially relieves.

ARSENICUM is particularly efficacious in many affections of the lungs, where the breathing is very much oppressed. Respiration is wheezing, with cough and frothy expectoration. Patient cannot lie down; must sit up to breathe, and is unable to move without being greatly put out of breath. The air passages seem constricted.

It is especially useful in asthmatic affections caused or aggravated by suppressed eruptions, like pneumonia from retrocedent measles, or even chronic lung troubles from suppressed eczema. I remember a case of asthma of years' standing to which I was called at midnight, because they were afraid the patient would die before morning. Found that her attacks always came on at 1 A. M. Gave ARSENICUM ALB. 30th, and she was completely cured by it.

The symptom by Rollin R. Gregg, "Acute, sharp, fixed or darting pain in apex and through upper third of right lung," is a gem, and has enabled me to cure a number of cases of obstinate lung troubles. In the last stage of pneumonia of old people, with gangrenous expectoration, if the other symptoms correspond, this remedy has often saved life. The burning is often found here as elsewhere. ARSENICUM is also one of our best remedies in pleuritic effusions.

ARSENICUM also affects profoundly the nervous system. To the characteristic restlessness, of which we have said so much, is added great prostration. This prostration is present in most diseases, both acute and chronic, where ARSENIC is indicated. For instance, in typhoids there is no remedy that prostrates more.

CARBO VEG. and MURIATIC ACID equal it, the difference being that the ARSENIC patient wants to move or be moved constantly, while with the other two remedies there is almost utter absence of any such show of life. Even if not confined to the bed, in acute or chronic diseases the patient is so weak that he is "exhausted from the slightest exertion;" must lie down. Sometimes this extreme degree of prostration comes on very rapidly.

Here is a picture that shows a condition of things in chronic trouble calling for this remedy. "From climbing mountains, or other muscular exertions, want of breath, prostration, sleeplessness and other ailments." This shows how weak the patient is, and this weakness may be coupled with various forms of disease. You may say it is common for sick people to be weak. True, but the ARSENICUM patient is weak OUT OF

PROPORTION to the rest of his trouble, or apparently so; and it is a GENERAL PROSTRATION, not local like the sense of weakness in the chest of PHOSPHORIC ACID, STANNUM and SULPHUR; or in the abdomen like PHOSPHORUS; or in the stomach like IGNATIA, HYDRASTIS and SEPIA. Now I do not see how I can make plainer the value of prostration as an ARSENIC symptom.

When we come to the tissues we find our remedy almost universally present. It attacks the BLOOD, causing septic changes, exanthemata, ecchymoses, petechia;, etc.

It attacks the VEINS; varices burn like fire, < at night. It attacks the serous membranes, causing copious serous effusions.

It attacks the glands, which indurate or suppurate. It attacks the periosteum. It attacks the joints; causing pale swellings, burning pains, etc.

It causes inflammatory swellings with burning lancinating pains. It causes general anasarca; skin pale, waxy or earth colored; great thirst (APIS none). It causes rapid emaciation; atrophy of children.

It causes ulcerations, constantly extending in breadth. The ulcers BURN like fire, pain even during sleep, discharge may be copious or scanty, the base blue, black or lardaceous.

Anthrax BURNING like fire; cold blue skin dry as parchment, peeling off in large scales. "Sphacelus," parts look black or BURN like fire. "Gangrene," better from heat (worse, SECALE).

"Parchment" like dryness, or dry scaly skin. The skin troubles of this remedy are mostly dry and scaly, and almost always burning. It is one of our best remedies for affections caused by retrocedent or suppressed exanthemata, also for suppressed chronic eczemas, etc.

But it is impossible and outside the scope of this work to mention by name all the affections of the tissues in which this remedy is useful.

Notwithstanding this, ARSENIC is not a panacea. It must, like

Study Guide

every other remedy, be indicated by its similar symptoms or failure is the outcome. Its great keynotes are Restlessness, Burning, Prostration, and Midnight Aggravation.

ARUM TRIPHYLLUM
(Jack-in-the-Pulpit)

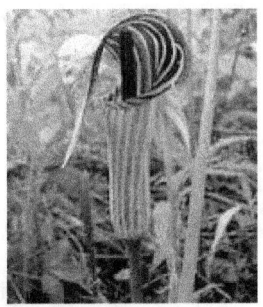

Acrid discharges and inflammations. Mucous surfaces destroyed, raw, bloody and burning. Scabs and cracks of the skin. Hay fever, impetigo and scarlet fever. Red tongue and or red rash. Wants to pick the nose and lips till they bleed. Dry lips. Itching and tingling of the lips, nose, palate and ears.

ARUNDO DONAX
(Reed)

Hay fever. Scalp itches and hair falls out. Roots of hair painful. Burning and itching of the palate and conjunctiva. Itching in the nostrils. Fissures in tongue. Cold sensation in the stomach. Craves acids. This remedy needs further proving to find out its emotional state and general symptoms.

Materia Medica

AURUM METALLICUM
(Gold)

Severe suicidal depression.

The patient tries to be perfect, or gain a feeling of self worth through being a workaholic.

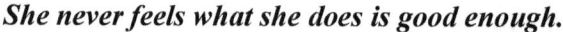

Feel better from accomplishment and praying.

She never feels what she does is good enough.

They feel in a pit of despair, when they look up there is no light.

They try everything to connect and feel worthy but as there is no way out and therefore they look for ways to commit suicide.

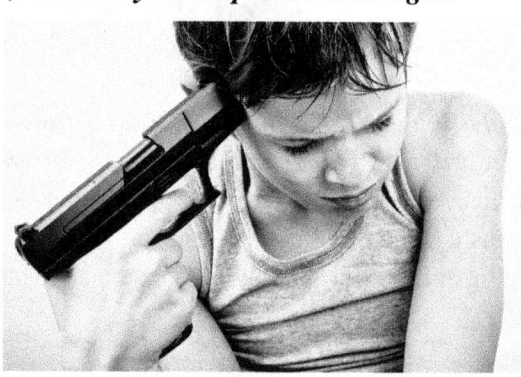

Cold and hard depression. Look for ways to kill themselves.

A quiet but heavy depression.
Those needing this remedy may experience the following physical and mental symptoms:
- OVERWORKING, DESIRE FOR PERFECTION, NEVER FEEL WHAT THEY DO IS GOOD ENOUGH – Self reproach
- *feeling hopeless*
- *feeling despondent*
- *constantly dwelling on suicide*
- *profound melancholy*
- disgust for life
- severe depression, *relieved by the thought of suicide.*
- feels herself utterly worthless, of no value, and reproaches herself

Study Guide

- physical pains make him suicidal

Ailments from situations like:
- grief, or disappointed love, or
- business failure

Amelioration from music and feels better in the evening.
Other typical behaviours and indications:
- a desire to pray
- pains worse at night
- chronic infections of the ear, sinus, throat, bladder
- headaches
- joint pain, chronic ulcers

Case 1: This 35 year old patient had a chronic bladder infection with ulceration of the bladder so severe that she was scheduled to have her bladder removed. At the last minute she decicided to not have this done; walked out of the hospital and called me instead. After Aurum her chronic bladder infection was cured, her depression also was relieved and she found her way out of poverty. Still better on a five year follow up.

2: In another case a patient came to see me on her way to commit suicide, she was planning to drink a bottle of vodka and then swim out into a lake and drown herself. She took the remedy about once a week for a month and was cured of this condition. She started to enjoy life and one can't describe the joy, relief and appreciation this brought to her.

Kent had a lot of experience with this remedy and says in these patients there is: *Self-condemnation, continual self-reproach, self-criticism, a constant looking into self; she does nothing right, everything is wrong, nothing will succeed, hopelessness.*

"Imagines he cannot succeed in anything, and he does everything wrong; he is in disunion with himself."

Imagines he sees obstacles in his way everywhere.

He is all the time imaging that he has neglected something, that he has neglected his friends.

He imagines that he deserves reproach in consequence of having neglected duty; he has neglected something, he is wrong, is wholly evil, has sinned away his day of grace, is not worthy of salvation; this is the train of thought that constantly runs through his mind.

The thought really becomes uncontrollable; he is absorbed in himself and sits and broods over it, and by brooding over it he only intensifies his present state and hatches new grievances, continues to worry over himself, thinks he is wholly unfit for this world, and then he longs to die.

He looks on the dark side of everything, constantly expecting bad news, looking for everything to go wrong. The future looks dark to him, and he wants to die; he never will succeed, for everything goes wrong that he turns his hand to.

His business is dark, his family troubles him, his friends annoy him; he becomes extremely irritable, easily angered, is worried over trifles, and easily excited.

Every little thing rouses him into anger and turmoil, he is always in a vexation. The Aurum state of mind is an insanity dreadful to look upon because of its turbulence and melancholy.

The remedy is full of rheumatic affections, not unlike such as are found in old mercurial cases; rheumatic affections with swelling of the joints; affections of the cartilages and bone, inflammation of the periosteum; thickening and induration of the periosteum. Indurations of glands; induration of the cartilages about the joints.

These are all of syphilitic and mercurial character. It is useful in old syphilitics when the bones are breaking down in any part of the body; the shin bones, nose bones, ear bones, any of the small bones.

Pains: Like syphilis and mercury, the complaints are aggravated at night, coming on in the evening and keep up all night. The pains are violent, they tear, the bones ache as if they would break, not in acute fevers but in old syphilitic bone troubles.

Knife-like pains in the periosteum. Pains in the joints rendering them immovable. Inflammation of the bone itself with caries.

Study Guide

It is not strange that the vascular coating of the bones, the periosteum, should be greatly affected because there is a strange vascularity, all over the economy, in this medicine.

"Pains drive to despair." The pains drive the patient out of bed at night and make him walk. This is seen in old syphilitic bone pains, and old mercurialized patients.

"Desire for open air." This patient ranks along with Pulsatilla as to temperature; but Aurum is not mild, gentle and yielding, he is obstinate, irascible, the very opposite of the Pulsatilla patient.

"Generally better from staying warm." This is in connection with the headaches.

"Cold water ameliorates pain in eyes. Averse to uncover, but he desires open air like Pulsatilla. Warm air aggravates the asthma."

Many symptoms disappear after washing, especially cold washing; but whenever the patient is suffering from great excitement, turmoil and vascularity, constitutional orgasm, pulsations, he wants the doors and windows open, wants to get out in the cool air; wants the clothing thrown off.

This state of excitement and pulsation is ameliorated by the open air. It has those flushes of heat so, common to women at the critical period, and these are followed by sweat, sometimes by chilliness.

Head: *In Aurum the pain in the head is very intense, maddening, often accompanied by a sensation as if air were blowing upon him; he looks around to see where the draft comes from when there is none; extremely sensitive.*

Often has to have the head wrapped up, although it feels hot, with a good deal of congestion and rush of blood to the head. The head is sore and feels bruised. Stitching, burning, tearing pains in the head; much throbbing in the head. The face is bloated, flushed and shiny with the congestive headaches. These headaches are often found in syphilitic subjects; often associated with cardiac disease. Pain in the back of the head associated with cardiac disease, with sluggish circulation, purple *face, duskiness of the skin. Exostoses as in syphilis.*

The skull bones are sensitive to touch; the periosteum is tender to touch. In old mercurialized cases with bone affections and necrosis of the skull, as in syphilis and mercury, the hair falls out copiously; the head becomes bald. (Kent)

This remedy affect many other body systems; information of which can be referenced in Kents materia medica.

AURUM MURIATICUM
(Gold Chloride)

Severe depression often as the result of grief, thinks about suicide.

Worse from sun and craves salt; these two symptoms show how it is different from Aurum metallicum.

Case 1: I had a very depressed patient come to see me. She was about 30 years old and had been suicidal since the age of 12. She had many Aurum symptoms such as being very religious, overly conscientious, pains at night and full of self reproach. Aurum metallicum did nothing but then because of the salt craving and being worse in the sun I gave her Aurum muriaticum 30c one dose. After this her debilitating depression was relieved. Then she got a very severe bronchitis with lots of salivation and told me she had an impulse to run through her sliding glass door. After Mercury 30c her infection was better overnight and her overall emotional state was even more improved as her impulses to do violence to herself also abated.

Aurum metallicum in general would have less ability to make contact with others while Aurum muriaticum will have a more

Study Guide

romantic contact or grief from a broken romantic contact.

Think about this remedy if you see Aurum symptoms and Natrum muriaticum symptoms in the same patient.

AURUM SULPH
(Gold sulphide)

In these cases you will see many Aurum symptoms and many Sulphur symptoms.

Case 1: A man in his 20's. He told me he was going to climb a high cliff that afternoon and jump. He was a cook, he had a young family. He was tall with red features and worse from heat. He had a chronic eczema. I gave him Aurum sulphur 30c one dose and advised him to call his family and go to the hospital. Instead he drove to the cliff, climbed up and sat there looking at the beautiful view.

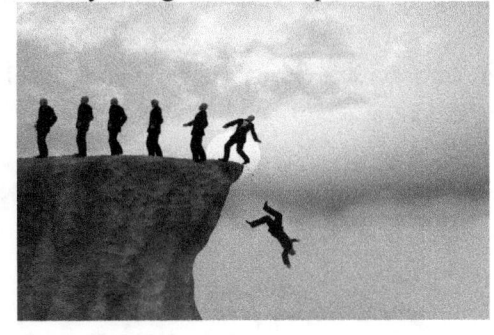

Then he fell asleep and woke up feeling much better; so he climbed down from the cliff and went home. When I saw him the next week I did not recognize him in the waiting room as his demeanor had changed so much. He now stood tall and with confidence.

He told me that the awful depression was totally gone and could not believe that he had almost ended his life and abandoned his family and children. He just sat there and shook his head in disbelief. His parents had divorced when he was ten and he had not been able to see his father.

He had blamed himself for the divorce; (all the Aurum remedies are for people who blame themselves, then feel they would be better off dead) even though he knew in his mind it was not his fault but he still mistakenly believed that if he had been a better child the divorce would not have happened. He went on to make a complete recovery in his depression and eczema.

BAMBUSA
(Bamboo)

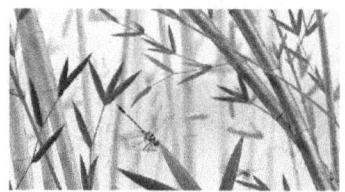

Rigid tension in the back. *Wants to be perfect; she folds the dirty laundry before she washes it*. Rigid beliefs. Anxiety to do everything and get everything done at once. There is not enough time to do it all. Desire and asking others for support and help. Frustration when not given help. Pains go from the spine and extend down the limbs. Tension and muscle spasms in the back and neck.

A remedy to think of when Nux vomica seems indicated but is not helping.

BARYTA CARBONICA
(Barium Carbonate)

SELF CONSCIOUS ANXIETY, irresolution. TIMID.

The child will want to hide behind their parent when a visor comes to the house.

Barium carbonate is a chalky substance that is used for x-ray studies of the gastrointestinal tract.

Study Guide

In homeopathic doses though it is used as a diluted medicine for EXTREME LOW SELF CONFIDENCE. Shy and can't grow into adulthood. (The Aids nosode is also listed for timidity and a childlike state).

This is a remedy that can be used for influenza, colds, ear aches, sore throats but especially for tonsillitis when the patient has the following symptoms:

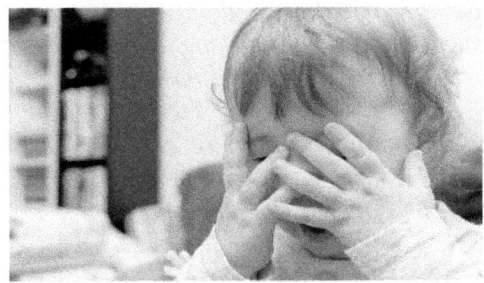

A feeling of LOW SELF CONFIDENCE. The person wants to retreat inward, they want others to help them with everything.

They feel it is difficult to make decisions, they ask others for an opinion. *Timid, shy and fearful.* Example: the child will hide behind the mother or father when a guest arrives. Fear they won't be able to complete their responsibilities. CHILDLIKE STATE.

For example a person has had a business failure, they feel overwhelmed by life, they want to go back to a time and a place where they were being taken care of.

A desire to be perfect so they will be accepted by others. May feel *self conscious in public places; feel as if people can see a small imperfection in how they look.* Self critical for no reason such as they feel they are too tall or their forehead is too large or their nose is the wrong shape. Believe there is something wrong with how they present themselves, when in reality they look fine and no one is noticing.

Swelling of the lymphatic glands below the jaw and neck area. Sensitive to cold and chilled easily. Normal thirst. Frequent colds and or <u>tonsillitis.</u>

Kent: *Lymphatic glands: The next grand feature of this remedy is its affinity for the lymphatic glands all over the body. The glands all over the body enlarge and indurate; the glands of the neck, the glands of the groin, the lymphatics in the abdomen are all affected-knotty chains form in the neck.*

With a few other things that we will put together shortly we will see in this patient a peculiar figure. It has emaciation-gradual dwindling in persons who have been fat, who have been well nourished.

It has an enlarged abdomen. It has been found suitable in marasmus, for children with enlarged glands, enlarged abdomen; emaciation of the tissues, emaciated limbs and dwarfishness of mind, and you have there the whole Baryta carb. marasmus.

The patient himself is chilly; sensitive to cold; wants to be well wrapped. Marked weakness with feeble pulse is a strong feature and he must lie down; he is worse standing and sitting.

The weakness is worse after eating. His pains are better from motion and in the open air. His complaints are aggravated by cold. The enlarged glands take on tenderness and congestion from being exposed. The tonsils gradually increase. The glands of the neck increase in size, and in hardness, from every cold and from becoming chilled.

"Swelling and induration of glands. Inflammation of glands with infiltration."

It brings on emaciation and dwindling of the whole body, except the abdomen, which gradually enlarges. These are phases not to be overlooked in the very beginning, because the symptoms only help to establish this basis and these troubles and tissue changes come on as ultimates.

Another grand feature in this remedy is the application of these things to more advanced years. We say this is a childhood state, this is the state of youth and arrested development.

Now it does not matter whether we have this arrested development in youth, in childhood, or at the advanced age of fifty. From some strange circumstance which we are not able to fathom we say the individual is taking on the, appearance of old age. Premature old age: We call it premature old age.

Baryta carb. has cured lingering complaints that have resulted from malaria, overwork, mental or physical, prolonged mental strain, when the appearance of premature old age was a prominent feature.

Study Guide

Old age creeps upon him too soon. There is but little difference between childhood and old age, and hence old age is called second childhood; but we always regret to see a man under seventy becoming childish, and yet we do see many becoming simple and childish. It does not mean merely imbecility, but childlike behavior.

The Baryta carb. child will be seen hiding behind the furniture when strangers come in; will hide as for shame of something or as if afraid. It imagines all sorts of strange things, that it is talked about, or laughed at. It does not seem to advance. It does not seem to do any good to teach it, for it does the same things over and over and remains untrained.

They either cannot comprehend, or they can not memorize, or they cannot maintain a thought, and you go over it and over it, and the mother wonders if that child is ever going to learn something, and the teacher reports that the child lacks capacity.

The teacher cannot comprehend it, the mother cannot comprehend it, but the homoeopathic physician should know all about it at once. If he knows his Materia Medica he should be well up in the development of a feeble child; those who are going towards rickets, who are feeble, who are always depending on somebody, fitted only for menial places.

Bashful. Timid. Easily frightened. Afraid of strangers. Other remedies have similar features, but it is a strong feature of this medicine. Withered face. Sickly countenance. It is the idea of hiding, the idea of timidity.

The child does not want to play, and it sits in the corner. Does not pay any attention to its hammer, if it is a boy; or its doll, if it is a girl. Sits and sits. Does not seem to be thinking; a lack of ability to think.

Children grow up without any distinctiveness, without any ability to perceive, and therefore fail to develop. Always borrowing trouble.

Like Caust., fear of something going to happen. Full of imaginations; imaginary cares and worries. Hatching up all sorts of complaints and grievances that may happen. A good deal like Ars.

Children in a constant whining mood; always whining.

Head: Troublesome headaches. Pressure in the brain.

A feeling of looseness in the brain, as if the brain fell from side to side or was rising and falling. A sensation of motion in the brain when moving the head or from sudden jarring.

Seems as if the brain moves to and fro to correspond to the motions of the head when the head is turned from, side to side.

Pressing headaches. Headaches ameliorated in fresh air, in the open air, and aggravated from heat. That is the opposite of its general state.

The Baryta carb. general state is aggravated from cold; he is sensitive to cold, and his complaints come on from becoming cold; but his headaches are ameliorated in cool air.

The Baryta carb. patient is often sensitive to the extremes of heat and cold. Hot weather will bring on complaints. Hot weather will cause the blood to mount to the head, and favors apoplectic conditions. (Kent)

BAPTISIA
(Wild Indigo)

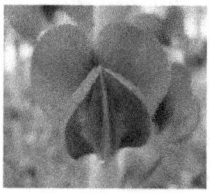

Low fever, septic infections with sore muscles and stupor. Feels bruised all over, (Arnica) pain to lie down and uncomfortable in any position. Face is purple or dark red. Delirium, confusion, mind wanders, can't think, muttering.

Tosses about in bed trying to get pieces together. Feels parts of body are scattered about.

Study Guide

Case 1: Schizophrenia, feels mind is broken into parts and can't get them back together. After Bapt his mental disorder vastly improved (Lorie Dack).

Pneumonia, heat all over with occasional chills. Feels will suffocate. Bad breath.

Boericke: *The symptoms of this drug are of an asthenic type, simulating low fevers, septic conditions of the blood, malarial poisoning and extreme prostration. Indescribable sick feeling. Great muscular soreness and putrid phenomena always are present. All the secretions are offensive-breath, stool, urine, sweat, etc. Epidemic influenza.*

Wild, wandering feeling. Inability to think. Mental confusion. Ideas confused. Illusion of divided personality. Thinks he is broken or double, and tosses about the bed trying to get pieces together. Delirium, wandering, muttering. Perfect indifference. Falls asleep while being spoken to. Melancholia, with stupor.

Head.--Confused, swimming feeling. Vertigo; pressure at root of nose. Skin of forehead feels tight; seems drawn to back of head. Feels too large, heavy, numb. Soreness of eyeballs. Brain feels sore. Stupor; falls asleep while spoken to. Early deafness in typhoid conditions. Eyelids heavy.

Face.--Besotted look. Dark red. Pain at root of nose. Muscles of jaw rigid.

Throat.--Dark redness of tonsils and soft palate. Constriction, contraction of œsophagus (Cajeput). Great difficulty in swallowing solid food. Painless sore throat, and offensive discharge. Contraction at cardiac orifice.

Stomach.--Can swallow only liquids, vomiting due to spasm of œsophagus. Gastric fever. No appetite. Constant desire for water. Sinking feeling at stomach. Pain in epigastric region. Feeling of hard substance (Abies nig). All symptoms worse from beer (Kali bich). Cardiac orifice contracted convulsively and ulcerative inflammation of stomach and bowels.

Abdomen.--Right side markedly affected. Distended and rumbling. Soreness over region of gall-bladder, with diarrhœa. Stools very offensive, thin, dark, bloody. Soreness of abdomen, in region of liver. Dysentery of old people.

BELLADONNA
(Deadly Nightshade)

Sudden onset of symptoms

<u>Eyes sensitive to light</u>

Redness and INFLAMMATION

Sudden and extreme anger. These are good natured people, but can suddenly become filled with rage, *they have a strong character, vivid, they can make a strong impression on you, they can be very obstinate.*

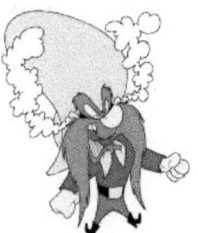

(Yosemite Sam Created by Friz Freleng, and Warner Bros)

<u>Steaming, explosive anger.</u> Yosemite Sam is a great example. His anger is sudden, extreme and out of control.

Case 1: In one case (my daughter) she was born with the most severe temper tantrums. Most of the time she was good natured, smiling and a happy baby but then when she felt a little hunger she would give the signal that I had about thirty seconds to get her bottle to her. Sometimes this was not possible and so her face would suddenly become bright red with anger. Then she would clench her fists and start to scream. The anger was so sudden and so intense that in less than a minute she would faint with anger. There was no way to comfort her or sooth her in these

episodes. After a couple of weeks of this I noticed that her *eyes were very sensitive to light,* she would also sleep on her back *with her hands under her head.* Based on these symptoms I gave her Belladonna 30c and within a few days the episodes of rage dissipated. She became very calm and patient after that. To this day she is a very patient and never had another temper tantrum.

Belladonna is one of the most important remedies for acute and chronic illnesses. It has the ability to heal many seemingly different pathologies. For example it can be the correct and curative treatment for an *acute headache with throbbing pain*, for a sore throat with swelling and redness, or for an ear infection with a raging fever. In all these examples and for all the other illnesses acute and chronic that need Belladonna there are a set of essential symptoms, that if present, make Belladonna a strong possibility to be the simillimum remedy that is a perfect match to the symptoms.

The important symptoms that need to be present are the following:
- EYES extremely SENSITIVE TO LIGHT, with all ailments this symptom will 99% of the time be present
- *Sudden inflammation*
- *redness*
- violent reactions, sudden anger
- intense symptoms
- *high fever with DRY SKIN and no perspiration*
- redness of face and eyes
- *flushing* and congestion producing a rush of blood to the head with heat radiating from the head, but with cold extremities
- sensations of pressure
- throbbing pains in the head and elsewhere due to hypertension

Symptoms become worse from:
- *exposure to light, sun, and or exposure of heat to the head*
- being bumped, stepping on the ground, a jar
- stooping; leaning foreward

Symptoms become better from:
- cold applications
- lying in the dark
- binding the head

Materia Medica

Generally, the personality of those needing Belladonna is vital and strong willed, obstinate, self determined and assurtive even if it takes some anger to make what they want known. This is in contrast to other remedies such as Pulsatilla, Magnesias, Carcinosin and the Aids nosose which are all remedies for tempraments that are yielding and have difficulty in standing up for themselves.

Photophobia has to be present; I would not use Belladonna if this symptom was not present.

If the patient has always had sensitivity to light and then develops an acute illness then Belladonna can still be used because, perhaps, they have needed Belladonna for a long time. Photophobia could be present in a mild influenza, the beginning of a sore throat, earache, headache, sinusitis or mild fever. It can also be present in a more severe illness, such as an ear infection that comes on every few weeks, high fevers with stiffness of the neck, more severe types of sinus infections or very high fevers with convulsions and hallucinations.

Other sure signs a patient could benefit from Belladonna:
- *Fever*, especially when there is *no perspiration*
- *radiant burning heat from the body*
- hot red face and hot head
- cold extremities
- *dryness of the skin*
- *the inflamed part shows redness, inflammation, intense burning swelling, pain, and it comes on rapidly*

Usually the person is thirstless (they avoid drinking water or only want one or two drinks a day) and often have throbbing pulsating pains such as headaches or pains in the ears.

There is sensitivity and pain to being bumped, to touch, to jerking or stepping with a jar. There is a tendency to constipation.

Symptoms are usually worse on the right side i.e. right sided sore throat, right sided ear infection.

Grinding teeth during sleep.

There is often flushing of the face, congestion, glassy appearance of the eyes. In the case of a high fever there can be a wild delirium, and dramatic symptoms such as disposition to bite, spit or strike and tear things. There also may be hallucinations, fear of imaginary things, sees monsters and hideous faces. Convulsions can come on suddenly with a fever, hot head and cold extremities.

Other symptoms that can indicate the use of Belladonna are intolerance to heat and sensitivity to the radiant heat of the sun. It can be used for sunstroke but usually Glonion is a better choice.

The patient can also be chilly, sensitive to drafts and the cold.
With children needing Belladonna, oftentimes the following symptoms are observed:
- ailments resulting from a fright, (Acon, Gels, Op, Stram)
- *anger, VIOLENCE*
- *obstinate and stubborn*: they won't change their mind and if you try to force them they will have a *temper tantrum*, scream extremely loudly and try to fight back

Even with the acute ailment, children will experience:
- much anger, striking, kicking, rudeness
- general defiant behaviour
- a dislike of being touched or examined
- waking up from frightening nightmares
- acute pains in the abdomen
- a worsening from having their hair cut
- sleep very deeply, often with involuntarily wetting the bed

Recommendation: Give one dose, (5 or 6 granules or 15 to 20 drops) of 30c potency and then wait one to four hours for a reaction. When there is a relapse then repeat the dose. It is safe to give one dose of a 30c a day for moderate symptoms to severe symptoms and one dose every two days for a mild set of symptoms.

Nash – Leaders: *We now come to consider what I call the trio of delirium remedies—BELLADONNA, HYOSCYAMUS and STRAMONIUM. Many other remedies have delirium, but these three deserve to head the list. BELLADONNA may also be called pre-eminently a head remedy. In most complaints where this remedy is indicated head symptoms preponderate.*

The BLOOD all seems to be rushing to the head. (AMYL NITRITE, GLONOINE, MELILOTUS.)

The head is hot while the extremities are cool. The eyes are red and blood-shot. The face is also red, almost purple red. The carotid arteries throb so as to be plainly visible. There is either great pain, pressure or sense of fullness, or an almost stupid condition.

The wild, terrible delirium, if present, may be found with pain, or even with no complaint of pain. In delirium the patient "imagines he sees ghosts, hideous faces and animals and insects." Fears all sorts of imaginary things and wants to run away from them; breaks out into fits of laughter or screams and gnashes his teeth; bites or strikes those around him; in short, performs all sorts of violent acts and is controlled with great difficulty. No remedy has more persistently VIOLENT DELIRIUM than BELLADONNA. One of the characteristic features of BELLADONNA in delirium as compared with the other two remedies is the decided evidence already mentioned of a surcharge of blood in the brain. When the throbbing of the carotids, the heat, redness and congestion of face and conjunctiva go away, the delirium subsides in proportion. BELLADONNA may have delirium with pale face as its alternate, but it is the exception. Even the upper lip is congested and swollen.

In inflammations, which LOCALISE, BELLADONNA is in the first stage as often the leading remedy as any other. It does not make much difference where they localize, whether in head, throat, mammae or elsewhere, if they come on suddenly, pursue a rapid course, are red, painful and especially throbbing. It is astonishing how many local inflammations, even a carbuncle or boil, will so disturb the general system and circulation, as to produce the general inflammatory fever, with the characteristic head symptoms calling for BELLADONNA, and no less astonishing how this remedy controls the whole condition, both local and general, when indicated. What! exclaims the believer in local applications, give BELLADONNA internally for a boil on the hand or foot? Yes, indeed, not only BELLADONNA, but MERCURIUS, HEPAR SULPHURIS, TARANTULA CUBENSIS, and many others, and you will not have any need for local medication at all. It is only in the first or congestive or active inflammatory stage that this remedy is in place; but, if properly administered then, it will often abort the whole thing and never leave it to finish all its stages, or if not, so modify as to make it comparatively insignificant.

BELLADONNA is one of our best remedies in the diseases of children, even vieing with CHAMOMILLA. They come SUDDENLY, almost without warning. This sudden and intense onset of fever is sometimes duplicated in CINA cases, but there is helminthiasis in connection with it. Child is well one minute and sick the next, and one very characteristic symptom in these cases is, the child is very hot, with red face and semi-stupor, but every little while starts or JUMPS IN SLEEP AS IF IT MIGHT GO INTO SPASMS. This condition is often found in children and then BELLADONNA is like "oil upon troubled waters." Remember BELLADONNA inflammations localize more than they do in ACONITE. I drew the difference between these two remedies in inflammations and inflammatory fevers when writing upon ACONITE. There is no use of confounding them. Some do so; but, in so doing, only exhibit their ignorance.

There are, in every remedy, symptoms of sensation, circumstance, constitution or modality which are peculiar both to diseases and remedies. These symptoms are not always easily accounted for. The attempt to explain them from a pathological standpoint is not always possible or even necessary were it possible. A simple acceptance of them as facts is often more sensible than to wait long to find the often unfindable. To act as a prescriber upon what we know is better than waiting, because we cannot explain or account for it. For instance, it is not easy to tell why "the pains of BELLADONNA APPEAR SUDDENLY AND AFTER A TIME DISAPPEAR AS SUDDENLY AS THEY COME," while those of STANNUM "GRADUALLY INCREASE TO A GREAT HEIGHT AND AS GRADUALLY DECLINE," or SULPHURIC ACID "BEGIN SLOWLY AND DECLINE SUDDENLY," or "GRADUALLY INCREASE AND SUDDENLY CEASE," but so it is, and the acceptance of these facts enables the homeopathic prescriber to cure his patient, whether he can explain them or not.

Guernsey says—"This medicine is particularly applicable, and in fact takes the lead over all others in cases in which QUICKNESS or SUDDENNESS of either SENSATION OR MOTION is predominant." To be sure all these symptoms have their pathological explanation if we could give it; but, acting on our law of SIMILIA, we can cure our *patients and are not left at sea, without chart or compass, because we cannot explain. We know that these symptoms are the natural outcry of the pathological state, and that the administration of a poison which is capable of setting up a similar outcry cures the patient. What else is necessary ? Either this is true, or Homeopathy is a humbug.*

The simple fact, abundantly proven, that the remedy having the symptoms corresponding to the symptoms of the patient, cures him, no matter what the pathology, where a cure is at all possible, is one of the greatest discoveries of scientific investigation. Long live the name of Hahnemann, the discoverer.

From our description thus far of this remedy you would expect it to be a good one for CONGESTIVE HEADACHES, and so it is, and not only so, but for neuralgic headaches. Throbbing pains, with the already described evidence of congestion of blood to the head. BELLADONNA headaches, whether congestive or neuralgic, are worse on STOOPING FORWARD, BENDING DOWNWARD, or LYING DOWN, anything that takes the patient out of the perpendicular. "WORSE ON LYING DOWN," in fact, seems to be a very reliable general characteristic.

The elder Lippe once told me of a case of suspicious enlargement or swelling and pain of the breast of long standing, which, as he expressed it, seemed likely to prove a case for the surgeon (cancer), which was entirely cured by a few doses of BELLADONNA, to which he was guided by this symptom of the pains being so much worse on lying down. Since then I have observed and verified this symptom in many cases of different kinds. I will not stop to give all the symptoms that might be present in BELLADONNA headaches.

No remedy has greater affinity for the throat. The BURNING, DRYNESS (SABADILLA), SENSE OF CONSTRICTION (constant desire to swallow to relieve the sense of dryness, LYSSIN), with or without swelling of the palate and tonsils, is sometimes intense. I once witnessed a case of poisoning in which these symptoms were terribly distressing.
There are two very characteristic symptoms in the abdominal region, viz.: "TENDERNESS OF THE ABDOMEN, AGGRAVATED BY THE LEAST JAR, IN WALKING, OR STEPPING, OR EVEN THE BED OR CHAIR, UPON WHICH SHE SITS OR LIES"; and "PRESSURE DOWNWARD AS IF THE CONTENTS OF THE ABDOMEN WOULD

ISSUE THROUGH THE VULVA, < MORNINGS." This last symptom is found under other remedies, notably LILIUM TIGRINUM and SEPIA. With BELLADONNA there is often associated with this pressure downward a pain in the back "AS IF IT WOULD BREAK." "STARTING AND JUMPING," or "twitching in sleep," or on going to sleep is characteristic.

So also is "SLEEPY, BUT CANNOT SLEEP," and "MOANING DURING SLEEP."

With BELLADONNA the head likes wrapping up or covering, takes cold when it is uncovered or from cutting the hair (SILICEA). (GLONOINE; can't bear hat on.)

Uniform, smooth, shining, scarlet redness of the skin, so hot that it imparts a burning sensation to the hand of one who feels of it, is very characteristic (H. N. Guernsey).

Convulsions with other symptoms of BELLADONNA are very frequently found under this remedy.

I have here endeavored to give an outline of this great remedy. A volume might be profitably written upon its virtues. No one remedy would be more greatly missed than this ... (Nash)

BOTHROPS LANCEOLATUS
(Yellow Viper)

This is one of the main remedies for *strokes*: embolic, thrombotic and hemorrhagic.

These patients are less bothered or not at all bothered by tight clothing about the neck. In all the other snake remedies this is usually a very strong symptom.

These people are not especially jealous or angry, they are more mild but excitable and communicative in a warm and friendly manner.

Materia Medica

From the book: <u>Snakes to Simillimum</u> (I highly recommend this text) by Farokh Master says of this remedy: *Stroke with araplegia and quadriplegia. Stroke with aphasia, paralysis. Eye symptoms: daytime blindness, retinal/conjunctival hemorrhage. Generally right sided.*

Loquacity or taciturn. Diagonal symptoms; such as left upper and right lower (Agar, Led, Rhus-t, Tarax) or right upper and left lower (Ambra, Phos, Sul-ac).

Fullness, sensation of swelling in various parts of the body; such as the head, chest and abdomen; this leads to persistent restlessness.

Problems of memory after ischemia strokes or TIA's. Makes mistakes in words and word hunting.

Speech disorders that range from slow, inarticulate, confused speech to aphasia as a result of ischemic insult to the brain.

Strong premonition (Anh, Med) with an uneasy restless feeling before developing strokes or thrombosis or hypertensive episodes. They walk about with a strong fear or sit very silently.

Gangrene. (Carb-ac, Helo-s) like dry, moist or gas gangrene. The gangrene spreads very quickly and involves huge areas with massive destruction of tissue including muscles, tendons, bones etc. The blood that oozes from the gangrene is dark, offensive and spurts out in jets (Lyc) from time to time. Gangrene and necrosis. Hemorrhage (black).

Worse after eating. i.e. after eating he gets a stroke or myocardial infarction.

Apprehension starting in the stomach. (Kali-c, Phos).

Conscientious about trifles. Restlessness more internal than internal before the stroke or thrombosis. Strongly opinionated personality with stubborn obstinacy.

Blackness of external parts. Caries and necrosis of bones. Lassitude and sluggish. Weakness and paralysis. Low grade depression. Black hemorrhage. Hypercholestremia.

Post surgical thrombophlebitis (Hippoz, Lycop-v, Vip).

Right sided affections especially the right cortex, liver, upper limbs and lower limbs. Sharp cutting pains that make him shiver, worse from motion.

Conductive system of the heart affected leading to frequent irregular and slow pulse (Kalmia, Verat-v).

Thrombosis; (Kali-mur, Vip). Varicose veins, phlebitis, arteritis, aneurism, hemorrhoids, embolism. Septicemia.

Weakness from diarrhea. Benign positional vertigo due to poor cerebral circulation, especially in older persons. (Ambra, Bar-c, Sin-n) that leads to persistent giddiness which is worse by carrying any load on the head, raising the arm above the shoulder, on exertion, on turning in bed; the room seems to turn around. (Con, Cycl).

Ailments from head injuries (Arn, Cic, Hell).

Low grade headache from a subdural hematoma. (Arn, Bell, Cocc, Op) and essential hypertension in old people. Migraines that are usually right-sided and settle in the occiput.

Blindness from retinal hemorrhage (Crot-h, Lach, Prun). Optic nerve atrophy.

Unable to swallow due to sense of constriction especially liquids (Lyss, Stam, Upa).

A sensation of apprehension in the stomach (Dig, Mez) before a cerebrovascular accident or onset of menses. Internal trembling of the abdomen. Excessive black vomiting - blood (Cad-s, Sec).

Severe inflamation, ulceration and necrosis or small bowels, leading to necrotizing colitis, ulcerative colitis, cancer of the colon, etc. Rumbling of the bowel. Urgent desire to evacuate. Craving for pepper, coffee, cheese, sweets and aversion to meat.

Septicemia due to gram negative organisms leading to nectotic wounds and gangrene.

Ascites, paralytic ileus, tympanites. Weakness from diarrhea. Black tary stools – melena – from hemorrhage of the intestines.

Bloody urine. Constant desire to urinate. No relief from emptying the bladder. Menorrhagia during menopause (Sabin, Ust). Pulmonary congestion with oppression of breathing with bloody expectorations.

Pulmonary edema, pneumonitis.

Dull pain in the heart on waking from sleep, extending to the left axilla (Lat-m) worse from 4 to 5 am.

Persistent high blood pressure even after the stroke (Fuma-as, Toxo-g).

Cyanosis – blue purple discoloration of the skin.

Necrosis of bones (Ang, Nat-sil-fl, Fl-ac) due to severe infections, like gangrene, oseomyelitis and septicemia.

BRYONIA ALBA
(Kudzu, Devil's Turnip)

PAIN worse from slight MOTION. Better from pressure. *Thirsty.*
It is a remedy that is indicated for joint injuries when the joint fluids dry up, stitching pains result and there is PAIN FROM ANY SLIGHT

Study Guide

MOTION of the joint, even very small motions cause an exceptional amount of pain. Emotionaly these people are *afraid something bad is going to happen*. To protect themselves they like to have stability in their lives, a large bank account and plenty of insurnace. Even the idea of change can bring on anxiety.

The use of Bryonia is not limited to the healing of injuries. Other tissues and organs in the body can have diseases that Bryonia is indicated for as well. In all of these illnesses the same basic symptoms are present. They include:

<u>*Aggravation from the least movement and the amelioration from pressure and remaining still.*</u> This symptom can be expressed in a variety of acute illness situations. If there is an ear ache the person will have the pains in the ear made worse from moving the head or the ear being pulled.

If there is a pleurisy (an infection of the lining that covers the lungs), pneumonia (an infection inside the lungs) or bronchitis (an infection of the airway leading from the trachea to the lung tissue), then the act of breathing causes severe pain as it causes these tissues to move resulting in friction and pain. As a result, the person will take very short, fast and shallow breaths to prevent this motion and friction.

Another way to prevent motion is to <u>*apply pressure*</u> on and around the area of infection. To accomplish this they may hold the chest when they cough, to prevent any excess motion of the lungs, lie on the painful side or desire to wrap something tightly about the chest.

In the situation of influenza there will be a headache that is worse even from small motions of the eyes or touching the hair. They may say something like, "If I move my eyes or brush my hair the pains in my head get much worse." I once treated a woman that had a continuous headache for four days. She sat in a very fixed position and moved very slowly. Any type of motion aggravated the headache. After a dose of Bryonia this acute headache was much improved.

In appendicitis the same symptom can exist. The patient will not let anyone touch or press on the abdomen. This guarding is another indication that motion aggravates. This can prompt one to ask some more

Materia Medica

questions to see if Bryonia is the remedy.

Other symptoms include - *excessive dryness of all mucous membranes.* These mucous membranes exist around every organ and are the inside lining for many other organs such as the respiratory system and digestive system. In a Bryonia illness therefore the mouth becomes very dry and there is an *excessive thirst for large amounts of cold water.*

The colon becomes dry and there is constipation. The respiratory organs become dry and so there is a dry cough. If the sinuses become infected there is also a lack of mucous.

Gradual onset of acute symptoms; such as the flu. (Gels, Eupat) The complaints of Bryonia develop over a few days. It is not the rapid onset as is seen in remedies like Belladonna, Aconite or Chamomile.

The emotional disposition is one of irritability, a desire to be left alone; he or she feels isolated and withdrawn.

At other times there can be anxiety, a restlessness to do something useful, to go home. Fear of the future, of poverty, of a business failure. Example: she feels insecure about finances and therefore desires to purchase extra insurance.

Fear of change. Desire for assured security and a stable financial position. Concerned about survival, working hard. Ailments from anger.

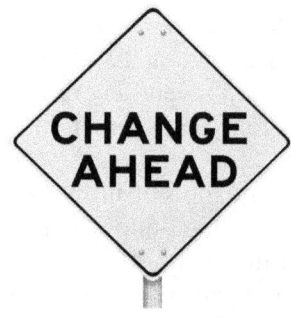

Life is full of change, Bryonia is fragile to this influence and it makes them sick. They will do what they can to prevent change as it produces insecurity and uncertainty.

Despair of recovery, fear of suffering. Capricious (often changing one's mind) and rejects things asked for (Cham). Delirium, speaks of business. Dreams of hard work. Suspicious, anger from contradiction. Aversion

Study Guide

and irritability to be touched, to have visitors. Refuses to answer questions. Wants things to be quiet. Mental dullness.

Local symptoms may include:
- oily perspiration
- tongue coated yellow
- weakness in the morning on rising
- desires cold drinks
- constipation with headaches
- constant motion of the mouth as if chewing something
- vomiting from slightest motion
- excessive paleness during the chill
- can't sit up from nausea and faintness
- nosebleeds at night, from suppressed menses
- dry painful cough
- mastitis, breast is heavy, hard, hot, painful
- joints red, swollen, stiff, stitching pains worse from motion,
- slow appearance of a rash in eruptive fevers, appearance of the rash ameliorates
- sciatica, the pains make her restless to move but more pain on motion
- vertigo from motion
- left sided headaches, worse when cough,
- dry cracked lips
- stool dry and hard
- colds that travel down into the chest
- stitching in the chest on coughing

Any symptoms that are *worse*:
- at 9 pm
- from warmth
- a warm room
- hot drinks
- jarring
- dry cold weather or wind
- taking a deep breath

Symptoms are *better* from:
- perspiration, and
- from sleeping on the left side

Case 1: 37 year old man came to me with autoimmune inflammation of the joints. He experienced severe pains in all joints; especially the shoulders and lower limbs. He can't hardly get out of bed in the morning as any motion makes the pains unbearable, he sits in a chair most of the day. He is a very successful business person owning a large company. Very frugal and careful with expenses. He writes down the length of each phone call and compares this with the bill when he gets his statement at the end of the month! If the bill is a few pennies wrong he calls the phone company to get it corrected. (Mind-anxiety- money matters, about: *Bryonia)*. After a year of taking Bryonia first 30c, then worked up to 10m he is all better and is not taking Cortizone or Methotrexate which was prescribed for him. His doctor had said he wold be taking these drugs for the rest of his life. After he has all better on asking about the phone bill he looked at me and smiled: "I don't worry about that type of thing any longer." Soon after he sold his company, retired and went to a world tour, seeming not to worry so much about spending money. It is now four years later and the joint pains have not returned.

In the situation of an ear infection the typical ear infections symptoms will be present plus the Bryonia symptoms listed above. That being pain worse from motion, better from pressure on the ear.

As one can see Bryonia is more than a cure for certain types of infections. When one can learn to evaluate the whole person and know the whole illness, then it can cure the acute illness and the whole patient.

Here is an example of materia medica from another of the past great masters in homeopathic prescribing E.A. Farrington. It is amazing in what detail he knew this remedy: *We find Bryonia indicated first of all in changes in the blood; in changes affecting its quantity, its quality and its circulation. For example, it is indicated in febrile conditions; in fevers of an intermitting type although not frequently; in those of a remitting type, very often ; sometimes too in synochal fever; and also in rheumatic, gastric, bilious, traumatic and typhoid fevers.*

The symptoms which characterize its fevers are in general these: There is an increased action of the heart, giving rise to a frequent hard tense pulse, very much as you find under ACONITE. There is actually an increase in the force and power of the heart's action. This action is augmented by any movement of the body, consequently the patient is anxious to keep perfectly quiet. Then you find that there is almost always intense headache with these fevers. This is usually of a dull throbbing character or there may be sharp stabbing pains in the head. This is almost always associated with sharp pains in or over the eyes. All of these parts are exquisitely sensitive to the least motion. The patient will avoid moving the eyes, for instance, because it aggravates the pain. The least attempt to raise the head from the pillow causes a feeling of faintness and nausea.

The mouth is very dry and the tongue is coated in the milder forms of fever as, for instance, in the synochal fever or in the light gastric type of fever. The coating on the tongue is white and is especially marked down the middle. The edges of the tongue may be perfectly clean. As the fever grows in intensity, it approaches more a typhoid type. Bilious symptoms predominate. This white tongue becomes yellowish and is associated with a decidedly bitter taste in the mouth. There are splitting headache, tenderness over the epigastrium, with stitches, soreness or tenderness in the right hypochondrium. As the typhoid symptoms increase, the tongue becomes more and more dry, but still maintains its coating.

If the fever is of an intermitting type, you will always find the chill mixed with heat, that is during the chill, the head is hot, the cheeks are a deep red and there is decided thirst, which is generally for large quantities of water at long intervals. In some cases, it may be a continuous thirst. The pulse is hard, frequent and tense. The sweat is provoked by the least exertion and has either a sour or an oily odor.

In typhoid fever, Bryonia is indicated in the early stages and by the following symptoms: There is some confusion of the mind; the sensorium is depressed but there are no perversions of the senses. During sleep there is delirium which is usually of a mild character. On closing his eyes for sleep, he thinks he sees persons who are not present. On opening them, he is surprised to find that he is mistaken.

Sometimes this delirium is accompanied or preceded by irritability. The speech is hasty, as you find under Belladonna. As the disease increases, some little heaviness almost approaching stupor accompanies sleep. The patient has dreams, which have for their subject the occupation of the day. Frequently with this delirium, the patient suffers from an agonizing headache. This is usually frontal. If the patient is able to describe it to you, he will tell you that his head feels as if it would burst. No better term than "splitting headache" could be used to describe it. It is congestive in its character.

The face is usually flushed and of a deep red-color. This is intensified like all the other symptoms of the drug, by any motion of the head and is often accompanied by nose-bleed. The epistaxis is particularly liable to come on at three or four o'clock in the morning, and is frequently preceded by a sense of fulness in the head. In very severe cases, you will notice that the patient puts his hand to his head as if there were some pain there, and his face is expressive of pain. Yet so stupid is he, that he makes no complaint other than that expressed by these automatic movements.

Another symptom to be noted in these typhoid fevers, is the dryness of the mucous membranes, especially those of the mouth and stomach. This is the result of deficient secretion. In no cases, is the condition more apparent than in typhoid states. The mouth is dry, as I have already intimated, and yet there may be no thirst. If there is thirst it seems to have the character I mentioned in speaking of intermittent fever. The patient drinks large quantities but not very frequently. After drinking water or while attempting to sit up, the patient has a deathly nauseated feeling and sometimes even vomits.

At other times he complains of a heavy pressure in the stomach, as if a stone were lying there. This symptom is no doubt due to the same pathological condition we found in the mucous membrane of the mouth. The secretion of gastric juice is deficient, consequently food lies undigested in the stomach. The bowels are usually constipated when Bryonia is called for. When they do move, the stools are large, hard and dry and either brown or black in color. They are expelled with difficulty owing to the atony of the rectum. Sometimes, in well-advanced cases of typhoid fever, you will find soft, mushy stools, calling for Bryonia. There is a symptom which sometimes accompanies typhoid fever at about the end of the first week of the fully developed fever, and that is a form of delirium in which the patient expresses a continual "desire to go home." He imagines that he is not at home and longs to be taken there in order to be properly cared for. This symptom is a strong indication for Bryonia and frequently disappears after two or three doses of the remedy.

Study Guide

In these febrile conditions, it is necessary to place Bryonia in its proper relations with its concordant remedies. First of all ACONITE. Aconite bears an intimate relation with Bryonia in all these types of fever except gastric, intermittent and typhoid fevers. Aconite has not in its totality any special relation to any of these, however incorrectly it may be given to lessen the temperature. The symptomatology of Aconite is opposed in every respect to that of typhoid fever. In gastric fever, it may be given in the beginning when there is the full pulse, hot and dry skin and restlessness, indicating that drug; but as the fever advances, it is then not indicated unless there are bilious complications. Then it is an all sufficient remedy.

The distinctions that you are to make between Aconite and Bryonia are as follows: In the first place, they hold the relation of Aconite and Bryonia and not Bryonia and Aconite; that is to say Aconite is given earlier in the case than is Bryonia. Aconite suits the hyperaemia, the congestion or even the chill which precedes an inflammatory fever. Bryonia is indicated later when Aconite fails.

The mental symptoms of the two drugs are so distinct that you ought not to confuse them. Aconite demands that the mind be excited, that the patient be restless, tossing about the bed, full of fears. He imagines that he is going to die. The Bryonia patient may suffer just as much as the one to whom you would give Aconite, but he is perfectly quiet. He is quiet because motion aggravates his symptoms. Early in typhoid fever and sometimes in rheumatic you may have Bryonia indicated by this symptom. The patient is restless and tosses about the bed impelled by nervousness, and yet he is made worse by the motion.

Still another remedy to be thought of in connection with Bryonia in these fevers is Belladonna, and particularly in the beginning of typhoid fever. Now there is really nothing in the symptomatology of Belladonna which would call for it in a well-advanced case of typhoid type of fever. Only in the beginning could you confuse it with Bryonia. In the first place it has erethism. Here you distinguish it by its delirium, which is of a violent character. The patient jerks his limbs and starts during sleep. He springs up from sleep in affright. As soon as he closes his eyes, he sees all sorts of objects and people, which disappear as soon as the eyes are opened. Belladonna then has more cerebral erethism, and more violence in its delirium than has Bryonia. With the Belladonna headache there are throbbing pains, and the patient may be obliged to sit up rather than keep perfectly quiet in order to obtain relief.

Another remedy to be compared with Bryonia is RHUS TOX. This is often indicated in typhoid fever. You all know the historic fact that Hahnemann during one of the war epidemics of typhus cured many cases with these two remedies. Since the days of Hahnemann, this use of these remedies has become universal. Remember, however, that they are not specifics. Each epidemic may so change in character as to require other remedies. Rhus tox. is indicated when there, is marked restlessness. The patient first lying on one side, changes to the other. For a few moments, he feels better in his new position. Then his side begins to ache and back he turns again. Like Bryonia, it has nosebleed, which nose-bleed relieves the patient's symptoms, and the headache I described to you last month as "a sensation as though a board were strapped tightly across the forehead." There are rheumatic aching pains through the joints and muscles of the limbs. The tongue differs from that of Bryonia. It is brown and dry and even cracked, and has a red tip. That is also an excellent indication for Sulphur. With Rhus tox., there is frequently diarrhoea from the very beginning. Bryonia usually has constipation.

I just referred to the symptom under BELLADONNA—"The patient sees persons and objects on closing the eyes, these disapear as soon as the eyes are opened." Both CALCAREA OSTREARUM and CINCHONA have this symptom. Under the latter remedy, however, it does not occur in typhoid fever, but after haemorrhage.

Next, I wish to talk about the action of Bryonia on serous membranes. Bryonia acts powerfully on these, producing inflammation. Hence we are called upon to prescribe it when the meninges of the brain and spinal cord, the pleura and the peritoneum, and the synovial membranes are inflamed. The indications for Bryonia in these serous inflammations are particularly to be looked for after exudation has taken place. There are sharp stitching pains, worse from any motion. The fever may still be high or it may have been partially subdued by the remedy which preceded.
Comparing ACONITE with Bryonia once more, you will see the same rule applicable here as before, Bryonia is indicated after and not before Aconite. Take for purpose of illustration a typical case of pleurisy. In the beginning of the disease when fever is high you select Aconite, but just so soon as the fever commences to decrease, and as effusion begins, as

indicated by the friction sounds, Aconite ceases to be of any benefit and Bryonia comes in as an all sufficient remedy. It is customary with some physicians to give Aconite for the fever and Bryonia for the pleuritic trouble. But this is useless. Bryonia is adapted to the whole case. It has not the same restlessness which demands Aconite. The patient is quiet and is full of pain. He lies on the affected side. Why? Because by the pressure thus exerted on the ribs, he moves the affected parts less than he would were he lying on the sound side.

When the meninges of the brain are affected, Bryonia is a valuable drug, but here, except in some rare cases, it follows BELLADONNA rather than Aconite. Belladonna ceases to be the remedy in meningitis, whether tubercular or otherwise, when effusion within the ventricles or beneath the membranes commences. It then gives place to SULPHUR in some cases, APIS in others and BRYONIA in still others. BRYONIA is indicated when meningitis follows the suppression of some eruption, as that of scarlatina or measles. The child's face is red, or else it is red and pale alternately. The child screams out suddenly as if it was in great pain, which it really is.

These pains are of a sharp lancinating character and are especially manifested on moving the child. There is marked squinting with one or both eyes. The bowels are usually constipated, the abdomen distended and the child has well-marked sensorial depression which seems to border on stupor. If you arouse the child and offer him drink, he takes it impetuously or hastily, just as under Belladonna. The latter remedy has more rolling of the head.

For sake of convenience we will next study the catarrhs of Bryonia and the effects of the drug on the lung structure. We find Bryonia indicated in nasal catarrh when there is either great dryness of the mucous membrane of the nose or (more frequently), when the discharge is thick and yellow. It is also indicated when the discharge has been of the character just indicated and has been suddenly suppressed. As a result, there is dull throbbing headache just over the frontal sinuses.
LACHESIS is also useful for suppressed coryza. But it has not so marked the aggravation from motion; nor has it that yellow discharge. The treatment of colds is a severe test of the skill of a physician. If you can successfully treat them you will well understand homeopathy. They are the most difficult class of cases we have to contend with. There are two

reasons for this. One is the patients are constantly exposed, and the other is that they are not watched sufficiently closely. If you are given the opportunity to watch the cases carefully, so that you may prescribe as the indications change, you will cure promptly.

We may also use Bryonia in pneumonia. The type of the disease in which it is indicated is in the true croupous form. Just as we found Bryonia indicated in pleurisy with effusion, so is it of use in pneumonia after the croupous exudation has taken place. Usually when it is called for there is also some pleuritis, hence it is applicable to pleuropneumonia. It is not indicated in the beginning of the disease because the exudation does not occur in that stage. It is indicated after Aconite, with the following easily understood condition. The fever still continues, but the skin is not so hot, the face so red and the patient so restless as when Aconite was indicated. The patient is more pacific, and his face and whole demeanor are expressive of anxiety.

I would have you discriminate between this condition and that calling for Aconite. It is not so much the mental anxiety that Aconite pictures as it is an expression of pulmonary oppression. That you MUST remember. The cough which under Aconite was of a dry teasing character, with frothy sputa, perhaps still remains troublesome but it is looser and more moist. There is very little expectoration yet but what little there is, is either yellowish or streaked with blood. Owing to the accompanying inflammation of the pleura, sharp pleuritic stitches are felt in the chest. They are worse on the left side. The patient complains of heavy pressure just over the sternum. The pulse is full, hard and tense. The urine is dark red and scanty.

Still another remedy that ought to be thought of along with Bryonia in pneumonia is ANTIMONIUM TARTARIOUM. It is indicated in pneumonia that begins as a bronchitis and extends downwards. It is especially suited to cases that begin on the right side, and that have these sharp stitching pains, high fever, great oppression of the chest, as in Bryonia. But it is called for more in catarrhal than in croupous pneumonia. Mucous rales are heard distinctly in the chest.

You should also recall SANGUINARIA and CHELIDONIUM.

Several other remedies than Bryonia have these pains in the chest walls.

GAULTHERIA has pleurodynia with pain in the anterior mediastinum. RANUNCULUS BULBOSUS is decidedly the best remedy for intercostal rheumatism; it has sharp, stitching pains and a sore SPOT in the chest, and these are worse from any motion or even breathing.

ARNICA is sometimes of use when the sore and bruised feeling of the chest predominates.

RHUS RADICANS is called for in pleurodynia when the pains shoot into the shoulder.

SENEGA acts best in fat persons of lax fibre. It is useful in cold when there are much pain and soreness in the thoracic walls, and much mucus within. There is hoarseness; the throat is so dry and sensitive that it hurts the patient to talk; the cough often ends with sneezing.
RUMEX CRISPUS has sharp, stitching or stinging pains through the left lung; it is indicated more in the early stages of phthisis. When the patient turns the left side feels sore.

TRIFOLIUM PRATENSE has hoarseness and choking spells at night with the cough. The neck is stiff; there are cramps in the sterno-cleido-mastoid muscles which are relieved by heat and friction.

In bronchitis Bryonia is indicated with this same pressure over the sternum; the dyspnoea is great; the cough is dry and seems to start from the stomach. Sometimes a little tenacious blood-streaked sputum is raised. The cough is worse after a meal, when it may even end in vomiting. During the cough the patient presses his hand against his side to relieve the stitching pains.

Returning now to the action of Bryonia on the serous membranes, we find it producing synovitis. The affected joint is pale red and tense. There is, of course, effusion into the synovial sac. There are sharp, stitching pains, aggravated by any motion. Bryonia is indicated in these cases whether the synovitis be of rheumatic or traumatic origin.
The nearest concordant remedy to Bryonia here is APIS, which is an excellent remedy for synovitis, particularly of the knee-joint. Sharp, lancinating, and stinging pains, and effusion into the joint, are further indications for the remedy. Apis seems to be preferable to Bryonia when this synovitis is of scrofulous origin, or at least appears in a scrofulous

constitution. Apis also has another kind of inflammation, which ends in thickening of the serous sac and of the tissues and cartilages about the joints, giving you the well-known white swelling.

You should also remember SULPHUR in these cases. This remedy supplements Bryonia and Apis, and urges them on when they fail to do their work.

We come next to the study of Bryonia in its action on the muscular system. It is one of the few drugs which produce a positive inflammation of the muscular substance; consequently, you expect to find the drug of use in muscular rheumatism. The muscles are sore to the touch, and at times swollen, and, as you might expect, there is aggravation of the pains from the slightest motion.

Bryonia may also be indicated in articular rheumatism. We find that the fever is not very violent, and the pains and swelling either shift not at all or else very slowly. The local inflammation is violent; that is characteristic of Bryonia. The parts are very hot, and dark or pale red. The pulse in these cases is full and strong, and the tongue is either uniformly white or, more characteristically, dry and white down the centre. The bowels are constipated. It is needless for me to say that the pains are worse from motion.

The difference between Bryonia and RHUS is principally this: Rhus is suitable for rheumatism after exposure to wet, especially when one is overheated and perspiring. Then, too, the Rhus patient finds relief from moving about. Rhus attacks the fibrous tissues, the sheaths of the muscles, Bryonia the muscular tissue itself. The difference between LEDUM and Bryonia may be described in this way: Ledum is useful for rheumatic or gouty inflammation of the great toe; instead of tending to copious effusion the effusion is scanty, and tends to harden into nodosities. In hot swelling of the hip-joint Ledum should be remembered as more successful than Bryonia.
ACTEA SPICATA has a special affinity for the smaller joints. It has this characteristic: The patient goes out feeling tolerably comfortable, but as he walks the joints ache and even swell.

VIOLA ODORATA has a specific action on the right wrist.

Study Guide

CAULOPHYLLUM is especially suited to rheumatism of the phalangeal and metacarpal joints, particularly in females.

In COLCHICUM we have marked aggravation in the evening; the affected joints are swollen and dark red. It is especially useful for weak debilitated persons. The urine is scanty and red, and burns in passing along the urethra; the pains are of a tearing or jerking character. The pains are superficial in summer and deep in winter. Bryonia has great oppression under the sternum, worse from motion ; sharp stitches in the cardiac region, pericardial effusion, with strong pulse. Colchicum has pericardial effusion, fulness and oppression while lying on the left side, compelling him to turn over. The pulse is small, weak, and accelerated. The Colchicum pains appear about the neck and shoulders, or, in a small part of th'e body at a time, and then shift quickly.

GUAIACUM is useful in chronic forms of rheumatism when the joints have become distorted by the concretions. It is also indicated in pleurisy during the second stage of phthisis with muco-purulent sputum.

Next we will study the alimentary canal. We have already spoken of its use here so frequently that its symptoms require but a passing notice. There are the dryness of the mucous lining throughout; the white coating of the tongue, the characteristic thirst, a feeling as though a stone or heavy weight were lying clogged in the stomach, the hard, dry, brown stool, passed with difficulty owing to the hardness of the fsecal matter, atony of the rectum, and intolerance of vegetable food. The symptoms are all worse in summer. It seems that the Bryonia patient cannot tolerate the heat" of the sun.

The liver also is affected. We find it congested, or even inflamed. The gastric symptoms just mentioned complicate the case. The peritoneum covering the liver is inflamed, consequently there are sharp stitches in the right hypochondrium, worse from any motion and better when lying on the right side. In jaundice from duodenal catarrh, you may give Bryonia, especially when the trouble has been brought On by a fit of anger. Although the patient appears hot, he complains of feeling chilly.

CHELIDONIUM is an admirable remedy for very similar symptoms to Bryonia; sharp pains in the region of the liver, shooting in every direction, up into the chest, down into the abdomen; well-marked pain under the scapula, even going through the chest like a rivet; and diarrhoea with either clay-colored or yellowish stools. It differs from Bryonia particularly in the character of the stool.

Bryonia is also similar to KALI CARB., which is indicated in bilious affections when there are these sharp pains in the right hypochondrium, shooting up into the chest, often there is sharp pain, coming from the lower lobe of the right lung. The difference between these pains and those of Bryonia is that these are not necessarily made worse by motion. YUCCA FILAMENTOSA is an admirable remedy for biliousness, with pain going through the upper portion of the liver to the back. There is bad taste in the mouth ; the stools are diarrhoeic and contain an excess of bile. A great deal of flatus passes by the rectum.

CHAMOMILLA, like Bryonia, is indicated in biliousness following anger. With Bryonia there is apt to be chilliness with the anger ; with Chamomilla the patient gets hot and sweats.

BERBERIS VULGARIS also has sharp, stitching pains in the region of the liver; but the pains shoot downwards from the tenth rib to the umbilicus.

The bowels, I have said, are usually constipated under Bryonia, but in some cases the reverse condition obtains. Bryonia is indicated in diarrhoea when the attacks are provoked by indulgence in vegetable foods or stewed fruits, and also by getting overheated in the summer time. The movements are especially worse in the morning after rising when beginning to move around, thus distinguishing it from Sulphur and making it akin to Natrum sulph. In other cases, the patient is seized with sudden griping pains, doubling him up, with copious pasty stools. Sometimes the stools are dark green, from admixture of bile. They have the odor of old cheese.

We next come to the action of Bryonia on the different organs. The mental symptoms have been pretty thoroughly described to you in speaking of typhoid fever. I will merely say here that the patients are irritable and easily angered. This is present with the bilious symptoms, with the headache, and with the dyspepsia, in fact, it is characteristic of the remedy.

Study Guide

The headache of Bryonia, I have also told you, is worse from any motion; even a movement of the eyeballs aggravates the pain. The pain begins in the occiput, or else in the forehead going back into the occiput. It is worse when awaking in the morning, and after violent fits of anger. The nearest remedy that we have to Bryonia here is GELSEMIUM, which has headache with this soreness of the eyes on moving them.

NATRUM MUR. has headache, with beating as from little hammers, with aggravation on moving the head and eyes.

With the occipital headache of Bryonia we should also compare PETROLEUM, which has throbbing occipital headache; and JUGLANS CATHARTICA for occipital headache with pains of a sharp character. CARBO VEG. and NUX VOMICA have occipital pains with bilious attacks.

On the external head, we find Bryonia developing an oily perspiration with a sour odor.

A similar symptom referred to the face is found under NATRUM MUR.

Bryonia is a valuable remedy in diseases of the eyes, not when the external coats of the eye are affected, however. It is to be thought of for metastasis of rheumatism to the eyes. The pains are violent and shoot through the eye-ball into the back of the head, or up toward the vertex. It is aggravated by any motion of the head or eyes. There is also a sensation of tension as if the eyeballs had been put on a stretch. Now you know from what I have said, that Bryonia is indicated in inflammation of the serous membranes with effusion.

Bryonia ought both symptomatically and pathologically be a remedy in glaucoma. The tension of the eyeball is greatly increased. Hot tears flow from the eyes. Photophobia and diminution of vision are present.
The toothache of Bryonia is of rheumatic origin and comes from cold. You will frequently find it in teeth showing no signs of decay. We are therefore led to presume that it is the nerve that is affected. More than one tooth may be involved and relief is momentarily obtained by firm pressure of the head against the pillow, or by the application of cold.

Toothache in children from decayed teeth, with relief from the application of cold water finds its best remedy in COFFEA.

KREOSOTE has neuralgia of the face with burning pains increased by motion and by talking, especially in nervous irritable persons whose teeth decay rapidly.

The characteristic urine of Bryonia is dark red without any deposit. The changes in its appearance are due to excess of coloring matters.

Bryonia has some action on the female genital organs. It is indicated in menstrual difficulties when the flow is dark red and profuse, but more especially when it has been suppressed and we have what has been termed vicarious menstruation.

Here you should compare PULSATILLA and PHOSPHORUS, especially if the suppression of the flow produces haemopytisis or haematemesis.

SENECIO if the patient has cough with bloody expectoration. HAMAMELIS and USTILAGO and MILLEFOLIUM for haematemesis.

Bryonia is indicated in the lying-in chamber. For years, I have been accustomed to using Bryonia for the so-called milk fever. I consider it indicated more than any one remedy because the symptoms are those of Bryonia. There is not very marked-fever, there is this tension of the breast with headache, tearing in the limbs and the patient is weary and wants to keep still.

In threatening mammary abscess, Bryonia is indicated when there are sharp stitching pains, tension of the breast, and pale red color to the swelling.

In incipient mammary abscess you should compare first of all BELLADONNA, which is useful when the symptoms are violent; redness shoots out in radii from the central point of the inflammation.

PHYTOLACCA is an excellent remedy when from the beginning the breasts show a tendency to cake. Especially is Phytolacca the remedy when suppuration is inevitable. When the child nurses pain goes from the nipple all over the body.

Study Guide

PHELLANDRIUM AQUATICUM is an excellent remedy when pains course along the milk ducts between the acts of nursing.

CROTON TIGLIUM, when there is pain from the nipple through to the back when the child nurses, as though it were being pulled by a string. Bryonia is to be remembered in measles. Here it is indicated principally by the tardy appearance of the rash. There is a hard dry cough which makes the child cry. The child doubles up as if to resist the tearing pain which the effort at coughing causes. There may be little or no expectoration. The eyes are inflamed. In other cases, the eruption suddenly disappears when cerebral symptoms appear. The child is drowsy. Its face is pale and there is twitching of the muscles of the face, eyes and mouth. Any motion causes the child to scream with pain. In other cases instead of these cerebral symptoms you have inflammatory diseases of the chest, bronchitis or even pneumonia.

In scarlatina, Bryonia is not often indicated, but when it is, you find some one or all of these symptoms to guide you. The rash has not that smooth character observed under BELLADONNA. It is interspersed with a miliary rash. The eruption comes out imperfectly and the chest and cerebral symptoms just mentioned are present. Now while all the senses are benumbed in these cases there are no absohite hallucinations of the senses as under Belladonna, the patients do not hear voices talking to them as under ANACARDIUM ; they do not awaken from sleep clinging to those about them, as with STRAMONIUM or CUPRUM.

When an eruption has been suppressed and the brain affected in consequence, you may also look to CUPRUM, which is the remedy when the symptoms are violent. The child starts up during sleep. There are decided perversion of the senses, and the spasms characteristic of CUPRUM.

ZINCUM is to be preferred if the child is too weak to develop an eruption. The eruption comes out sparingly. The surface of the body is rather cool. The child lies in a stupor, grating its teeth, it starts up during sleep. Squinting and rolling of the eyes are observed, and there is marked fidgetiness of the feet.

IPECAC. is to be thought of when the chest is affected from the recession of the rash of measles, when there is difficulty in breathing, cough, etc.

It may not be cholera that you need to treat, the fever may have a different name but the sensations, modalities and general symptoms oulined above for each remedy will still be relevant and guide you to the correct remedy.

CALCAREA CARBONICA
(Oyster Shell Calcium)

Key Symptoms: *Soft nails* – almost all who need this remedy have very soft brittle nails, they can be paper thin and or break very easily.

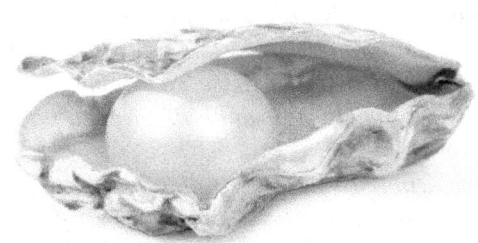

Obesity- these people easily put on weight very easily but can't lose it easily even with diet and exercise. (Effect of Carbon).

Extra perspiration – they sweat easily and especially on the head and neck at night. (Sanicula).

Chilly – they are cold easily and like to stay warm.

Responsible – they like to work hard and stay very responsible.

This is one of the most important medicines used in homeopathy. When indicated based on the totality of the symptoms, it can treat a variety of acute and chronic ailments.

It is frequently needed by newborns and children for the acute illnesses and symptoms listed below. The symptoms that most often are present to justify the use of Calcarea carbonica in children are: PERSPIRATION ON THE HEAD AND NECK WHEN SLEEPING. Cold damp hands and feet.

Sensitivity to cold. If the child is less than eight years old, the they can be less sensitive to the cold; such as play in cold water etc. Over the age of 8 all persons needing Calc-carb will be chilly and feel the need to be kept warm.

Obstinate children, strong will power, anger if you try to move them or change their mind. (Ferrum remedies, Cuprum remedies, Bell, Cham).

Responsible children, want to help out, worry about other people in the family. Worry about other peoples opinion of them. Anxious concerning security. Very curious and intelligent children. May have fear of the dark, ghosts, heights. Nightmares. Strong sense of duty.

Tendency to chronic infections. This remedy will get to the root cause of recurrent infections, such as frequent colds and flus. It follows Belladonna well. Chronic sore throats, tonsillitis, especially the left tonsil. Chronic ear infections. Swollen and hard lymphatic glands.

Other keynote symptoms are:
- Intolerance or allergy to milk
- Craving for eggs and sweets
- Out of breath easily from walking up a hill
- Difficult to loose weight
- Soft and brittle finger nails
- Difficult and painful dentition (new teeth coming in)
- Late learning to walk
- Fontanelles (soft spots on the head in newborns) are late to close
- Slow repair of bones
- Leg cramps

I have often given Calcarea carbonic for the above symptoms. Perhaps one of the reasons for this is the fact that as this medicine is made from calcium it has an effect on all the systems in the body that use calcium. This includes the bones, muscles, nervous system, and the immune system. Early in life these systems are under rapid development and the healing system that keeps this development in homeostasis often needs to be reinforced.

Here is the information from Allen's Keynotes: *Disposed to grow fat, corpulent, unwieldy.*

Children with red face, flabby muscles, who sweat easily and TAKE COLD READILY in consequence.

Large heads and abdomens; fontanelles and sutures open; bones soft, develop very slowly.

Curvature of bones, especially spine and long bones; extremities crooked, deformed; bones irregularly developed.

Head sweats profusely while sleeping, wetting pillow far around (Sil., Sanic.).

Profuse perspiration, mostly on back of head and neck, or chest and upper part of body (Sil.).

Difficult and delayed dentition with characteristic head sweats, and open fontanelles.

During either sickness or convalescence, GREAT LONGING FOR EGGS; craves indigestible things (Alum.) ; aversion to meat.

Acidity of digestive tract; sour eructation, sour vomiting, sour stool; sour odor of the whole body (Hep., Rheum.).

Girls who are FLESHY, PLETHORIC, AND grow too rapidly.

Menstruation TOO EARLY, TOO PROFUSE, TOO LONG LASTING; with subsequent amenorrhoea and chlorosis with menses scanty or suppressed.

Women: menses too early, too profuse; feet habitually cold and damp, as if they had on COLD DAMP STOCKINGS; continually cold in bed.
THE LEAST MENTAL EXCITEMENT causes profuse return of menstrual flow (Sulph., Tub.).

Fears she will lose her reason or that people will observe her mental confusion (Act.).

Lung diseases of tall, slender, rapidly growing youth; upper third of right lung (Ars upper left, Myr., Sulph.); oftener the guide to the constitutional remedy than Phosphorus (compare, Tub.).

Diseases: arising from DEFECTIVE ASSIMILATION; IMPERFECT OSSIFICATION; difficulty in learning to walk or stand; children have no disposition to walk and will not try; suppressed sweat.

Rawness of soles of feet from perspiration (Graph., Sanic.); blisters and offensive foot sweat.

Longing for fresh air (when in a room) which inspires, benefits, strengthens (Puls., Sulph.).

Coldness: general; OF SINGLE PARTS (Kali bi.); head, stomach, abdomen, feet and legs; aversion to cold open air, "goes right through her"; sensitive to cold, damp air; GREAT LIABILITY TO TAKE COLD (opposite of Sulph.).

Sweat: of single parts; head, scalp wet, cold; nape of neck; chest, axillae, sexual organs; hands, knees; feet (Sep.).

Pit of stomach swollen like AN INVERTED SAUCER, and painful to pressure.

Uraemic or other diseases brought on by standing on cold, damp pavements, or working while standing in cold water; modelers or workers in cold clay.

Feels better in every way when constipated. Stool has to be removed mechanically (Aloe, Sanic, Sel., Sep., Sil.). Painless hoarseness, < in the morning. Desire to be magnetized (Phos).

CALCAREA IODATUM

Lots of Calcarea cabonica symptoms and lots of Iodum symptoms. Obesity worse from heat and hypoglycemia. Hurried, or restlessness all the time. Hyperthyroid. Or thin and lean; difficulty to gain weight. Hot blooded. Anger or impulses. Can be overweight and *worse from hot and cold.*

Materia Medica

If you see many Calcarea carbonica symptoms but the patient is worse from heat, thin and hurried then think of this remedy.

CALCAREA PHOSPHORICA
(Calcium phosphate)

RESTLESS discontent – DESIRE for CHANGE or desire to leave the house. Never happy to stay at home. (Opposite to Bryonia).

This remedy is useful for chronic colds, swollen tonsils, slow dentition, headaches, rheumatism, stomach problems and bone diseases. The symptoms that can help you to identify this remedy are:

The child is often RESTLESS and wants to leave the house, go outside or visit with others. He or she wants to travel to another country. For people who have a feeling of discontent with a craving for something new or a change in ones life circumstances.

The baby may have colic after every feeding and or intolerance to milk. The child often craves bacon, ham, smoked meat or hot dogs. There may be temper tantrums, children who can't stay focused, slow to learn.

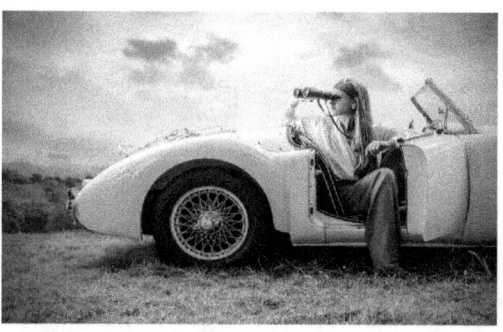

Tall thin children, (Phos element) picky eaters and difficult to gain weight. May have growing pains.

Case 1: One year old child. She gets up in the morning and immediately is in a whining and frustrated mood. She points through the window as if to say: "let me go out, let me go out there." She is angry while eating her breakfast but finally gets to go outside, move about in her stoller, look at the flowers and play with the cute boy down the street. After Calc-phos 30c a few doses she became content and happy both at home and going out. The discontented feeling was totally alieviated. Her great, great grandfather had tuberculosis in his 20's. The only way to explian this is through the model of epigenetics. That being susceptibility to illness is passed from one generation to the next and is a function of gene expression.[1]

George Vithoulkas, with his many years of experience seeing thousand of patients a year, wrote in his <u>Materia Medica Viva</u> about Calcarea phos:

Deficient or poor nutrition is required to produce the classic Calcarea phosphorica picture, especially on the physical level. This picture encompasses the basic structural and developmental pathology described in earlier texts, whose symptoms include: rachitis; emaciation; bone diseases; the non-union of fractured bones; anaemic states; slow or difficult convalescence after acute diseases. Specifically in babies: the non-union of sutures, open fontanelles, late learning to walk, late learning to talk, late dentition and troubles incident to this period.

Fifty or one hundred years ago, case descriptions of Calcarea phosphorica children treated by earlier homeopaths were abundant in our literature. Nowadays, in Western countries, the remedy is not indicated as often because nutrition has greatly improved. In developing countries, however, the classic picture can still be frequently encountered.

Similar to the effect of malnutrition, unexpectedly hearing bad news causes an imbalance in the organism and makes the individual sick. Apart from the predisposition that a child inherits from its parents, there are other causes that trigger a Calcarea phosphorica state. These include psychological stresses experienced in everyday life, e.g. grief, anxieties, insecurity, anger, contradiction, insults, etc., with the most devastating effect being wrought by the sudden hearing of bad news. This is one of the great key-notes of the remedy. This kind of shock cannot be tolerated by the organism so predisposed and brings about a deep imbalance and disease.

For example, a Calcarea phosphorica individual receives a telephone call informing him of a car accident involving a close relative. He becomes overwhelmed and cannot cope. His organism reacts to the information by getting excited, by having palpitations and fainting spells. He perspires profusely, especially around the neck and head and wants to fan this area all the time. What began as a temporary imbalance then turns into a

---

[1] See the web site: EpigenMedica.com for more on this topic.

chronic condition. He is afraid of hearing anything bad and becomes distraught from any kind of unpleasant news. Even the mere idea that he may encounter something unpleasant is unbearable.

The pathological consequences of such a shock can affect the mental, emotional, or physical level, or all simultaneously. An individual that was previously patient and balanced now becomes fearful, fretful, afraid of the dark, and afraid to be alone. These people become oversensitive; they cannot stand to see others suffer, a feeling that assumes pathological proportions.

Irritability and anger develop. This remedy rages and swears almost as much as Nux vomica. The provings describe symptoms such as: 'Grows very violent if his opinion is differed from, or if contradicted, so that he is vexed afterwards not to have been able to control himself.' Or: 'Violent, irritable, and snappish; it affects him most to hear that someone has done wrong; indignation rises in him, and he would like to avoid conversation.'

There is a tendency to become very critical of oneself and others, which may induce these violent and irritable states. Coffee has an aggravating influence. Not only may it cause nausea, heartburn, confusion of the head, and headache, but it may also produce or increase intense ill-humour and irritability.

The possible consequences of hearing bad news in a Calcarea phosphorica individual are described in the provings in this fashion: 'Unpleasant news make him beside himself; he cannot think of any serious thing, cannot collect his thoughts, and gets into a general sweat about it.' Phatak also says that numbness and a crawling sensation can come on after bad news. This indication probably has its basis in the following proving report: 'Very much out of humour, does not want to talk a word, prefers not to be asked and to be left alone, after disagreeable news. — Very restless sleep, tosses about much. — In the morning after waking, the extremities are 'asleep', especially hands and feet (the day after disagreeable news).' The vexation that comes from bad news may also produce depression, a feeling as if lame, an inability to work or even to walk, and diarrhoea.

It is interesting to note that Calcarea phosphorica is seldom indicated for romantic disappointments. In these situations people usually have some sort of warning, either spoken or implied, of the impending separation.

Study Guide

This opportunity for preparation mitigates the suddenness of the shock that otherwise might have provoked a Calcarea phosphorica condition.

Calcarea phosphorica is often indicated for ailments caused by grief, especially when the grief is profound and is precipitated suddenly. A sudden insult that is left unanswered can bring about a state of Calcarea phosphorica. In this case one may mistake the patient for Staphysagria.

Changes of weather, especially to cold and to wet, often cause severe symptoms. Calcarea phosphorica develops rheumatic pains that are worse in the winter (due to the cold weather), disappear in the spring and return in the autumn. Another modality of rheumatism observed in Calcarea phosphorica is that special times for aggravation are in the autumn and when the snow is melting, i.e. in the spring. This is a valuable and well-confirmed symptom.

Getting wet in the rain often brings on rheumatic pains in the shoulders, chest and extremities; the pain moves about all over the limbs and rump. A kind of dull pain from damp, rainy, cold weather has been observed in the lower limbs, as well as a feeling as if lame and beaten in the buttocks and other parts.

Discontent and Restlessness: *A psychological theme central to Calcarea phosphorica is that of discontent. These people never seem to be satisfied with themselves. Their inner discontent renders them aggressive and extremely peevish, causes them to complain and more specifically, to moan and groan.*

This characteristic is most readily witnessed in children. They may suffer discontent for a number of reasons (bone pains, teething difficulties, etc.) and moan and whine constantly and for extended periods of time. Parents typically complain that the moaning grates on their nerves. Mothers of Calcarea phosphorica children typically describe their child as a 'moaning child', thus summarising the whole situation in one word and providing the practitioner with the true essence of the case. Calcarea phosphorica should be the first remedy considered for children who moan in their sleep; in adults, the main remedy is Aurum.

I recall the case of a four-year-old boy. He had fallen and sustained a head injury. For no ascertainable reason, he moaned, groaned, and shrieked for seventy-two hours straight. His father carried him about and took him for walks around the block, but with little effect. Chamomilla did nothing for this child, while Calcarea phosphorica immediately put him into a restful sleep from which he awoke with no residual problems.

We can compare Calcarea phosphorica's dissatisfaction to that of Tuberculinum. Both experience discontent and the resulting desire to travel. Tub.'s dissatisfaction, however, is active and pertains to his locale. These people are unhappy with their surroundings and consequently develop an urge to travel, hoping to alter their environment and situation. They search for another set of conditions or circumstance that will excite them and provide them with strong mental stimulation.

In comparison, Calcarea phosphorica has an indefinable inner and passive discontent. At its core, is a discontent with themselves more than with others, although they may exhibit great irritability, anger, and censorious behaviour toward others. As Calcarea phosphorica is a realist and not one to engage in flights of fancy, his inner discontent constantly brings him back to reality and to his organism that works at a slow pace, to his inability to think, to his feelings of dullness and to his lack of joy. This even further intensifies his suffering, as Calcarea phosphorica's symptoms are definitely aggravated by thinking about them.

It is not surprising, then, that the desire to travel while listed in our repertories along with Tuberculinum, has an entirely different meaning. Calcarea phosphorica does not have the desire to travel per se, nor the excitement of seeing new places that Tub. has. Calcarea phosphorica just wants to be 'off somewhere', to change the place where the person is at the moment 'just for the sake of changing it'. The act of travelling, the altering of impressions, focus and goals distracts him from his inner discontent and restlessness, and thereby ameliorates him. For example, if he leaves his home, not for any major reason, but even just in order to visit a friend in another town, he feels better while travelling. Once he's arrived, however, his discontent returns and he wants to go home again. Calcarea phosphorica and Ignatia share a feeling of being better while travelling.

At this point, I feel it necessary to insert a warning. It is unfortunate and confusing that several authors, based on my description of essences, describe in their teachings or writings the personality traits of their clients, instead of their psychopathology. Only the mental/emotional pathology, not

Study Guide

the personality need be taken into consideration when prescribing a remedy. That which has changed in the mental/emotional sphere after the appearance of the disease is of interest to the homeopath. If, for instance, in our case, there is a curious person who likes to meet people from other countries and is asked the question whether he likes to travel, he may answer yes—but this is not pathology!

Although Calcarea phosphorica and Tuberculinum children have superficial similarities, especially the strong desire for smoked meats, bacon and sausage and the desire to travel, it is important to discriminate between the way they express their dissatisfaction. This is done by noting whether the expression of dissatisfaction is active or passive. The Calcarea phosphorica child, when hurt or displeased, withdraws and begins to complain and moan from morning until night. Nothing satisfies the child; it seems to be unaware of what it wants. The Tub. child, on the other hand, is more prone to act out its dissatisfaction by taking action - by becoming malicious or by trying to hurt others. Were a mother to say, "My child is very nasty," one would not consider Calcarea phosphorica.

Indignation is another key-note of this remedy. When insulted, Calcarea phosphorica does not stay in order to fight back, but rather leaves with a sense of indignation. It is interesting that they can even become indignant at unpleasant dreams. This is another point where they resemble Staphysagria. Staph., however, is sweet and mild and accepting, while Calcarea phosphorica is vehement, angry, censorious and displeased with others and themselves. Though the symptom is the same, the context is different.

Sluggishness: *Without knowing what exactly is wrong or why, Calcarea phosphorica patients realise that something is awry with their system. They may be functioning at their optimum when they suddenly find themselves becoming tired more easily. They feel sluggish. They start to lose interest in pursuing their daily activities, whether it be work or play. Their minds are duller, less vital. In order to mobilise their minds, they need stimulation, either mental, i.e., a good conversation, or physical, such as a good strong coffee. They are unable to explain the reason for their vague discontent. They only perceive that they are no longer easily excited nor enthusiastic about life, and that they are tired and do not comprehend things as readily as before.*

The sluggishness on the mental level can be termed a 'mental flabbiness', and parallels the physical flabbiness that characterises this remedy — similar to what was written in my description of Calcarea carbonica. In Calcarea phosphorica people, the ability to reflect is very compromised. (This is exactly the opposite of Chamomilla, where the ability to reflect is quite active.) Mental tasks require far more time to complete than they did previously. Mental exertion becomes very difficult and may even provoke a headache. Indeed, Calcarea phosphorica is one of the major remedies for headaches in school children (compare Natrum carbonicum). Calcarea carbonica is the major remedy for headaches from physical rather than mental exertion.

The increasing deficiency in the area of the intellect assumes various forms, among them are the following: the memory begins to lack precision (a prover reported that he was unable 'to remember common symptoms of common remedies'), or is lost so that one does not remember at all what one has done, or what one should do. The operations of the intellect begin to lack the accustomed acuity. Ordinary intellectual operations are performed only with difficulty. Words get confused (a prover found himself writing throat for tonsils, red for swollen etc.) or are written twice. It becomes increasingly difficult to distinguish among things and notions under consideration. Mental 'stamina' begins to suffer; the individual is unable to sustain prolonged mental efforts.
Exertion-Exhaustion

As a result of their mind being sluggish, Calcarea phosphorica people dislike mental exertion. In fact, these people dislike performing work of any kind; if they do not work at all, however, they feel they have been neglectful and suffer even more discontent. If they are successful in stimulating themselves to work or are roused by somebody else, they feel better for having made the mental effort. They briefly experience a sense of satisfaction for having done some useful labour. The sluggishness, however, eventually reasserts itself and the discontent and nagging sense that something is wrong return, and progressively worsen. If these people direct their attention to their symptoms —to the difficulty they have concentrating, to their loss of memory, etc.—they feel much worse and their dissatisfaction increases. Similar to Oxalic acid, and as mentioned earlier, Calcarea phosphorica patients are worse from thinking about their symptoms and complaints.

Study Guide

At a more advanced stage, their inability to comprehend can progress to the point where they begin to do silly things. They make silly jokes or say silly things that are inappropriate to the situation. Their comments might be understood were they presented as jokes, but they are often made in all seriousness and with little awareness of the impression created by them.

Calcarea phosphorica's emotions suffer from sluggishness as well. Their emotions move with difficulty; they are indifferent. The emotional indifference, while somewhat similar to that of Phosphoric acid, is not nearly as profound.

Sighing: *Sighing is a well-known key-note of Calcarea phosphorica. One might mistake a Calcarea phosphorica case for Ignatia because both remedies sigh frequently. Calcarea phosphorica's sighing, however, is primarily of a physical origin as opposed to Ign.'s psychological etiology and seems to be a consequence of physical pathology rather than psychology. Calcarea phosphorica cases have a weakness of the respiratory apparatus such that there is a need to take a deep breath. The deep involuntary inspiration that ensues sounds like sighing.*

The sighing does not commence after an experience of grief, though such an episode may aggravate it, and usually appears for no apparent reason and much earlier in the case than Calcarea phosphorica's emotional symptoms. A psychological shock, like grief, may produce other symptoms, such as those previously mentioned under the heading 'Bad News' 'in the Essential Features'. This is different from Ign.'s sighing, which results directly from an incident of grief, and can be traced back to that experience.

Sympathetic and Fearful: *Calcarea phosphorica individuals are typically sensitive people. Before they reach the state of inner discontent, they are quite open and outgoing. Though they are shyer than Phosphorus, the phosphoric element contributes to their sociability. Their feelings can be rather easily hurt, and when this happens they tend to develop an aversion to company; they become sulky and angry.*

Both the qualities of desire for, and aversion to, company are observed, but at different stages of the pathology. The sympathetic moment can take a pathological form, but it is seen at an earlier stage of pathology than the inner discontent that is so striking in the more progressed stages.

Calcarea phosphorica is also very sympathetic toward other people's suffering and many times can become considerably anxious about others (again displaying their phosphoric nature). These ailments, together with some fears like the fear of thunderstorms, of the dark, of dogs, of cats, of being alone that are all key-notes of both Phosphorus and Calcarea carbonica, are encountered frequently in the Calcarea phosphorica child.

In the sexual sphere, we have a polarity. On the one hand, Calcarea phosphorica's general weakness may make them less prone to seek out sex. On the other hand, some Calcarea phosphorica individuals, especially women, possess a very strong sexual drive, some to the point that they suffer from the intensity of the drive. This 'nymphomania' is most intense before menses. Also, having an orgasm sometimes gives Calcarea phosphorica extra energy, resulting in a feeling of general well being, a good appetite, and a desire for work after coitus.

The Calcarea Phosphorica Child: *The general makeup of the Calcarea phosphorica child has frequently been described in homeopathic literature, especially cases where the cause is malnutrition. A good example of such a case is a child who is pale, thin, scrawny, very underweight, mentally and physically underdeveloped, slow at learning to walk (or has lost the ability), hardly able to talk, has tottery legs, a head that is inclined to wobble, a belly that is flabby and prominent or flabby and sunken, is subject to bronchitis and tonsillitis, has a very unstable nervous system, and is very restless. Remedies that should be compared are Baryta carbonica, Borax, Calcarea carbonica, Magnesia carbonica, Medorrhinum, Natrum muriaticum and Phosphoricum acidum.*

Problems with the formation of bones and/or an inclination to bone diseases and bone pains, often indicate Calcarea phosphorica,. The remedy should be considered when the head bones are slow in forming or do not keep pace with the growth of the child, when the fontanelles don't close early enough, or even reopen. Clarke differentiates: 'Calcarea carbonica has an open anterior fontanelle; Calcarea phosphorica has both open, especially the posterior.' The skull is often thin and soft, gives way under the pressure of a finger or seems to crackle like paper. There are pains in the skull bones, especially in the region of the sutures.

Another indication of the remedy is the so-called 'growing pains' (due to delayed closure of the epiphyses) in fast growing children, which appear especially at night. These children grow very quickly, but the assimilation of nutrients to support such rapid growth is deficient; thus we see skeletal and dental problems. A number of pathologies that have been cured or favourably influenced by this remedy are: lateral curvatures of the spine (scoliosis); hydrocephalus, acute or chronic; rickets, frequently with diarrhoea (cholera infantum), in emaciated children; caries, easy decay of the teeth, especially of the first teeth; late or slow dentition, in connection with a host of teething complaints which include cough, diarrhoea and spasms, especially without fever. Symptoms associated with spina bifida are reported to be favourably influenced by Calcarea phosphorica. Enlarged tonsils and adenoid growths are often seen and have also responded well.

An important symptom, though not to the same degree as in Calcarea carbonica, is a profuse night sweat around the head.

Great sensitivity is also exhibited to cold and to jarring. Hering describes: 'A child of fifteen months, with a big head and open fontanelles... violent screaming, grasping with hands in great agony towards his mother; cold sweat, most in face, whole body cold.'

Concerning the mental makeup, some important traits have been described before. The discontent, with the typical moaning (especially during sleep) and the restlessness, is the core of the mental and emotional pathology. Patients tend to be peevish, fretful, and ill-humoured. Boericke describes them as follows: 'Anaemic children who are peevish, flabby, have cold extremities and feeble digestion.' Babies turn over all the time, cry a lot, are restless, constantly kick and move their extremities. Trying to console them by picking them up does not work; on the contrary, it makes them feel worse and may cause a suffocative attack with a cyanotic face and extreme restlessness. This aggravation from lifting the child from its bed is just the opposite of Borax, where downward motion brings on symptoms.

Anxieties and fears are also frequent. They are often related to bodily symptoms (i.e. abdominal pains, chest and respiration symptoms, teething problems). Calcarea phosphorica children tend to be timid and shy; they tend to start or to develop convulsions from fright or other external influences.

On the intellectual level, the growth process of these children is also frequently disturbed. Their memory is poor, and mental exertion is often dreaded; prolonged mental efforts are difficult to sustain and often bring on symptoms (like the headaches in school children mentioned earlier, or a kind of dull sluggishness with the desire to be alone). Mental retardation with bodily hyperactivity is an indication that has been confirmed more than once by many homeopaths including Stiegele, who saw favourable results even in more advanced stages of this syndrome (after cerebral polio).

The food desires are very unusual and strong. 'Craving for fat bacon', or, as Margaret Tyler puts it, for 'ham rind', is a symptom that has been well-verified in children; however an aversion to ham has also been observed. Smoked meat is frequently the favourite food. We also see desire for sausages, for potatoes and farinaceous foods, and for indigestible things, which refers to things that the little patient cannot digest, such as fat bacon in cases of cholera infantum, or to slate pencils, clay or such things. An aversion to ham, however, has also been observed. Children's appetites frequently increase, and the child wants to eat (or nurse) all the time; this often occurs in emaciated children, who despite this do not 'put on flesh'. We also see nursing children who refuse their mother's milk; this, however, is due to the milk being spoiled and tasting salty, not to any problem with the child. (Vithoulkas)

Case 2: A boy of 12 had just lost his father in a construction accident. He could not sleep and his mind had become paralyzed by grief. He was very tall and slender, he had always been restless with discontent. Sighing often. After a dose of Calcarea phos 30c he recovered from the grief in a week. I could not believe it if I had not seen if for myself as he displayed an even mood, eating and sleeping well, mind clear, peaceful and philosophical about the tragedy but positive about the fond memories he had about his father.

CALCAREA SULPHURICA
(Calcium sulphate)

JEALOUSY** – **jealous of siblings, of partner, for parental attension, or friends; it can take many forms and be displayed in many ways.

With Calcarea sulphurica there is like Sulphur a great need for validation and attention, but this is even stronger in this remedy.

Study Guide

Case 1: Child of four years. He would try and push the parents apart when they talked to each other as if to say: "You can't take your attention away from me, you can't talk to each other and exclude me even for a minute." In this way it is much like Lachesis and Hyoscyamus. But we see also many Calcarea and Sulphur symptoms to help us find the correct remedy for jealousy. After Calcarea sulph his jealousy is better, his speech is better (Calcarea – slow to learn), his skin eczema is better (Sulphur – itchy skin), and he is less angry overall.

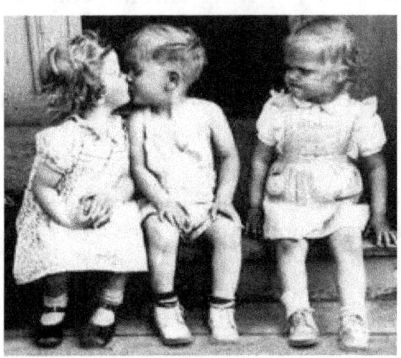

Anger when no respect shown – the ego is like that of Sulphur, they want recognition to be respected, they need constant praise and to be shown admiration. Children who constanly say: "Look at me, look at me, see how I can jump or go down the slide..." Teenagers who like to be on the front stage of life, admired by everyone.

This medicine is made from a combination of calcium and sulphur. It will, therefore, have characteristics of the remedy Calcarea carbonica and Sulphur with some symptoms that are unique to it. It is also similar to Hepar sulphur in many of the physical symptoms.

The physical symptoms that point to a need for Calcarea Sulphuricum are:
- Recurrent otitis media (middle ear infections) with chronic yellow discharge from the ears
- Abscess of the external ear, with blood and puss
- Mastoiditis (infection of the bony cavities around the ear)
- Chronic stuffy nose
- Chronic cough, croup, abscesses of the lungs
- Productive yellow mucous from the lungs

- Boils that open and drain yellow pus for days and weeks

The main symptom that makes it possible to differentiate it from Calcarea carbonica and Hepar sulphur is a **sensitivity to heat and an aversion to getting too warm**. Both Calcarea carb and Hepar sulpur patients are sensitive to the cold with Hepar being the most averse to cold.

Usually Calcarea sulph is for lingering chronic complaints. The Calcarea person can be obstinate and stubborn. The sulphur element adds a degree of egotism and selfishness to their character leading to JEALOUSLY which is often found in a person needing Calc sulph. Not as much suppressed anger or insecurity as those who need Hepar sulph.

Acne, allergies, eczema, impetigo, sinusitis. This is a good remedy to use when most of the symptoms are like Calcarea carbonica but there is an aggravation from heat, the child throws off the covers at night, the complexion is more ruddy, red and full blooded and they are more selfish.

CAMPHORA
(Camphor Tree)

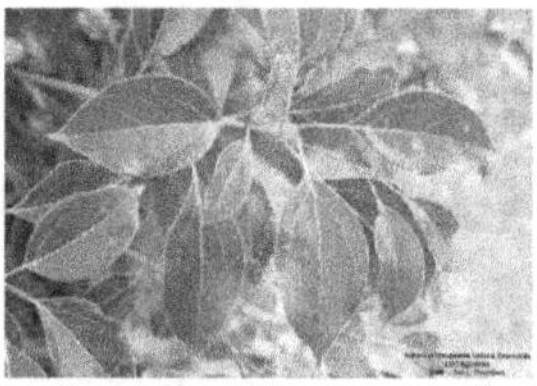

Feels hot and cold at the same time in the extreme. Body is icy cold but wants to uncover. Flu with chills, collapse in vitality. Cold sweat, sneezing. Feels alone, neglected, forsaken. Depression from being abandoned.

Boericke says of this remedy: *Pictures a state of collapse. Icy coldness of the whole body; sudden sinking of strength; pulse small and weak. After operations, if temperature is subnormal, low blood pressure, 3 doses camph. 1x, 15-minute intervals. This condition is met with in cholera, and here it is that Camphor has achieved classical fame. First stages of a cold, with chilliness and sneezing. Subsultus and extreme restlessness. Cracking of joints. Epileptiform convulsions. Camphor has a direct relationship to muscles and fascia. In local rheumatic affections in cold climates necessary. Distention of veins. As a heart stimulant for emergency use of Camphor is the most satisfactory remedy. Drop doses on sugar as often as every five minutes.*

It is characteristic of Camphor that the patient will not be covered, notwithstanding the icy coldness of the body. One of the main remedies in shock. Pain better while thinking of it. Very sensitive to cold and to touch. Sequelæ of measles. Violent convulsion, with wandering and hysterical excitement. Tetanic spasms. Scrofulous children and irritable, weakly blondes especially affected.

Case 1: Flu with extreme weakness. Can barely get up to walk around. Collapse of energy. Sore throat, achy all over. On the fourth day the patient woke up at 4 a.m. with a sensation of heat and coldness at the same time all over the body. The patients said: "I could not descide whether to cover or uncover but in the end I had to uncover. **Plan:** Camphor 30c one dose. A few hours later the body temperature was back to normal and that same day made a full recovery in vitality and all other respects.

Nash has this to say about Camphor: *The great characteristic around which the whole action of CAMPHOR seems to revolve is: "GREAT COLDNESS OF THE EXTERNAL SURFACE, WITH SUDDEN AND COMPLETE PROSTRATION OF THE VITAL FORCES." It is no wonder Hahnemann headed his trio (CAMPHOR, CUPRUM and HELLEBORE) of cholera remedies with CAMPHOR. If we were to sum up the same condition in one word it would be COLLAPSE. No remedy comes nearer to CAMPHOR than the last of the trio, viz., VERATRUM ALBUM, but CAMPHOR has the collapse with painless stool or even no stool at all, while VERATRUM has the collapse seemingly as a consequence of the very profuse evacuations of stomach and bowels. Both have great external coldness, but VERATRUM has a very marked appearance of COLD SWEAT upon the hippocratic face, especially forehead. CUPRUM leads the trio, when the CRAMP in stomach and extremities is the most prominent symptom.*

These remedies are indicated when these characteristic symptoms

Materia Medica

appear, not only in cholera, but in any disease. There is one peculiarity in the coldness of CAMPHOR, viz., THE PATIENT WILL NOT BE COVERED, OR OBJECTS TO IT, NO MATTER HOW OBJECTIVELY COLD HE IS. SECALE coldness or collapse is exactly like this, and even in gangrena senilis it proves a great remedy on the same indications. The signal success of Dr. Rubini, of Naples, in treating five hundred and ninety-two cases of cholera with CAMPHOR verified the prediction of Hahnemann beyond question.

Collapse with cold surface and aversion to heat may come on in retrocedent exanthema, or in the later stage of so-called cholera infantum, in pneumonia, or capillary bronchitis, from exposure to intense cold or traumatic shock. Indeed it does not matter from what cause except death. CAMPHOR is the first remedy to be thought of, and according to susceptibility or strength of the patient the dose must be varied from tincture to highest potency. (Nash)

CARBO VEGETABILIS
(Vegetable Charcoal)

Desire for a fan when sleeping – summer and winter. Wants a fan often when sitting at home. These people need the air to be moving as they can't oxygenate their blood properly. Tend to gain weight easily and can't loose weight. With this symptoms there are many pathologies that will yield to Carbo-veg.

Case 1: Hay fever, he wants the fan on all night. After Carbo-veg 30c he is much better in one day. Took remedy once a week for a month. Next year no hay fever.

Desire to be fanned- feels better from being fanned.

Case 2: Cough, post nasal catarrh, sore throat, hot flashes, weakness, eyes burn, anxiety in a closed in room, she wants fresh air, windows open and fan on. Short fuse and anger. Frequent headaches. Depression for six months. No sex drive. Tearful all the time. Can't concentrate at work, feels overwhelmed easily, bloated and gassy, fear of fire, psoriasis on scalp. The only symptom that was helpful in solving this case was the desire to be fanned. After Carbo-veg 30c she is much better two weeks later in all of her above symptoms. Depression a lot better, happier, no anxiety, sex drive came back, etc.

Nash say of this remedy: *Vital force nearly exhausted; complete collapse.* (Acetanilidum – fainting; Lauro – fainting, blue).
Blood stagnates in the capillaries; venous turgescence; surface cold and blue.

Haemorrhages (nose, stomach, gums, bowels, bladder or any mucous surface), with indescribable PALENESS of the surface of the body.

Mucous membranes break down, become spongy, bleed, ulcerate and become putrid.

Excessive flatulence, pressing upward, stomach and abdomen.
Hunger for oxygen, decarbonized blood; cries, "fan me, fan me hard!"

Anaemic, especially after acute diseases, which have greatly depleted the patients; chronic effects.

Persons who have never fully recovered from the exhausting effects of some previous illness; has never recovered from effects of typhoid, weak digestion; the simplest food disagrees; eructations give temporary relief.

Bad effects from loss of vital fluids (CAUST.); haemorrhage from any broken-down condition of mucous membrane.
Looseness of teeth, easily bleeding gums.

In the last stages of disease, with copious cold sweat, cold breath, cold tongue, voice lost, this remedy may save a life.
Coldness of the knees, even in bed (APIS); of left arm and left leg; very cold hands and feet; finger-nails blue.

Persons who have never recovered from effects of some previous illness or injury; suppression by QUININE or drugging; typhoid or yellow fever.

CHINA is its great complementary.

In our remarks upon CHINA we said that for flatulent conditions the choice lay often between it, CARBO VEG. and LYCOPODIUM. CARBO VEGETAHILIS also ranges alongside CHINA for debilitated states. The weakness of CARBO VEGETAHILIS is not surpassed by any other remedy. This, with ARSENICUM and MURIATIC ACID form a trio of remedies which according to well-known indications has snatched many a patient from the very jaws of death. Picture of CARHO VEG.: VITAL FORCES NEARLY EXHAUSTED,

COLD SURFACE, ESPECIALLY FROM KNEES DOWN TO FEET; LIES MOTIONLESS, AS IF DEAD; BREATH COLD; PULSE INTERMITTENT, THREADY; COLD SWEAT ON LIMBS. This is truly a desperate condition. Then add to these symptoms, BLOOD STAGNATES IN THE CAPILLARIES, CAUSING BLUENESS, COLDNESS AND ECCHYMOSES; the patient so weak he cannot breathe without being constantly fanned. Gasps: "Fan me! Fan me!" CARBO VEG. has saved such cases. This is a picture of a case of typhoid fever, and in one case we saw added still to this, haemorrhage of dark, decomposed, unclotted blood; could not clot on account of its broken down condition; blood oozing from gums and nostrils, and an indescribable PALENESS, not only of the hippocratic face, but also of the skin of the whole body, yet CARBO VEG. restored to health, and in an aged woman at that.

I have here, as faithfully as I can, portrayed the wonderful power of this remedy in such a desperate case. Of course no remedy can raise the dead, no matter how strong the indications before death; but no remedy can come nearer than this and the dominant school know little or nothing about it, and never can until they will consent to use it in the homeopathic form and according to homeopathic indications.

The sphere of this remedy is not by any means limited to low or weakening states in connection with acute diseases. To give an idea of its use when indicated by the symptoms in chronic ailments, I can do no better than quote from Henry N. Guernsey: "No truer remark was ever written than that CARBO VEGETABILIS is especially adapted to cachectic individuals whose vital powers have become weakened. This remark is made particularly clear when considered in the light of those cases in which disease seems to be engrafted upon the system by reason of the depressing influence of some prior derangement. (PSORINUM.) Thus, for instance, the patient tells us that asthma has troubled him ever since he had the whooping cough in childhood; he has dyspepsia ever since a drunken debauch which occurred some years ago; he has never been well since the time he strained himself so badly (RHUS TOX., CALCAREA OST.); the strain itself does not now seem to be the matter, but his present ailments have all appeared since it happened; he sustained an injury some years ago, no traces of which are now apparent, and yet he dates his present complaints from the time of the occurrence of that accident; or again, he was injured by exposure to damp, hot air and his present ailments result from it.

It will be well for the physician to think of CARBO VEGETABILIS in similar cases which are numerous and may present very dissimilar phenomena, as these circumstances being suggestive of CARBO VEG. it in all probability will be found to be the appropriate remedy, which the agreement of the other symptoms of the case with those of the drug will serve to corroborate." This is from the pen of one of the best prescribers that ever lived, and I feel justified in quoting it entire.

This remedy seems to affect deeply the whole alimentary tract, and the same broken down, weakened condition appears. The GUMS BREAK DOWN, BECOME SPONGY, BLEED ON TOUCHING OR SUCKING THEM, OR BECOME RETRACTED FROM THE TEETH, LOWER INCISORS, and are painfully sensitive or sore on chewing or even pressing the teeth hard together.

The stomach also becomes weak. Acidity and pyrosis is frequent; the plainest food disagrees, fat foods especially. Here CARBO VEGETABILIS succeeds when PULSATILLA fails.

The most marked and valuable place for this remedy is in its power to relieve complaints from EXCESSIVE FLATULENCE IN THE STOMACH. "Great accumulations of flatulence in the stomach." "Stomach feels full and tense from flatulence." Great pain in stomach on account of flatulence, worse especially on LYING DOWN, should always call attention to this remedy. All this may occur in different affections

Materia Medica

ranging from a simple dyspepsia to incurable cancer of the stomach. In the latter case, and even in cases not so serious, we may have added BURNING IN STOMACH.

This flatulence is also generated in the abdomen, but, in the CARBO VEGETABILIS cases, is most troublesome in upper part; yet may extend so far as to cause great meteoristic distention, especially in typhoid fevers, dysenteries, etc. It is a remedy of inestimable value in haemorrhage from any broken down condition of mucous membranes. This action upon the mucous membranes does not stop with the alimentary tract, but attacks those of the respiratory tract also. Beginning with the larynx, it causes and cures great hoarseness, which is characteristically WORSE IN THE DAMP AIR, ESPECIALLY OF EVENING. It may be very bad even (if the air is damp) in the morning; but morning hoarseness is oftener reached by CAUSTICUM.

This condition may go on extending and increasing until it reaches the bronchia. This is particularly true in case of elderly people of broken down constitutions, venous system predominating. It is a great remedy for the bronchitis of old people; also for asthma of the same, in very desperate cases where the patient appears as if dying. Here the choice must be sometimes made between this remedy and CHINA.

In the chest there is sometimes "BURNING AS FRONT GLOWING COAL," and again, "weak, fatigued feeling in chest," where the choice may fall between it and PHOSPHORIC ACID, STANNUM and SULPHUR. It has been found very efficacious in desperate cases of pneumonia, and comes in quite naturally after TARTAR EMETIC has failed to assist the patient to clear his lungs of the great quantities of loosened mucus, when cyanosis and paralysis threaten from weakness. Its sputa then is apt to be foetid with cold sweat and breath and the characteristic WANTED-TO-BE-FANNED CONDITION.

Before we leave this remedy I want to emphasize its power over haemorrhages, which may occur from lungs, nose, stomach, bowels, bladder or any mucous surface. No remedy can take its place in broken down, greatly debilitated constitutions where the surfaces from which the blood oozes seem too weak and spongy to hold the blood in them. Their vitality is gone with the patient's nervous vitality. The patient's face and skin is VERY PALE, even before the haemorrhage has occurred. (Nash)

Study Guide

CARCINOSIN
(Cancer Nosode)

There are a few main symptoms that are usually present in the patient who needs this remedy. This includes:

PERFECTIONISTIC tendencies. They are trying to make a perfect home, a perfect garden, do perfect work for their employer; but it is too much for them and so they become anxious about it or break down under the stress of their own expectations.

FEAR OF REPRIMAND – they are very sensitive people, it takes very little criticisms or scolding to make these people feel mortified. They can suffer for years from being told they did something wrong and try to be perfect so as to never be scolded again. **Guilt** from being wrong (Aids).

YIELDING - their identity is not strong. They do what others tell them to do or expect of them. They find it very difficult to say 'no' and can't act in a selfish manner. (Opposite to Bell, Ferrum, Lach) They often work for others for free, become a slave because saying 'no' may lead to criticism.

SYMPATHETIC – they can feel the suffering of others and want to do all they can to help others especially those in their family. They do more for others than for themselves, (Mag-phos).

FASTIDIOUS – they want everything to be clean and perfect.

DESIRE to make things look beautiful. Love to dance and be with friends.

Forgiving others very easily and can't say no. No boundaries.

These people are happy to serve others.

This all adds up to a person who lays them self down and *allows others to walk all over them.* In

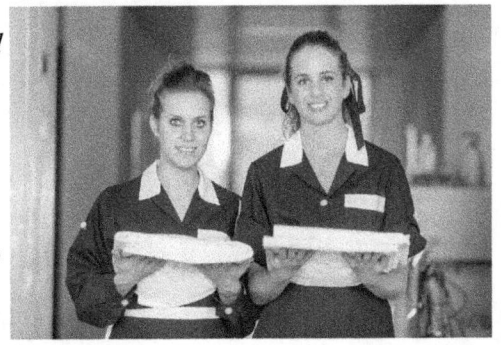

138

fact they will say: *"Go ahead walk on me"*. It is normal to make sacrifices for others at times but these people do it for years with family, at work and with friends.

They never seem to get very angry about it as they make excuses for other people to be mean and selfish or abusive toward them. Over time letting others treat them this way erodes at their own individuality as they don't make very many choices out of self interest; like finding ones own vocation, choosing a sport, choosing a belief system or choosing a new friend or life partner; all of which are examples of a healthy balanced person assuring their individual identity. They are too easily controlled by others but this is mostly because they are too yielding and can't seem to stand up for themselves.

History of domination from others. They can carry a heavy burden of guilt, if they do something for themselves or go against what others want they feel guilty and give up.

The human condition was never meant to be perfect.

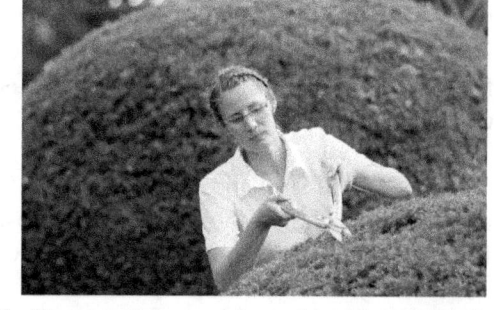

This is a common remedy in our society. This remedy can treat a wide variety of acute and chronic ailments if it fits the nature of the patient and general symptoms. It is indicated for people who are *mild* in character, *giving too much to others, too generous,* <u>*she can never say no to anyone.*</u>

He can not get angry when he should, instead he suppresses his anger and therefore they no longer feel any anger. This remedy is listed for being offended easily but I have not seen this in the patients I have treated.

Grief with weeping and sympathy for the person who is no longer with them. They are able to express their emotions and cry easily, (Opposite to Natrum muriaticum).

They feel guilt too acutely. For example; how they fell short of the expectations from others. They may say to themselves: "I should have done more to help them when they were sick, it was my fault they died so soon."

Case 1: I gave this remedy to a person who felt guilty about wasting dirty dish water. So she left it in the sink until she had new dishes to wash. After using this remedy for a month she could let the water drain out right after doing the dishes without any more guilt feelings.

Case 2: Another time I used it for a boy who could not play with other children, he was too serious, grief stricken and depressed. Instead of being a normal child; he felt an obligation to help his grandfather work on chores around his farm, that is all he wanted to do. He had watched his mother die of cancer in their home and felt he had to try and save her. Here again we see that this child was full of obligation and his sense of duty was too strong. After Carcinosin his depression lifted, he could play again with his friends and no longer felt obligated to help his grandfather with everything.

These persons easily experience feelings of guilt, they feel they can never do enough for others and as a result, cannot find a way to say no when others ask them for help.

They are too yielding in general; it is very difficult for them to stand up for themselves. They can too easily be dominated by others. These are usually life long traits but after taking this remedy their character will change and all or most of the physical symptoms will improve.

They put up with abuse for too long to please their family or some other person. Instead of being assertive they worry they are not doing enough to help the abuser. They lay themselves down so that others can walk on them. And all too often others do take advantage of them, control them or abuse them.

They seem to find it difficult never get angry toward the abuser or seem to feel no anger at all. Instead he or she will feel empathy for the abuser. 'Well I know he is not nice to me and is beating me up at times but he had a bad childhood.'

Generally the people who need this remedy are perfectionists and try to accomplish too much. Fear of making mistakes, fear that they are not measuring up.

The house has to be clean and neat all the time, especially if people come to visit. The garden has to be in order; they need to look good all the time.

They are too worried about what others will think of them. They try to please others all the time and don't take any time for the things they need to do for themselves.

Too nice and too compliant. Their friends will tell them: "By gosh don't be so submissive and stand up for yourself ….." But they can't seem to muster up the strength to do this. They put up with things for too long and never get angry. Small children experience a terrible fear of a reprimand, so try to do extra tasks to help their parents. People who never develop a strong identity or follow a path of self-determination.

They are very outgoing, excitable, friendly, helpful, sympathetic, soft and gentle. They love music, to socialize and to help others.

Confirming symptoms: women with breast tenderness before their menses, love of thunderstorms, biting of nails, very neat and tidy. Children who sleep in the knee chest position. Love of animals, to dance and a desire to travel.

Carcinosin has the capacity to cure many chronic ailments too numerous to mention and can be used as long as the symptom picture above is present. This remedy can treat any type of chronic infection, headaches, stomach problems, joint pains, asthma etc.

CARDUUS MARIANUS
(Milk Thistle)

Liver pathology from alcoholism or toxicity. *Varicose veins in the legs, hemorrhoids and esophageal varicies*. Edema. Tender liver and gall bladder. Cirrhosis of the liver. Even in herbal doses we can see this remedy have the same effects on the liver.

Study Guide

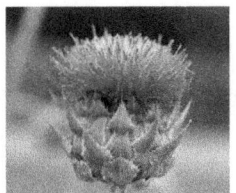

Case 1: I treated a 42 year old alcoholic. She was in the hospital; her liver and kidneys had stopped working and her family were told that she was going to die in the next day or so. The father called me to see what I could do. After each dose of Carduus 30c she improved and her blood tests improved along with the lessening of her symptoms. After I saw her in person a few weeks later she told me her craving for alcohol was no longer present. She was able to go back to work.

Nash says of this remedy: *This is one of the most important liver remedies, if a homeopathic author can be excused for the expression. There are many pains, pressing, dragging, drawing, burning; worse from motion. The patient is very sensitive to cold, and is subject to attacks of bilious vomiting at regular or irregular intervals. The author has cured many violent sick headaches ending in vomiting bile, and cases in the habit of taking calomel, with this remedy (SANG.). Dropsical effusions with liver diseases. It is useful in haemorrhages and jaundice, when symptoms agree.*

Sadness, irritability and weeping. Congestive headaches; pressing pains coming periodically. Fullness and heaviness in the head.

Sensitiveness of the scalp to cold air. Pressing outward of the eyeballs. Yellow sclerotics. Burning in margins of lids. Burning inside of the nose. Epistaxis.

Taste bitter, insipid, or wanting. Foul tongue. No desire for food. Nausea, and vomiting mucus, then bile. Painful retching, and then vomiting sour greenish fluid. Drawing pains from left to right in the stomach. Burning in the stomach. Vomiting blood, very black.

The most important of all the liver symptoms. Dragging pain in right hypochondrium when lying on left side; like AM., MAG. M., NAT. S. and PTEL. Pressing, drawing, stitching in right lobe of liver. This remedy establishes a healthy flow of bile, and thereby cures the condition that favors the formation of gall stones.

It has many times broken up the tendency to gall stone colic. Portal congestion and hemorrhoids. Sore, bruised, hard liver; sometimes the left lobe, but oftener the right. When complicated with lung and heart symptoms; with expectoration of blood.

Drawing, stitching or burning pains in the abdomen. Distended abdomen. Cutting pains.

The stool is black. Stool hard and knotty. Clay-like, bile-less stool. Burning in rectum and anus. Itching piles. Bleeding piles. Inveterate constipation. (Nash)

CAUSTICUM
(Potassium remedy from Hahnemann)

Anxiety for others. Most people in society are concerned about their own lives and that of their family. *For Causticum people, the circle of empathy is much wider; it extends and includes a genuine concern for the issues that affect society in general, such as what is unjust in society, politics, who is in special need of help, the environment and animals.* They don't just think about the issue, but what makes this remedy indicated is that *they join a group and fight for what is just in a very systematic manner.*

They are quite inspirational people to interview because their lives are so interesting, and they are so much less selfish than the average person. (Most opposite remedies in this respect is Arsenicum). A strong keynote symptom, especially for women is *weakness of the bladder – involuntary urination - when cough or sneeze. Restless legs in the evening or when in bed.* Lots of ear wax.

Phosphorus is also very empathetic but the main concern is with family and friends or who-ever is right in front of them at the time. *For Phosphorus the empathy is much more spontaneous, then the next day it is another person who they become involved with. Causticum has a deeper insight into things, they think about the issue for a long time, come up with an idea then go to work for many years to help solve it.* Kali Phos is closer to Causticum in this respect.

This remedy is indicated for grief of long standing. Ailments from worry. *Fear something bad is going to happen.* Paralysis such as Bell's Palsy, multiple sclerosis. Arthritis. Cough on waking. Feels better when it is raining.

Nash says of this remedy: *In the first place it has GREAT WEAKNESS, such as characterizes the potash salts generally. It is with CAUSTICUM "FAINT-LIKE WEAKNESS, OR SINKING OF STRENGTH, WITH TREMBLING." In this it resembles GELSEMIUM, and it has another symptom, in connection with its general weakness which resembles GELSEMIUM, viz.: "DROOPING OF THE LIDS." SEPIA, CAUSTICUM and GELSEMIUM is the trio having this peculiar symptom in a very marked degree. Now, the weakness of CAUSTICUM progresses until we have "GRADUALLY APPEARING PARALYSIS;" indeed, PARALYSIS is common with CAUSTICUM and attacks in a general way the right side (LACHESIS THE LEFT), but it also has local paralysis; as, for instance, of the VOCAL ORGANS, MUSCLES OF DEGLUTITION, OF TONGUE, EYELIDS, FACE, BLADDER and EXTREMITIES.*

On the other hand, it has all grades of nervous twitchings, chorea, convulsions and epileptic attacks, even progressive locomotor ataxia. I can only name these diseases here, but will notice further on the symptoms and conditions which appear in connection with them.

Neuralgic affections are also common with this remedy and are generally of an obstinate character. CAUSTICUM has helped me out in such cases when other seemingly indicated remedies failed. One of our oldest and most eminent writers on Materia Medica, Charles J. Hempel, sneered at the multiplicity of symptoms of this remedy, as found in the "CHRONIC

DISEASES," but the clinical test has proven it to be a remedy of great use and wide range.

On the mind it exerts a very depressing influence in keeping with its general action on the nervous system. MELANCHOLY MOOD; SADNESS, hopelessness; is apt to look on the dark side of everything. This melancholy may come from care, grief or sorrow. It often comes from long-lasting grief or sorrow, and should be remembered here alongside IGNATIA, NATRUM MURIATICUM and PHOSPHORIC ACID. (Nash)

CHAMOMILLA
(German Chamomile)

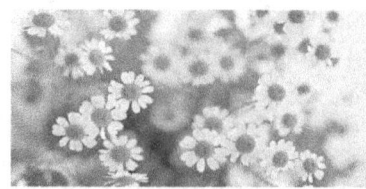

Study Guide

Pain with irritability. Perspiration at night, wants to uncover.

FUSSY, IRRITABILITY, whiny, CONTRARY and CAN'T BE PLEASED. (Cina, Ip, Rheum) *The more the pain the more the child is angry and whining.*

You can see from the picture how helpless the child is from the pain. Often the pain is the result of an ear infection.

The core symptoms that differentiate it from other remedies are:
- *Thirst for many drinks of water or juice*
- *Perspiration when sleeping*
- Kicks *the covers off at night*
- VERY IRRITABLE CHILDREN

He or she cries easily, extremely loud crying, *inconsolable*, difficult to please, aversion to touch from strangers, whining and crying for almost no reason, restless, wants things then throws them away, wants to be constantly carried or rocked vigorously, fussy, impatient, insulting, violent anger, aversion to be looked at, anger at trifles, contrary, capricious, restless, always complaining, demands things and discontented.

A mild and contented child is a good reason <u>not</u> give Chamomile. Just as in Belladonna the sensitivity to light is the main keynote symptom, in order to prescribe Chamomile the person should be in a state of <u>*irritability.*</u> It is like they have been spoiled, now they are selfish and want everything for themselves and if not appeased will start to whine and scream about it. The ego of a child has to eventually let go to see that they are in fact not the center of the universe. That is why this remedy is most often needed from birth to age five.

If this pathological state is strong enough to continue into adulthood then this is one remedy that we can use for borderline personality disorder. The ego is still unfortunately firmly in control. The adult Chamomilla will demand total attention and obedience from their partner; and for example threaten suicide if they do not get their way or try to kill their partner out of selfish anger because they felt betrayed for a trivial reason such as; 'he left to go to work and did not make my breakfast just the way I wanted it'.

In most Chamomile cases there will be the typical state of a child in a state of *unendurable pain* usually and as a result of an ear infection. The nervous system is over-sensitive and overwhelmed by the pain. Usually the child can't sleep from the pains in the ear. When it is the correct medicine, the child will go to sleep and wake up in the morning almost completely better and with a new found ability to see that other's needs can be taken into account and this can be an interesting and enjoyable part of life.

Other symptoms that a person needing Chamomile will often include: *One cheek red* and hot, *the other pale* and cold.

Diarrhea that is hot and green (looks like chopped eggs), and burns the anus.

Numbness of the suffering parts, which is worse at 9 a.m. or 9 p.m. Colic, sudden sharp pains in the abdomen from trapped gas, fuss, whine, then arch the back, kick and scream. Especially complaints that come on after anger, with red cheeks and hot perspiration.

Pain and irritation of the gums from teething, worse from warm drinks, waking often with irritability from the pains. Earache sensitive to cold wind, better from wrapping up the head warmly.

Generally, the person is worse from heat, they will kick the covers off when they are sleeping, burning soles of the feet at night. Profuse perspiration at night, on waking the sweat ceases and returns again on falling asleep.

The children often have a desire to be carried and rocked. They will stop crying only when they are carried and moved about vigorously. If you see a parent holding their child and jumping up and down you now know why.

Other conditions Chamomile will treat are colic, diarrhea, especially during teething, and sleeplessness from teething. Nose stopped up, congested, with hot drainage. Rattling mucous in the chest. Asthmatic respiration. Violent rheumatic pains driving him out of bed, compelling him to walk about. Ear infections in adults from suppressed anger.

In older girls and women, dysmenorrhoea (painful menses) - she wants to quarrel (a way to get attention), is impatient and irritable. The menses may be dark and clotted with labour-like pains.

During childbirth Chamomile is indicated by an extreme intolerance to pain. The labour pains may be unproductive, shooting upward. Chamomile is one of the main remedy to consider for the after effects and withdrawal of narcotics. (Coffea, Op, Nux).

Chamomile is listed as a treatment for milk allergy, therefore it is a good idea for the cow's milk and dairy products to be replaced by soy milk, or rice milk until this remedy has had some time to work.

Recommendations: a child or adult with one of these very painful ear infections can be given one dose a day until he/she is 80 per cent better and then one dose every three or four days for another week.

In summary no one likes to be around a chamomile patient, who is restless, outspoken and in such an 'ugly mood.' An obvious thirst, perspiration and diarrhea are the symptoms that can help to tell it apart from Belladonna.

Chamomile is one of the most effective treatments for ear infections and far superior to any antibiotic therapy. One can expect the patient to be better within 24 hours.

It can be used for otitis media (middle ear infection) and otitis externa (infection of the ear canal) in adults and children. If the ear infection returns after a few weeks, check for food allergies by eliminating processed foods, sugar, sweets, wheat and eggs. Give acidophilus if any antibiotics have been used. Chamomile is a wonderful remedy when indicated.

Take one dose of the 30c and wait three hours to see if there is a reaction. If the patient is improving the remedy does not have to be repeated. If the symptoms start to return then repeat the remedy and then after this dose has no more benefit or is not holding then give a higher potency.

CHELIDONIUM MAJUS
(Greater Celandine)

Liver pathology. **Cold hands and especially cold fingertips. Pain from the gall-bladder refers to the right scapula. Pain under the inferior angle of the right scapula.** Allergy to dust. Jaundice. Tongue yellow with imprint of the teeth. Stool hard round balls. Rheumatic symptoms. Headaches.

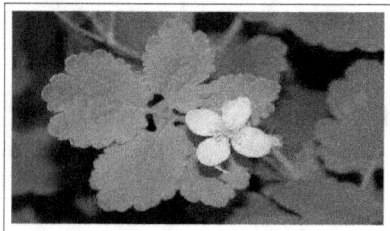

Pain under the right scapula.

Cold hands and feet. Icy cold fingertips. Allergy to dust.

I have used this remedy quite a few times. I have not seen it treat a specific type of emotional ailment. I can only say they were all hard working people, family oriented, responsible, polite and easy to get along with.

Kent says of this remedy: *Skin: The skin is likely to be sallow, and gradually increases to a marked jaundice in connection with these complaints. Semi-chronic gastritis, with jaundice.*

"Gastro-duodenal catarrh. Congestion and soreness in the liver, with jaundice. Right-sided pneumonia, complicated with liver troubles, or jaundice."

This remedy seems to act throughout the system, but almost always along with it the liver is involved, and it is suitable for

Study Guide

what the old people and the doctors called "biliousness." The patient is generally bilious, has nausea and vomiting. Distension of the veins. Yellowish gray color of the skin. (Kent)

CHOCOLATE

This is a new remedy proving by Jeremy Sherr. He has also studied: Hydrogen, Triticum, Germanium, Diamond, and many others:(http://www.dynamis.edu/provings/). All of his provings are worthy of careful study.

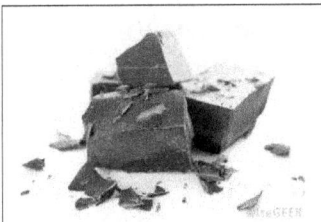

Critical, mean.

Feels forsaken.

Very short hair. Drill sargent at home.

Chocolate is most similar to Sepia in many respects. *They are both often intolerant, unfeeling, angry and display no affection or sympathy for their children or spouse.*

He or she will angrily correct members of family. *Harsh and hateful toward others* like we see in Nux vomica, Kali iod and Borage. Act like a drill sargent toward others.

Want everything perfect and in order.

Yell and scream at others. Feels alone and forsaken (most likely their family left them as they could no longer take the abuse).

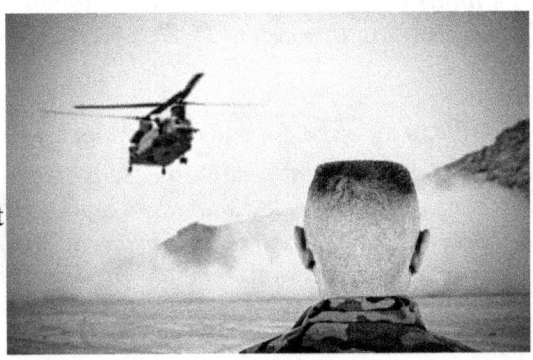

Demand too much from themselves, *work too hard and have a nervous breakdown.* They treat themselves as they treat others i.e. too harshly, too much discipline, not enough play or rest.

Desire to cut their hair very short. Fear to leave home as they fear having an accident. Children who say: *"I hate my parents"* when in fact they have very nice parents.

CINA MARITIMA
(Worm-seed)

This remedy is most similar to Chamomilla; the child is angry but worse from touch, wants to be carried then and wants to be put down again – *capricious* (Cham).

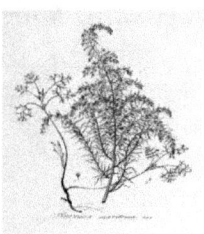

Grinding of teeth during sleep. Eyes sensitive to light.

Cina is pre-eminently a child's remedy, but it is suitable for conditions in adults that are seldom thought of. A marked feature running through is TOUCHINESS, mental and physical.

The child wants something, but does not know what. The child is aggravated by touch and even by being looked at, and is worse from seeing strangers. The skin is sensitive to touch. The scalp and back of the neck, the shoulders and arms are so sensitive, that it is almost a soreness as if bruised. The hyperaesthesia is both mental and physical. The old routine of giving Cina for worms need not go into your notes, for if you are guided by symptoms the patient will be cured and the worms will go.

This patient is disturbed by everything, worse after eating even a moderate meal. The child takes a moderate supper and dreams all night, jerks and twitches in sleep, rouses up in a fright, talks excitedly about what he has dreamed, thinks it is real, and sees dogs, phantoms, and frightful things he has dreamed about. The dream is prolonged into the wakeful hours. Screams and trembles, with much anxiety on waking; whines and complains. While this little patient is aggravated by being handled yet he wants to be carried and kept busy, like CHAMOMILLA; although not so intensely irritable as that remedy, yet he must be carried. At first on taking him out of the crib he screams when taken hold of; the first touch aggravates.

This aggravation from touch and sensitiveness runs through the convulsions and fevers, with delirium, glassy eyes, drawn mouth and white ring around the nose and mouth. With a disordered stomach he has convulsions after eating, with the head drawn back and glassy eyes. The stomach is sour and the child is always spitting up sour milk and belching sour wind. The child smells sour. The mother says that "Baby has a worm breath," but the same odor is present when there are no worms. In the convulsions there are loss of consciousness and frothing at the mouth.

Hallucinations of smell, sight and taste, in the delirious state, after taking cold, or on waking from sleep; wakes up with the delusion. Things taste and smell differently. The senses of taste and touch are exaggerated or perverted.

In some cases of internal hydrocephalus, not with enlarged skull, but with increase of the fluid in the ventricles and central canal of the spinal cord, the patients take on Cina symptoms. Rolling of the head; frequent headaches; sensitiveness to jar; cannot be touched or tapped along the spinal cord without headache; always worse in the sun; the head is hot and the feet are cold in the sun. Cina will cure some of these cases. They cannot stand any kind of disturbance; it produce; a convulsion. They cannot

Materia Medica

be punished because they go into convulsions. If the ITER A TERTIO AD GUARTURN VENTRICULUM is closed they will be incurable, the internal pressure will go on and they will die from it. Such congenital states are incurable.

Dull headache with sensitiveness of the eyes. Headache before and after epileptic attacks and after intermittents. Before and during the headache sensitiveness of the skull. Cina children cannot have the hair combed, and the Cina woman must have her hair down in head and nerve complaints.

There is coldness of the extremities and also some itching of the skin, but the head symptoms are predominant. From slight disturbances of the mind he cannot digest, and he has diarrhea. The complaints are aggravated in summer; the heat affects the brain, arrests his functions, and on comes diarrhea with green, slimy stools or white stools, and the child vomits.

It is pre-eminently BRAIN in Cina; the orders are not received from the brain and so stomach symptoms develop, and worms hatch out. If he is cured the healthy gastric juice will chase the worms out.

The child turns his head from side to side, The pains are sometimes better from turning the head from side to side. You will see this in sensitive women, who must have their hair down; ROLLING the head relieves, not SHAKING as in the text, that is too violent.

All sorts of colors before the eyes. Objects look yellow. It is useful in sensitive women, sensitive nervous women, who are always worse from using the eyes, and get pain in the head and eyes from sewing. It is like RUTA in that respect, symptoms of eye-strain. It is not so much indicated in young people but more when presbyopia is beginning in middle-aged women, and there is the effort to strain the eyes on fine work or print. Rubs the eyes and can then see more clearly. On rising from the bed blackness before the eyes; different colors, especially yellow. Strabismus when worms are present, depending really on brain trouble because the worms are dependent upon that.

Study Guide

Face sunken, pallid, wings of nose drawn in. Blue ring or gray streak around the mouth. "A sure sign of worms," the mother says. Child rubs its nose with the hands or on the pillow or on the nurse's shoulder. Child bores into the nose until the blood comes. The sickly aspect is striking, but it is representative of brain trouble, central trouble. The brain symptoms are the highest and most important. If frightened, whipped, or scolded, the brain is disturbed and the stomach disordered. They get indigestion and breed worms; white or blue appearance about the mouth, grinding of the teeth during sleep. Before the child has teeth it has a chewing motion, a side to side movement. Sensitiveness of the teeth to the cold air and cold water.

Bleeding from the mouth and nose. Inability to swallow liquids; they gurgle down the oesophagus — before and after convulsions. When the head symptoms are present, the milk or water gurgles down the esophagus with a gurgling cluck. This is present in diarrhea and vomiting with brain symptoms.

ARSENICUM and CUPRUM are also prominent in gurgling down the esophagus when swallowing. Choreic movements extend to the tongue.

The child or adult is not relieved by eating, is still hungry. The stomach is loaded and yet he is hungry. After vomiting you would expect there would be an aversion to food, but there is in Cina the same empty, hungry feeling. When there is gnawing in the stomach after eating, or when the child has taken all it can hold yet cries for the bottle, or empties its stomach by spitting up and vomiting the food and then reaches out whining and crying for more, think of Cina. Shuddering when drinking wine as if it were vinegar.

Abdomen hard and bloated. Very often the Cina child will flop over on its belly and get to sleep in that way. If it is turned on the side it wakes up again. While in the mother's arms it will go to sleep with the abdomen resting on the mother's shoulder, but when she puts it on the side in bed it wakens. If you had a child with copious, gushing, violently foetid stool, ameliorated by lying on the abdomen, and it would have another stool if lying any other way, PODOPH. would be the remedy. That would not be Cina. The Cina stool is not very copious, and often white.

Gagging cough in the morning. Short, hacking cough at night. Spasmodic cough. Whooping cough.

Oversensitiveness to touch; trembling, spasms, chorea. Spasmodic yawning. Child cannot sleep unless on the belly or in constant motion. (Kent's – Materia Medica)

Case 1: Five year old. He has epilepsy, multiple seizures a day. He can't walk because his muscles won't develop. Very angry if his father leaves him to go to work. He can't talk either. He sleeps sitting up - (keynote for Cina); if his parents try to lie him down he wakes up! At Children's hospital near Seattle he was found to have a rare genetic disorder. After Cina 30c for a few weeks he is all better; no more seizures, walking and learned to speak. Two years later on follow up he is still better.

Compare this remedy to Artemisia vulgaris; they are both in the same botanical family, both treat seizures and have some of the same chemical constituents:

Essential Oil from **Cina**: Artemisia maritima L. Constituents: α-Pinene, Camphene, β-Pinene, 2,3- Dehydro-1,8-cineole, α-Terpinene, 1,8-Cineole, Santolina alcohol, γ-Terpinene, β-Thujone, Chrysanthenone, Some p-mentha-dien-ol, L-(-)-Camphor, L-Borneol, Terpinen-4-ol, α-Terpineol, Z-Chrysanthenyl acetate, Bornyl acetate, α-Terpinyl acetate, Z-Chrysanthenyl propionate, E-geranyl acetate, β-Caryophyllene, Aromadendrene, Elixene, Cis-Davanone, Artemone.

Artemesia Vulgaris Constituents trans-Thujone was determined as the first major constituent in one oil (20.2%) and cis-thujone as the second dominant compound in one oil (12.9%).

Chrysanthenyl acetate prevailed in one oil (23.6%). 1,8-Cineole was the predominant constituent in two oils (16.7 and 17.6%). Among the other major compounds were sabinene, β- pinene, artemisia ketone, caryophyllene. Eighty one identified components formed up 81.9–96.8% of the total oil content. Oxygenated monoterpenes made up 17.1–48.7%, while sesquiterpenes 17.1– 44.1% of the oils. (Chemical composition of essential oils of Artemisia vulgaris L. (mugwort) from North Lithuania)

CINCHONA
(Peruvian Bark – China)

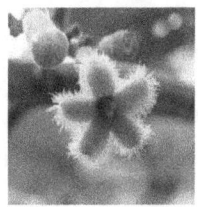

The first proving made by Hahnemann was Cinchona. In his own words: *I made the first pure trial with cinchona bark upon myself, in reference to its power of exciting intermittent fever.*

With this first trial broke upon me the dawn that has since brightened into the most brilliant day of the medical art; that it is only in virtue of their power to make the healthy human being ill that medicines can cure morbid states, and indeed, only such morbid states are composed of symptoms which the drug to be selected for them can itself produce in similarity on the healthy. This is a truth so incontrovertible, so absolutely without exception, ...

Here is the beginning of this proving done by Hahnemann from his <u>Materia Medica Pura</u> – (Six Volumes and 61 medicines). It is worth reading it in its entirety. Here is a small sample of this proving:

First vertigo and giddy nausea, then general feeling of heat. (Comp. With 1, 3, 4, 5.).

Vertigo in the occiput, when sitting. [Fz.].

Vertigo; the head tends to sink backwards, worse when moving and walking, diminished by lying down (aft. a few m.). [Hrr.]. 5.

Constant vertigo, the head tends to sink backwards, in every position, but worse when walking and moving the head (aft. 6 h.). [Hrr.]. Stupidity.

He is long in collecting his thoughts, is much disinclined for movement, and more disposed to sit and to lie.

Confusion of the head. [C. E. Fischer, (Effects of china in agues.) in Hufel Journal, iv, pp. 652, 653. 657.]

Confusion of the head, like vertigo from dancing and as in catarrh. (Comp. with 11 and 49.). 10.

Confusion and emptiness in the head and laziness of the body as from watching at night and sleeplessness. (10, 15, 21, comp. with 6, 8, 11, 12, 13, 14, 16 and 23.) (aft. 1 h.).

Confusion of the head, like a catarrh. § (aft. 9 d.). [Ws.]. Confusion of the head in the forehead. [Hbg.].

Confusion of the head, as after a debauch, with aching in the temples. [Hbg.].

A cloudiness spread all over the head, for half an hour. (aft. ¾ h.). [Htg.]. 15. Stupefaction of the head, with aching in the forehead (aft. ¼ h.).

A dull feeling in the lower part of the head behind, as from awaking from sleep. [Bch.]. Heaviness of the head (at noon vertigo rises up into the head, without pain). (17, 20, comp. with 6, 8, 11, 12, 13, `4, 16 and 23.).

Study Guide

Heaviness of the head (18, 19, 22, see 17, 20) [J. E. STAHL. (As) in various works, particularly in his Diss. Problem. De febribus.]

In summary some of the most important symptoms we can learn from this proving: *Great sensitivity to light touch better from hard pressure.* Socially it is the same, they don't like superficial interaction; they prefer serous conversation and deep meaningful experiences. They feel their life has no significance or meaning so *they fantasize about heroic deeds, about being something special* (Coca).

He makes many plans, and thinks over their accomplishment; many ideas force themselves upon him at once. [Hrr.]

He has many ideas, undertakes to carry out all sorts of things, builds castles in the air (aft. some h.). [Wth.] (Hahnemann- MM Pura).

These thoughts can be so intense that they prevent sleep. They may get involved with many projects in order to take away this feeling of being mundane and bored with life. *If they can't accomplish things then they will complain that others are on purpose obstructing them which brings great offense.*

Discontented; he thinks himself unfortunate, and fancies he is opposed and tormented by everybody *(aft. 5 h.).* (Hahnemann).

They can feel so bitter and angry about life it can make their mouth feel dry and bitter. Touchy and irritable, discontented.

Contempt for everything. (Comp. with 1121.) (aft. 1 h.).
(Hahnemann)

Liver and gall stone problems. *Bloating, distension.* Worse from tea, milk, fish and fruit. Boericke, Kent, Farrington and Nash can add to your knowledge of this remedy.

Materia Medica

Case 1: 25 year old female. Aversion to get married as she is severely irritated when her fiancée holds her hand or touches and caress her arm.

In the proving we find the same information: Worse by light touch:

Excessive, almost painful sensitiveness of the skin of the whole body, even of the palms of the hands. (Comp. with 540, 754.). (aft. 10 h.). (Hahnemann).

It makes her so irritable that she can't be around him.

Extremely disposed to be vexed, and to take every occasion to get cross; afterwards quarrelsome and disposed to vex others, and to make reproaches and give annoyance to others (aft. 2 h.). (Hahnemann)

She has digestive issues with bloating. Her grandfather had chronic malaria. After Cinchona 30c once a week her irritability, and skin sensitivity are all better and she gets married.

COCA
(Leaves from Erythroxylaceae Coca)

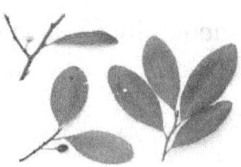

The mind is over stimulated like we see in Coffea, Ginseng and Kola. With all of these remedies we see people who love to work long hours. Ginseng does not care what work they do as long as it can last ten or more hours a day. Kola loves to work as well but likes to do two things at once. Coffea loves work but thinking about work keeps them awake at night and they develop heart problems.

With Coca they have to do something special; almost superhuman that no one else can accomplish. We see this trait in people who train for the Olympics. If the person is balanced it will not be a symptom. If they depend on this trait for their happiness then it becomes a symptom.

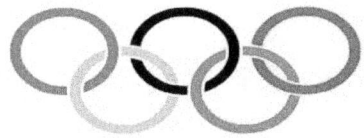

Case 1: 40 year old. Arthritis, he was the main person in charge of building a sky-scraper. He was confident and had over worked for many years. After Coca his arthritis was all better.

Case 2: In another patient he was 85 years old but wanted to hike a mountain every day! His main complaint was bladder infections *which only happened when he ascended to a high altitude.* In the repertory we find this symptom: General, *ascending aggravates* and there we find Coca in red letters. So these people are like Argentum nitricum; *they like to get on stage or accomplish some great thing* but then when they reach this height they can panic and loose all confidence or suffer in some physical way such as altitude sickness.

Coca can have a lack of confidence but (if for example they come from a good family) can easily compensate so that the person feels they can accomplish superhuman feats of strength. For example she is training to be an Olympic down-hill skier. He wants to find a cure for cancer and stays up all night, not eating or taking care of himself. *These people can taste the excitement of success, they are driven and they can become addicted to the adrenalin.*

If the nervous system breaks down they can become paranoid and or experience some of the following symptoms: *Melancholy from nervous exhaustion. Hypochondriasis. Amenorrhea. Dysmenorrhoea.*

Bashful, timid, ill at ease in society. Sadness, irritability; he delights only in solitude and obscurity; frequently he gives proof of obstinacy. Remarkable aversion to exertion of any kind in consequence of nervous exhaustion.
Loss of energy.

Slow in finding the words to express himself at times. Mental depression with beginning of atrophy. Overpowered by an indescribable anxiety. Feeling of anguish increased with failure of every effort to strive against the weariness; torment only diminishes with perfect rest. Stupidity. Brain feels so muddled that he cannot read understandingly. Gentle excitement, followed by wakefulness. Peevish temper. Want of will power; shakiness and mental depression. (CONSTANTINE HERING, M. D.)

Case 3: Chronic bronchitis. Cough is better from lying down (Cough, lying, amel: Coca). Depression if he does not work (Coca). Feels he has to do something special all the time (Coca) Mind: delusion, great person, he is: Coca). After Coca the cough is better in a few days. All strength returns.

Case 4: Female in 70's. She is feeling weak and out of breath all the time. Depression since she can't go door to door teaching the Bible. *She wants her strength back so that she can do Gods work.* After Coca 30c she feels much stronger, her lungs and heart are stronger and she goes back to work.

The remedy **Cocaine** is similar to Coca but is refined into the

Study Guide

pure drug. These people are *often paranoid and have many suspicious theories.*

Case 1: A women comes to see me for the sensation of worms under her skin. She tried to dig them out and brings me some worm tissue to show me. After Coca 30c she is much better and no longer mentions the worms but now is full of grief over her brother who died a number of years previous. This is a big step of progress, she is now strong enough to feel the grief. This gives us a hint about Coca. *When a person can't process a shock they can go into a fantasy world; with suspicious delusions.*

Case 2: A women in her 80"s calls me because aliens are breaking into her apartment and stealing things. They are also tipping her apartment building over and she is afraid it is about to fall. She is also afraid to drink milk. She is quite sweet in her demeanor and tells me all of this with great sincerity; staring at me me with great conviction as if to say: "what are you going to do about it?". After Coca 30c she is much better and looks back on her ideas with some embarrassment, reminding me not to repeat them to anyone. *As a child while on a school field trip she was raped at a dairy farm and then forced her to drink milk.* This trauma made her feel that drinking milk could get her pregnant. *Again we see a big shock followed by paranoid ideas.*

COCCULUS INDICUS
(INDIAN COCKLE)

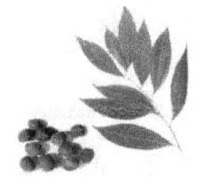

In a first aid situation we can use this remedy for a hit on the head or a **concussion**. (Arn, Hell, Nat-s) In these cases the person will feel *light headed, vertigo and nausea*. Often they will feel weakness in the neck and that their head is heavy.

This is a common remedy. We can use it for nausea from riding in a car or sea-sickness when the nausea is *worse from the smell of food or even thought of food*.

These people are very *sympathetic* toward others. They worry about their family easily and will want to stay up all night and take care of them. In the morning they feel they can't think, feel dizzy and nausea because they did not get enough sleep. Again this nausea is worse from the smell of food cooking.

As teenagers they fall in love easily and if they have a grief they again can't sleep and the same symptoms result. If they get a flu, mononucleosis or some other illness it can develop toward paralysis such as multiple sclerosis.

This remedy is for mild, gentle and kind people. I have never seen a person who needs this remedy that is in any way aggressive.

In all of the situations above the patient can't tolerate loss of sleep. It makes them sick right away to loose sleep, they have to have 8 or 9 hours of sleep a night. Nausea and vertigo from the loss of sleep.

Weakness during menses she can't stand up. When there is paralysis there is numbness of the hands and feet. Worse from alcohol it makes them feel more confusion.

This is an excellent remedy for so many ailments that affect the mind, stomach, nervous system and muscles. They are mild, sincere people who worry and care too much for others; so much

Study Guide

so it makes them sick.

After a grief they suffer terribly with worry, sadness resulting in a breakdown of the nervous system. Confusion, loss of memory and physical weakness are the result.

COCCUS CACTI
(cochineal Scale Insect)

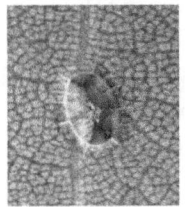

Cough better from cold drinks and worse from warm drinks. Better also from cold air. Cough with thick stringy mucous.

Cough with retching and vomiting like Ipecac. Tickle in larynx. Sensation of a crumb behind the larynx. Kidney pathology with edema like Apis. Kidney stones, red brick dust urine.

Cuprum and Causticum also have a cough that is also better from cold drinks.

COFFEA CRUDA
(Coffee Bean)

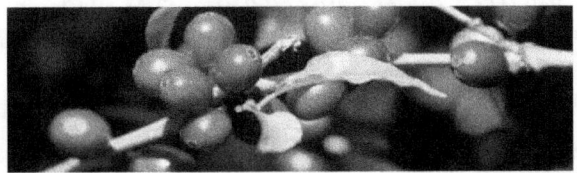

Materia Medica

Sleepless from good news or from being too excited. Sleepless; he can't stop thinking about all the wonderful things he is going to do the next day. People who work too hard, they give their time away, *generous to a fault* and eventually their heart gives out. Skipped beats, irregular heart action.

Nash has this to say about Coffea: *All senses more acute; reads fine print easier; smell, taste and touch acute; unusual activity of mind and body; full of ideas, quick to act, no sleep on this account, etc.*

Affections from sudden surprises, especially joyful surprises; very emotional.

Pains insupportable, drive to despair; exasperation, tears, tossing about in agony; great sleeplessness.

Headache, from over-mental exertion, thinking, talking ; one-sided, as from a nail driven into the brain (IGN., NUX); as if the brain were torn or dashed to pieces; < in open air.

Jerking toothache; relieved by holding ice water in the mouth; returns when water becomes warm.

COFFEA CRUDA, like CHAMOMILLA, *acts strongly upon the nervous system. Indeed in nervous troubles, where the patient has not been addicted to the coffee habit, it often takes precedence. If on the other hand he is a coffee drinker,* CHAMOMILLA *is the remedy. .... The* COFFEA *patient is a subject of very great general exalted sensibility. See Hering's characteristic cards.* "ALL THE SENSES MORE ACUTE, READS FINE PRINT EASIER, SMELL, TASTE, AND TOUCH ACUTE, PARTICULARLY ALSO IN INCREASED PERCEPTION OF SLIGHT PASSIVE MOTIONS." "UNUSUAL ACTIVITY OF MIND AND BODY." "FULL OF IDEAS, QUICK TO ACT, NO SLEEP ON THIS ACCOUNT." "LIVELY FANCIES, FULL OF PLANS FOR THE FUTURE."

These symptoms portray, as plainly as words can, the nervous conditions calling for this remedy.

It makes one think of CHAMOMILLA, but the mind of CHAMOMILLA IS NOT THERE. On the other hand, it makes one think of ACONITE, but the fear of death is not there.

Hering used to recommend ACONITE and COFFEA in alternation in painful inflammatory affections, where the fever symptoms of the former and also the nervous sensibility of the latter were present, and I know of no two remedies that alternate better, though I never do it, since I learned to closely individualize.

COFFEA is especially adapted to mental shocks, such as SUDDEN SURPRISES, ESPECIALLY JOYFUL SURPRISES, EXCESSIVE LAUGHTER AND PLAYING, DISAPPOINTED LOVE, NOISES, STRONG SMELLS, etc. It is also adapted to VARIABLE moods; FIRST CRYING THEN LAUGHING, THEN CRYING AGAIN.

COFFEA also vies with CHAMOMILLA and ACONITE as a PAIN remedy. "PAINS INSUPPORTABLE, DRIVE TO DESPAIR." "EXASPERATION, TEARS, TOSSING ABOUT IN GREAT ANGUISH." Here again we would not give COFFEA in an habitual coffee drinker, but CHAMOMILLA rather.

The particular localities where these pains mostly occur are in the head, where the pain is generally one-sided, feeling "AS THOUGH A NAIL WERE DRIVEN INTO THE HEAD." IGNATIA has a similar headache, and it generally occurs in hysterical subjects. Then the choice may have to be made between these two remedies.

Prosopalgia, which is often traceable to bad teeth, and COFFEA has a very peculiar toothache, in the fact that the tooth is easy as long as he HOLDS COLD WATER UPON IT. Remember CHAMOMILLA toothache is often caused by taking WARM things into the mouth, but is not relieved by taking cold things like COFFEA.

Dysmenorrhoea, with excessively painful colic. If there are large BLACK CLOTS and COFFEA does not relieve, follow with CHAMOMILLA.

Pains threatening abortion, or after-pains, or very severe unbearable labor pains are often relieved by this remedy. In short, for pains anywhere, which seem intolerable, and there are no other especially leading symptoms, COFFEA is to be remembered.

The same over-excitability, so characteristic of this drug, causes great SLEEPLESSNESS, and COFFEA has won to itself great credit as a SLEEP remedy. In my experience and observation, it works best here in the 200th potency. And there is no more beautiful verification of the truth of SIMILIA than just here, for it CAUSES GREAT SLEEPLESSNESS in many people when taken in large quantities.

Cough and sleeplessness after measles (a very common occurrence) is wonderfully relieved by it, and it is sleep, not narcosis, and never injures or sickens the patient like the STUPOR of the opium preparations. (Nash)

Case 1: 45 year old with heart problems. He says he can't make everyone happy as he has to go to work two jobs and have a family. He can't sleep, he is totally exhausted. After Coffea 30c he is more balanced and his heart feels well again.

COLOCYNTHIS
(Bitter Cucumber)

Indignation with stomach cramps that make the patient bend double.

Suppressed anger, anger that is held up inside. Subluxation and dislocation of joints.

Study Guide

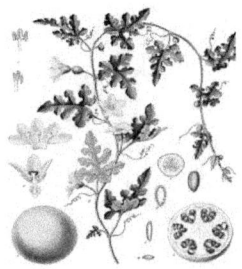

Case 1: After she gave birth her ribs dislocated due to too high prolactin. The pain was unbearable and went on for years till she came to see me and was given Colocynth. She was brought up in foster homes and treated unfairly. I have no doubt she was not treated right and it left her with emotional and physical pain (anger and indignation) that was unbearable.

Nash says of this remedy: *Disinclined to talk, to see friends, impatient, easily offended, anger with indignation; colic or other complaints as a consequence.*

Colic, terrible; they seek relief by BENDING DOUBLE or pressing something hard against the abdomen.

Dysentery-like diarrhea; renewed after least food or drink, often with the characteristic colic pains.

Frequent urging to urinate, scanty; urine sometimes thick, foetid, viscid, jelly-like.

Crampy pain in sciatic nerve, from hip down posterior portion of thigh; > from hard pressure and from heat; < in repose, driving patient desperate. Tendency to painful cramps, with all pains.

Modalities: < evening, anger; after eating; > from coffee; BENDING DOUBLE and HARD PRESSURE. No remedy produces more severe colic than this one, and no remedy cures more promptly. (Nash)

CONIUM MACULATUM
(Poison Hemlock)

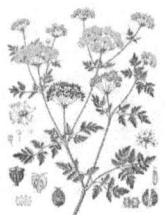

Hardening of tissues, vertigo turning from turning over in bed, swelling of the prostate with feeble stream.

This remedy is similar to Hyoscyamus. They become *overly sexually dependent* on their partner. But in Hyoscyamus there is jealousy and anger when their partner leaves in contrast to Conium where there is resignation and the development of severe physical ailments such as senility, cancer and paralysis.

Without sex the Conium patient can easily become susceptible to such ailments as prostate swelling, breast tumors and mental confusion. The *vertigo typically comes on when they turn over in bed or move the head too quickly*.

In women they have swelling and a lot of pain in the breasts before menses (Calc-carb).

Socrates took this poison. It can produce an ascending paralysis, weakness and trembling.

No interest in anything, rigid ideas and mental confusion.

Perspire on falling asleep. Indurated glands. Soft tissue get hard and hard tissues get harder. May be difficult to interview them as they are not proud of how selfish they are and the extent of their material needs. They don't really want to open up and tell the whole story.

Case 1: An elderly man came to see me. He had just married to a much younger women. He had a lot of hip pain with no modalities. I suspected cancer and after some test it was found he had bone cancer. For the pain I gave him Symphytum which allowed him to stop the Morphine. Then his prostate became swollen and so he could not urinate. After Conium 30c the prostate returned to a normal state and this remedy kept him going for many months. He was able to leave the hospital and go home again. He stayed on Conium but with other complications that I could not solve he eventually died of cancer.

Here is an example of the materia medica by George Vithoulkas from his <u>Materia Medica Viva:</u> (12 Volumes so far). I highly recommend this series. I went to many of his seminars back in the 80's and 90's. He would show us video after video of cured cases. It was a wonderful way to learn case taking and materia medica. Many of these videos are still available through his courses. (www.Vithoulkas.com)

In his own words George says of this remedy: *The idea of paralysis - the one we know from Socrates' death by the 'noggin of hemlock' real paralysis <in the average patient who needs Conium> comes only as an end result, and this may take a very long time, twenty years, thirty years, or more. Conium suffers with a gradually progressing weakness and paresis, and gradual is the key word here.*

The idea is much more that of sclerosis, of becoming hard, especially the glands, which become swollen and indurated. A gradually progressing weakness with the formation of indurations during the decline, is the picture of Conium pathology.

Mental Paralysis and Induration. This process develops on all three levels. On the mental level, we observe a gradual decline of the intellectual capacities.

The patient becomes more and more dull; he has more and more difficulty in comprehension.

Thinking is slowed down, memory becomes weak, and the patient becomes forgetful. His five senses lose their acuity, and his reserves slowly ebb away. A frequent and characteristic symptom is an inability to sustain mental effort over any length of time.

All these symptoms can also be found in other remedies; but the characteristic here is the snail's pace of the progress. It happens so gradually that the patient is not aware of the process himself. After some years he may go back in his memory and say, 'What is happening to me?' But it takes him years to see the declining process. Nor is this decline observed by the people around him, especially those who are in contact with him every day. The process develops too slowly and undramatically.

Even when he finally feels that something serious and deeply disturbing is going on, he will often say nothing to anybody, because no one else seems to have noticed anything. Finally a kind of stupefaction takes over, and now he feels that this state is definitely leading him into a serious condition of degeneration, of imbecility and premature senility.

Conium produces as it were areas of sclerosis, of callus in the brain. It seems to be a remedy that is very set in its thinking, to the extent that it becomes superstitious. Conium is the main remedy in superstition or 'superstitious thoughts'. It is like an induration in a certain area of the brain.

The patients tend to have compulsive thoughts and to execute compulsive actions, but only in a separate arena of their mental lives. The remainder of the brain is working beautifully, and they are otherwise normal people, performing their tasks, holding their jobs, and fulfilling all their social functions, but in this separate mental arena they have some fixed ideas which they cannot get rid of.

Those superstitious obsessions may be more or less harmless in themselves. They might think, 'If I don't touch the corner when I go around it, something bad is going to happen to me'. Or, 'I mustn't step on the cracks between the slabs of the pavement, and if I do, I will suffer some misfortune'. These ideas may make life intolerable for the people around them.

I remember a case in which the wife related that her husband would not take off his trousers to go to bed until everything was absolutely quiet outside. If he could hear a car, he was unable to take off his trousers. So he waited until he couldn't hear the car any more, and then he started pulling off his trousers.

But soon the noise of another car came, and he couldn't continue taking off his trousers: he had to wait for absolute quiet. This man was a manager in a bank, he had a responsible position, and he was normal in every other way, but he could not be talked out of this obsession.

Of course, there was more to it that. He admitted that his memory had begun to fail, and that his concentration was not the same as it had been. He could not read as much as he used to, because he was slower to comprehend. All of these functions came back after the remedy, Conium 10M in a single dose, and the compulsive action has disappeared.

Conium's fixed ideas often (but not always) center around needing absolute quiet, as in the case above, and problems with strangers. This is especially true regarding toilets. They often cannot urinate or pass stool if there are people near the bathroom. And they can get terrible constipation because of that, especially when they are traveling, because there are nearly always people around. It is beautiful to see how such behavior is taken away by the correct remedy.

Emotional Paralysis and Induration. On the emotional level, we again witness this gradual paralysis with induration. The emotions are gradually weakened and paralyzed until it is impossible to bring them to the surface, to 'move' them. The final state is a condition of complete indifference and apathy, when they find no interest in anything. And when they have gone so far, they are no more able to show emotion when it is needed or appropriate to the surroundings.

If they get a present, they cannot be happy, and they are also unable to cry when they would like to; their feelings may still be there but they are petrified and indurated, they cannot be moved. Then they become gloomy and unhappy; they do not want company and they feel unable to communicate with anybody.

But this indifference doesn't develop quickly, and again it takes a long time until the pathology has gone this far. Before that state of indifference, there is a stage where patients are worried because they feel that something is happening with their mental condition. They are worried about their health, they wonder what is happening in their mind, how all this will end. They become anxious, and in this state they do not want to be alone. In Conium the aversion to company is not a very strong feature.

How can we speak of induration presented on the emotional level? It manifests as a kind of insensitivity. Conium people are not sweet persons, they are hard, 'down to earth', materialistic and practical people. As the doctor you will see that they are demanding. They will be loyal to you as long as they feel you can help them and as you are not hurting them. But if there is a stage where, in their opinion, you are not helping them enough, they will immediately let you know, demanding their 'rights'.

Conium people are materialists in a different fashion to Platina. They don't have the extreme egotism and haughtiness of Platina, they don't think that they are 'big'. Rather, Conium's attachment is to the material world around him, his property, his habits, his family.

Conium says: 'This is mine. This table is mine. This is my house'. Once any of this is taken away from him, there is a definite morbid, pathological reaction, and this is often accompanied by an induration on the physical level, a tumor which is usually malignant.

These symptoms after a 'material loss' can occur very suddenly, even immediately, at quite another speed compared to the slow and gradual paralysis of the remedy. If, for instance, the patient's house burns down and many valuable things are lost, he can develop symptoms very quickly, especially hard tumors, even cancer, and in such a case Conium will often be indicated.

Suppression of Sexuality. The biggest material loss for Conium is the deprivation of regular sexual activity. The moment they lose regular sex with their partner, problems start. The body may function well as long as there is a regular release on the sexual level, a release of the hormones at regular intervals with a specific partner.

This is what they need to feel in balance, otherwise the balance is lost. Therefore you will often see Conium indicated in women who have lost or separated from their partner and do not have a new love affair.

Female Conium patients depend on the regular sexual activity they are used to, and if the husband dies, the woman does not easily start a new affair. Because of this failure to release the hormones, problems will arise, which can go from vertigo, which is usually the first to appear, to trembling and weakness.

It can go as far as developing severe problems, even cancer, and especially cancer of the breast or of the uterus. Cancer of cervix uteri is also often seen. The idea is that a hard tumor develops, mostly of the glands, but it can be anywhere.

Conium is the main remedy for the gland that is affected greatly by sexual activity in man: the prostate. If a suppression of sexual urge in a Conium man is present, the first gland that is affected is the prostate, it can swell and even cause prostate cancer. Moreover, Conium is an important remedy in indurated and malignant swelling of the testes.

Also we may see hypochondria in unmarried men with very strict principles of sexual morality: 'Hypochondriacal complaints, especially in unmarried people who are strictly abstinent in sexual matters'.

Here the comparison with Platina is again very interesting. Conium people have a strong sexual urge, as do Platina, but the difference is that Conium are not oversexed, they are more on the practical side. They don't think of sex day and night, like Platina, rather they look upon sex as something they just need from time to time to release their hormones; they are people without illusions, matter of fact in their approach to sex.

You have to understand the mentality: they feel that the good things which we can enjoy in life are given to us, it is our right to enjoy them. They do not tend to have bad feelings, feelings of guilt or doubt, neither do they tend to hypersexual behaviour.

We can say, they know exactly what they want: sex and the release of orgasm is what they need to keep their organism functioning, that is the idea, and they take it as a fact or, as it were, their right.

But if this outlet stops suddenly, once this 'right' is taken away from them, then there is a kind of dizziness, which they constantly complain about, they say that their head is never clear. They start trembling, shaking all over and a feeling of paralytic weakness eventually takes them over. The dizziness can become really severe, and Meniere's Syndrome may develop. Things seem to be turning around them.

The worst situation is when they lie in bed and want to turn to the other side; this movement aggravates them terribly. (This should be differentiated from the similar symptom in Silicea, where the vertigo in bed only arises from turning to the left.)

On sudden motion, for example on turning the head to look behind them, everything seems to turn around them. They complain about the head problem, it is nearly indescribable for them: they do not say vertigo, instead they use words like a buzzing inside the head, a noise, a dizziness, or similar terms.

In a recent case from Argentina (quoted in Klassische Homoopathie 5/93), a 57-year-old man got 'vertigo, worse when turning around in bed, with a feeling as though the brain had gone to sleep'. This came on after his wife had (in his words), 'condemned him to celibacy'.

In other cases, patients start to tremble and feel as if paralyzed all over; even mentally paralyzed, unable to perform any duties, with problems in concentrating; unable to stand mental effort for any length of time.

Conium are also fixed on their sexual patterns, not at all flexible. They are not oversexed, and they do not tend to promiscuity or extramarital relationships. On the contrary, when they make a decision to keep with one partner, they will stay together until the partner dies.

Typical symptoms will be: complaints of swollen glands, the head is not clear and there are headaches, even very severe headaches, or headaches together with vertigo. The patient starts trembling and feels weak. With this picture you might prescribe Gelsemium, Cocculus or Carbo vegetabilis. But once you have the information about the loss of a partner and the abrupt end to sexual activity, then there is only one remedy that will help and this is Conium.

Of course, such a history also happens to other people who do not need a remedy, but where other organisms can manage this interruption and can balance themselves, it will be Conium who, almost invariably, will develop pathological symptoms.

Further Mental Symptoms. Some proving symptoms to show how the Conium pathology affects the intellect: 'Dullness; difficulty in understanding what he is reading, with confusion of the head'.

'Dullness, like stupefaction; difficulty in understanding what he

is reading'. 'Want of memory'. 'Forgetfulness and weakness in head'.

'Unable to correctly express oneself by talking, with difficulty of recollecting things'. 'Inability to sustain any mental effort'.

There are often states of difficulty in concentration and absence of mind, even insensibility and confusion, especially after awaking from a midday nap.

There are many emotional symptoms where anxiety, gloomy thoughts, fears and peevishness dominate. They correspond to the state where the patient begins to feel his decline (see above), but they can also appear in other situations.

For instance: 'Deeply absorbed in thought, he meditates anxiously about present and future, searching for solitude'. 'Hysterical anxiety'. 'Ill humour and gloom'. 'Constant ill humour and peevishness'. 'Peevish mood; does not know what to do; time passes too slowly'.

From a proving by Robinson: 'She feels peevish, vexed, and easily put out about trifles'. Where these symptoms dominate there may be a rather contradictory attitude toward human company, as is manifested in this proving symptom: 'Shuns people and their approach, and at the same time dread to be alone'.

In the context of the menses, there are also states of sensitivity, tearfulness and restlessness. 'Before the menses, aching in all limbs, with tearful mood, restlessness and anxious worry about trifles'. Or: 'She is easily moved by trifles, moved to tears'.

In the Chronic Diseases, we even find a veritable weeping fit which later transforms into vertigo and weakness: 'Paroxysm: alone at home, she feels an inclination to weep; after yielding to it, the weeping changes to a loud sobbing; afterwards flickering before the eyes and indistinct vision, so that she had to hold on to something when walking; afterwards weariness in all limbs and a dull headache'.

A number of mental symptoms corresponds with the stage of indifference, apathy, emotional paralysis and petrefaction: 'Very ill-humoured, every afternoon, from 3 pm to 6 pm, as though a great guilt weighed upon him, with paralyzed feeling in all the limbs, indifference, and taking no interest in anything'. 'Morose mood; everything about him makes an unpleasant impression upon him'. 'Disinclination for work'. 'No pleasant feelings whatsoever'.

Conium has successfully been used in depressive states, and it is easy to see that the depressive element prevails in the remedy. There is on record a cured case of a woman who fell into a 'very unhappy mood' every 14 days. She had no desire to dress, to eat anything, to talk or to see her children.

The periodic recurrence of this unhappy state may be a hint that Conium could also be indicated in cyclic manic-depressive states. And though the depressive symptoms preponderate, we still see proving symptoms like this: 'He is averse to being near people, and to the talk of those passing him; is inclined to seize hold of and abuse them'.

A cured case, fragments of which are very often quoted in literature, shows that Conium can be useful when there is an alternation of marked manic and depressive stages:

'A 16-year-old boy... became mentally ill... It was peculiar that he was alternately in a depressed mood for 10 days and then again in an excited mood for 10 days. He is silent for 10 days, sad and worried, picks his fingers, lies in bed most of the time, does not like to answer questions, with more frequent urination during the night. Confused feeling in head, often sits as if he were in a dream. Eats and drinks but has a stool only every third day; weak memory. Timid, cannot be persuaded to any work.

Sleep very restless. Then very excited for 10 days, vehement, domineering, quarrelsome, tends to scold. Likes to wear his best clothes, makes useless purchases and then cares very little for them, wastes or ruins them; does not want to work, prefers to play; picks quarrels, does not tolerate contradiction. Continuously picks his nose which bleeds easily'.

Conditions of Weakness. As mentioned above, the Conium weakness increases very gradually, year after year, finally amounting to complete paralysis, and this process may take many years. Conium is an important remedy in chronic recreational drug users; not for the acute consequences of high doses of cocaine, for instance, but for people who are more careful with drugs.

They take small doses of drugs, they enjoy them little by little for many years, and very gradually they keep going into a state of loss of power on all levels, mental, emotional, and physical, so slowly that it is hard to perceive. After many years, the mind is totally paralyzed, they cannot think any more, imagination is exhausted, all energy is lost. In chronic drug users who do not take large or strong doses of narcotics, Conium will be indicated if there is such a gradual loss of power.

I include alcohol as a recreational drug here; Conium is in any case sensitive to alcohol and is easily affected by it. Hahnemann writes: 'The least quantity of spirituous drink intoxicates him'. Headaches are aggravated from alcohol, and the characteristic process of weakening and decline may be sped up by alcohol. But we have to know that underneath there is a predisposition; alcohol and drugs may catalyze and intensify the process, but they are not the deepest reason for the pathology.

On the physical plane, the weakness of Conium especially manifests in the urinary and genital systems. In spite of the intensity of the sexual desire, the sexual powers are weak, and there is often impotence. Men tend to have ejaculation praecox, and women may also get orgasms without even touching their partner. To quote Hahnemann's own delicate phrase: Emission even while frolicking with a woman'.

I once treated a female patient who used to flirt with priests. She liked to make them excited, and she would have a complete orgasm while she was flirting with them, without ever touching them. This symptom made me think of Conium. You may wonder why I call this a state of weakness. But in fact this is how I understand it: the sexual organs are weakened, almost paralyzed, and they are unable to hold back the release of the orgasm. A little stimulation, then orgasm happens, and that is it.

A keynote for Conium is interrupted urination. People in a Conium state will be urinating and the urination suddenly stops, in the middle of the flow. They wait a moment, and it starts again, stops again and so on, three, four or five times, before the urinary tract is empty. 'The discharge of urine suddenly stops during urination and only continues after a while'.

Such a symptom may point to a weakness of the bladder in expelling the urine, but sometimes also to a stenosis of the urethra or to the swelling of the prostate. If the urethra is narrowed because of an enlargement of the prostate gland, Conium may be indicated as well. If the urethral stricture is caused by inflammation and cicatrization, you should also think of Thuja and Medorrhinum when other symptoms agree.

An interesting modality: complaints of the extremities which respond to Conium are relieved by letting the affected limb hang down. This modality is indeed a strange, rare, and peculiar symptom that should call Conium to mind. As Kent puts it: 'Conium differs from a great many medicines. It is common for pains and aches to be relieved by putting the foot up on a chair; by putting them up in bed. But the patient with rheumatism, with ulceration and the other strange sufferings of the legs, will lie down and permits his legs to hang over the bed up as far as the knee'.

An ulcer on the foot that is painful even when lying in bed, is ameliorated by hanging the legs down from the knee. We may comprehend this peculiar symptom by knowing the pathology of the remedy, especially from the case of Socrates, who observed that its actions started by paralyzing first the lower extremities. It is therefore possible that Conium restricts the blood flow in the lower extremities, causing problems thereafter.

The Conium Vertigo: Vertigo is one of the most prominent features of the remedy. It may occur on rising from bed or from a seat, or on walking, on going downstairs, when lying, etc. But the most characteristic modality is vertigo on turning in bed. Also on moving the eyes or the head, especially in sideways motion. In this kind of vertigo Conium is the main remedy together with Belladonna, especially when the vertigo occurs when turning around in bed. Clarke mentions a case of lumbago with the symptom 'cannot turn over in bed without being dizzy' that was cured with Conium.

You may also compare Cocculus, because the Conium vertigo frequently has to do with an accommodation weakness of the eyes, as in Cocculus.

Nash reports a case where a patient seemed to have all the symptoms of locomotor ataxia. The striking symptom was that he could not, when walking, turn the head or the eyes the least bit sideways without staggering or falling. When he went out with his wife, he always walked in front of her or behind her, but never by her side! This strange behaviour made Nash think of Conium.

Some more proving symptoms and cured symptoms relating to the Conium vertigo:

Vertigo, in the morning, on rising from bed. Very dizzy while walking. Vertigo, like turning in a circle, on rising from his seat. Vertigo, worse when lying down, as though the bed were turning in a circle. Vertigo on becoming erect after stooping, as if the head would burst. Vertigo on looking around, as though the patient were to fall sideways.

'On raising my eyes from the object upon which they had been fixed to a more distant one the vision was confused, and a feeling of giddiness suddenly came over me. So long as my eyes were fixed on a given object the giddiness disappeared...

'Another prover even staggered when walking, but as soon as he closed his eyes, '... I could now walk straight and steady, and, what was more, without any feeling of giddiness'.

Generalities: Glandular induration as a result of contusion.

Conium has acted very well even in mammary cancer which developed after a blow against the breast, in cancer of the lip after long-time pressure by a tobacco pipe, etc.

Lassitude and weakness, even amounting to fainting. A striking symptom is a tremulous weakness after every stool that ceases in the open air. 'Sudden relaxation (a kind of paralytic weakness) while walking' has also been cured by Conium. But usually the weakness will develop very slowly and deeply, as discussed above. 'So weak that she has to lie down; sick and weary in the morning in bed, with ill-humour, sleepiness and pains in the stomach'.

The paralytic states of Conium usually begin below and proceed upwards (as in Socrates' death); this direction of development may also manifest in other Conium symptoms.

They are affected by cold and exertion. Conium patients tend to have complaints from over-lifting.

They are particularly sensitive to complaints from walking in the open air where exertion and cold may combine: 'Great liability to catch a cold, even in a room, after a walk in the open air, during which he had perspired'. 'Walking in the open air makes her weary, and the air affects her'. Extreme exhaustion, sudden relaxation, ill humour and other complaints appear after walking in the open air.

Warmth will usually ameliorate, particularly warmth of the sun. 'Chilly with trembling in all limbs, and therefore she has to remain constantly in the warmth of the sun'. Bright light, however, will often disturb the patient very much, and excessive photophobia is a striking symptom of Conium.

Two strange symptoms that can be understood as keynotes: Perspiration as soon as one closes the eyes. This symptom permitted Lippe to cure a 80-year-old man who suffered from hemiplegia.

'The clothes lie upon chest and shoulders like a load'. Conium may be indicated in mononucleosis infectiosa, especially in the glandular form (if the symptoms agree, of course). Other remedies frequently indicated in this disease are Iodium and Mercurius.

Head: 'Violent headache with vertigo, from which she suffered for three or four days; she was sad and silent, just sitting there the whole time'. Sick headaches with vertigo and an inability to urinate. There are also headaches with unsatisfactory and too small stools.

Constant sensation of confusion and stupefaction in the head. 'Constant dullness of the forehead, in the region of the eyebrows and the root of the nose'. Alcohol aggravates, even when mixed with water and drunk in very small quantities. 'Even watered wine rises to his head'.

Great sensitivity of the brain, especially to jar. 'On shaking the head, headache from the forehead to the occiput, as if something were loose in there'. 'On every step a snapping in the vertex, without pain'. 'Forcing and griping in the forehead, seemingly coming from the stomach, with much sensitiveness of the brain; the brain is shaken even by a noise or by talking'. There are also headaches from over-study.

Sensations of heaviness in the head, especially in the occiput, arising when sitting bent forward and ceasing when raising the head.

Strange sensations: 'Numbness, with sensation of coldness, of one side of the head'. Sensation in the right half of the brain as of a large foreign body. Hot spots on top or back of head, worse from excitement or overwork.

Study Guide

Often there are severe headaches from within outward. 'Headache, as if the brain were too full and the skull would burst, in the morning, on waking'.

Sticking pain in top of head and forehead, from within outward. Very severe occipital pains on every heartbeat, 'as though the occiput were pierced with a knife'. Throbbing headache, felt in the forehead.

On the other hand, there is also a sensation of 'giddy constriction of the brain' or a headache 'as if externally contracted' above the os frontale, or else a headache 'like a compression from both temples, after every meal'.

Drawing in the head, as soon as one goes out in the cold air; relieved on closing the eyes. With this, there is a sensation of 'great weakness in the head and the whole body'.

Tearing pains in occiput and back of neck, but also in the orbits, with constant nausea, urging to lie down.

Headaches with blindness or disturbances of vision, also with a sensation as if something like a fringe was falling over eyes.

Falling hair.

Eyes: The most important symptom is a weakness of the eye muscles, and particularly of the accommodation of the eyes, sometimes amounting to paralysis. The remedy may be indicated in presbyopia, as Hahnemann already presumed in the Materia Medica Pura. 'Far-sightedness; could distinctly see rather distant objects'.

'Affected with a weakness and dazzling of my eyes, together with a giddiness and debility of my whole body, especially the muscles of my arms and legs, so that when I attempted to walk I was apt to stagger like a person who had drunk too much liquor'.

Double vision occasionally occurs, as well as squinting, etc. Conium affects all the muscles in the region of the eyes, producing difficulties with every kind of motion of the eyes, on looking around or behind, turning the head, etc. 'Eyes feel as if pulled outward from nose'. And: 'He could hardly raise the eyelids, which seemed pressed down by a heavy weight'.

Weakness of vision may be cured with Conium, but also many other disturbances of vision. For instance: Sees before his eyes dark spots and coloured stripes, or clouds and bright spots, or else bows, sometimes playing in all rainbow colours; red vision.

'Fiery zigzags, moving through each other before the sight, on closing the eyes at night'.

Excessive photophobia, frequently without any signs of inflammation in the eye. Dazzling of the eyes from light of day, even in the room. Photophobia may be coupled with lid spasms. From a classic case: I frequently saw the most excessive photophobia with spasm of the lids. After hard efforts to separate the lids it finally succeeded, and a flood of hot tears spurted out, but cornea as well as sclerotica proved free of any inflammatory process'.

Disturbances of vision that are caused by injury, as for instance: ophthalmia after injury by a wood-chip, with dimness of cornea; dimness of the lens (cataract) after a blow against the eye, etc.

Much and constant dilatation of the pupils. Burning in the eyes, and especially of the inner surface of the eyelids. Pressure in eyes, worse when reading.

A biting pain in the inner canthi as if something caustic had come in, with lachrymation. Itching beneath the eyes, rubbing does not ameliorate but leads to a burning biting pain.

Repeated manifestation of styes, especially if styes became indurated A strange symptom from Bonninghausen: cold feeling in eyes when walking in the open air.

Study Guide

Ears: In Meniere's disease it is the first remedy to be thought of.

Much accumulation of earwax, even obstruction of the external meatus, with partial deafness. Conium may act curatively, especially when this complaint is coupled with pain in the liver region.

Something comes before the ears on blowing the nose and they feel stopped. Or else: painful sensitivity of hearing, noise startles him.

Noises in the ears: ringing, buzzing, humming, throbbing. Tinnitus. Tearing and stinging pains in and around the ears. Or else: drawing stinging pain, from within outward, in the ear.

Swelling and induration of the parotid gland, with painful tension of the skin.

Nose: Tendency to bore or pick in the nose, which bleeds easily.

Epistaxis when sneezing. Excessively acute sense of smell. Burning at the nostrils.

Stitching and sore pain in the nasal septum, also on tip of nose.

Too frequent sneezing, or obstruction of nose, which may become chronic. 'Obstructed nose for years' (Hahnemann).

Discharge of pus from the nose, mingled with blood.

Before the menses, pain inside in root of nose, aggravated by blowing nose and pressure.

Face: Eruptions in face, itching; pustular or vesicular; gnawing ulcers in face. Blisters at the upper lip, at the margin of the red portion, painful. Indurated tumours on cheeks and especially on lips, also as a consequence of pressure or contusion (tobacco pipe). Malignant tumours of the lips. Hardening and enlargement of the submandibular glands. Tearing stinging face-ache, directly before the ear; or a drawing pain from the jaw to the ear, or else painful tension near the ear. Facial pains that mostly occur at night.

Mouth: Drawing toothache, extending through the temples, aggravated by eating cold things, but not by cold drinking.

Drawing, jerking or gnawing toothache, with a sensation as if the teeth were loose, especially on mastication.

Tongue swollen, stiff, and painful, with difficult speech and articulation. Paralysis of the tongue.

Saliva tasting sour, or bitter taste in mouth. Throat: Bitter taste in throat.

Constant inclination to swallow, especially when walking in the wind. Strange rising in the throat, with a sense of stuffing as if something were lodged there. This may be a hysterical symptom (globus hystericu): 'Pressure from pit of stomach upwards into oesophagus, as though a round body were ascending'. Or else: 'Fullness in pit of throat, with fruitless efforts to belch'.

Respiration, Chest and Cough: Irritation to cough in the larynx, especially in this form: dry spot in the larynx, where there is a crawling, and almost constant irritation to dry cough. There may also be itching, tingling or scraping in throat, provoking dry cough.

Conium cured a 13-year-old boy who had a 'clapping noise' in the larynx with the act of expiration. The noise was distinctly audible and was usually preceded by marked spasmodic twitching of the right facial muscles.

Difficult inspiration, also with air hunger; with a sensation as if the chest couldn't expand enough, or else with a feeling of constriction of the chest; especially in the morning on waking and in the evening in bed.

Study Guide

Cough that occurs almost exclusively when first lying down, immediately after assuming a lying position; has to sit up and cough it out, afterwards he has rest.

Cough which is triggered by lying down and deep breathing; especially in the evening and at night.

Loose cough, but nothing can be expectorated; has to swallow the mucus which is detached by the cough. Conium is often indicated in obstinate dry cough remaining after influenza or a cold.

Cough which is followed by vomiturition. 'Night cough continued without any intermission until gagging and vomiting occurred'.

A sharp thrust directly through the chest, from the sternum to the spine. Stitching pains in the sternum and in the whole thorax are frequent with Conium.

'Violent stitches in side, as if a knife were plunged into it, causing loud moaning'. Or else: violent stitches in the right side of the chest about the nipple, on every inspiration while walking, relieved by hard pressure with the hand. Dry cough, excited by the slightest exposure to cold air, even by putting arms out of bed {Hepar).

Heart: Palpitation of the heart after stool, with intermission of heart beats. Violent palpitation: after drinking , when rising from bed.

Stomach: With many Conium complaints, there is loss of appetite. But Conium has marked desires: for salt and salty food; for sour food; for coffee. Milk does not agree. Bread tastes bad and 'does not go down'.

Empty eructations are frequent. They can start in the morning and continue all day. Usually they are odourless and tasteless, but there is also 'putrid eructation'.

Much nausea after every meal, with inclination to vomit and often enough with real vomiting. Conium may be indicated in vomiting in pregnancy.

Violent spasmodic pains in the stomach, especially if coupled with a tendency to constipation. From a cured case: 'Feeling as though the stomach contracted, as though a heavy weight were pressing upon it; she thinks she cannot tighten her clothes, and believes the stomach cramp would never stop, it only remits sometimes but increases again, making her sufferings intolerable'.

Contracting stomach pains, together with feeling of coldness in stomach and back; sensation of soreness and rawness in stomach.

In excessive stomach pains, e.g. in the context of a perforating ulcer or even cancer, Conium has been given with good results; the pains and the general state of the patients were markedly ameliorated. In one case the pains were gnawing and appeared mostly two or three hours after a meal and during the night, in another case they had a burning and cramping character and extended as far as the back and the shoulders. But the most remarkable modality was, 'pains relieved most in the knee-elbow position'.

Abdomen: Distension of abdomen, the belly is often hard and tense, with flatulence. 'Hardness and severe bloating of abdomen, in the evening after eating, the umbilicus protrudes which makes her sleep restless'. Swelling of the mesenteric lymph nodes.

Rapid bloating of the belly especially after drinking milk. Cutting in the abdomen precedes the discharge of flatus.

A strange concomitant symptom: 'Distension of abdomen, like flatulent colic, in the evening, with coldness of one foot' (compare Lycopodium). Stitching pains in the liver region, sometimes with intervals, or painful tearing there. Swelling of liver with pressive pain and accumulation of ear-wax, causing partial deafness.

Painful tension about the hypochondria, as from a constricting band. Pressive-tensive pain in the left hypochondrium, extending to the left side of the hypogastrium. Oppressive contraction of the hypogastrium. Contractive pain in lower abdomen, like after-pains. Pinching pains in the abdomen, as if diarrhoea would come on. Spasmodic or bearing-down pains, like menstrual colic or labour pains. Sore feeling in belly when walking on stone pavement. Trembling of the whole abdomen.

Rectum and Stool: Conium has some very characteristic and unusual symptoms in this region. The symptom 'Discharge of cold flatus' seems to be unique in the materia medica. Clarke reports that in a case of severe diarrhoea where the stools felt cold Conium was successfully given.

However, there is also the opposite sensation that is much more 'normal'.

'During stool, burning in the rectum' and 'Heat in lower portion of rectum' (but not in the anus!).

Conium has been useful in constipation with ineffectual urging or with unsatisfactory stools. Sometimes violent stomach cramps in combination with the constipation. Hard stools, only every other day. 'Constant urging without any stool. Frequent unsuccessful urging'. Several stools every day, but in very small quantities.

The remedy may also be indicated in diarrhoea, especially if watery or liquid stools are mixed with hard particles and are discharged together with noisy flatus. 'Frequent diarrhoea; stools like water, with many eructations, and copious passage of urine'. Watery diarrhoea, intermingled with undigested food.

The attacks of weakness after stool are very characteristic, too. After every stool, tremulous weakness, that ceases in the open air. And: after stool, palpitation of the heart, with intermission of heart beats.

Stools coated with blood. Involuntary discharge of stool during sleep. Stitches in the anus when not at stool.

Urinary Organs: The best-known symptom in this region has been quoted above:

'The discharge of urine suddenly stops during urination and only continues after a while'. Frequently there is also cutting in urethra during urination with it; also burning during or after micturition. The problems with urination may have their cause in a weakness of the bladder but also in hypertrophy of the prostate gland. Frequent urging to urinate and strangury; with burning in urethra and feeling of heat during micturition.

Frequent urination at night. 'Has to get up at 2 o'clock to urinate, several nights successively'. Dribbling of urine in old men. Turbid, whitish and viscous urine.

Urine is more easily discharged while standing, but in the beginning almost nothing is discharged even when standing; later on, however, the urine flows freely.

Male Genitalia: The ill effects of sudden loss of a sexual partner in both sexes are discussed extensively above.

Sexual weakness: impotence; erections absent, incomplete or of too short duration. Depression and weariness after coition.

But sexual desire is indeed present. Intense sexual desire with lack of sexual potency is characteristic. 'Vivid sexual desire, without erection'. Frequent discharge of prostatic fluid, on every emotion, on straining for stool, etc.; also with itching of prepuce. Nocturnal ejaculations without erotic dreams. Spermatorrhoea; with intermittent discharge of urine.

Swelling and induration of the testicles, especially after contusion; cancer of testicles. Cancer of the prostate. Cutting pain in the urethra at the moment of ejaculation.

Violent pain of testes. 'Pain as though a knife was cutting through the middle of the scrotum, between the testes upward as far as the root of the penis; with frequent short repetitions'. In his Dictionary, Clarke reports a case of contusion of the testes with very similar pains; Conium C200 relieved in 5 minutes! There is also pressive, pinching and tearing pain in the testicles.

Female Genitalia: In this region, Conium has particularly caused and cured indurations and hard tumours with stinging, shooting pains. It has been frequently used in mammary and uterine cancer, and in induration and enlargement of the ovaries as well. Some proving symptoms: 'Hardness of the right breast, with painfulness to touch and nightly stitches with it'. 'Stitches, as with needles, in the left mammary gland'. Conium proved especially useful, in hard tumours after a blow or beating against the mamma.

Moreover, Conium is indicated in many complaints in connection with menstruation. Some symptoms caused and cured by Conium that occurred before the menses: aching in limbs, tearful mood, restlessness and anxious worry about every trifle; anxious dreams; pains in mammae, especially on every jar; dry heat in whole body, but without thirst; stinging pains in the liver region, more at night while lying down and especially on inspiration; flatulence; pain inside in the root of nose.

Dysmenorrhoea with violent uterine cramps. Some descriptions: 'Grinding pain is felt above pudendum; the abdomen becomes inflated, the pain affects the chest and stitches are felt in left side'. Pressure downward and drawing in the thigh or stitching pain in the vagina. Contractive pain in the hypogastrium disappearing on walking in the open air. Concomitant symptoms: great fear when alone, but dread of strangers or company; stitches in mammae; headache; eruption all over body, consisting of small red nodules that burn violently after scratching and disappear with the end of the menstrual bleeding.

Moreover, Conium has effected a cessation or suppression of the menses, and so it has acted curatively in amenorrhoea and complaints from amenorrhoea, and in too scanty menses as well. If the 'premenstrual' symptoms mentioned above occur every four weeks but the bleeding is totally absent, there is a good chance that Conium is indicated. 'Menses stopped by putting hands in cold water'.

In a recent case, this symptom permitted the cure of a patient whose menses stopped after the first day. She had prepared beans in cold water before. Now she suffered with pain and congestion in abdomen, back and mammae (which was not the case otherwise). The cause made the therapist think of Conium, and the remedy brought the menses back and made the pain disappear (Sharma, Klassische Homoopathie 6/92).

Leucorrhoea which is preceded by much abdominal pain and a weak and lame feeling in the small of the back; afterwards lassitude and exhaustion. 'Leucorrhoea of a white acrid mucus, which caused burning'. 'Thick, milky leucorrhoea, with contractive labour-like colic coming from both sides'. A discharge of bloody mucus is also reported. Conium may also be indicated in vomiting of pregnancy; in complete insomnia and extreme exhaustion for days after childbirth, with excessive photophobia; in oozing of milk from the breasts long after weaning of the child, but also in dwindling of the mammae. 'The female milk glands shrivel from Conium so that the most beautiful bosom looks like an empty fold of the skin' (from Heraclides). Severe itching deep in the vagina.

Violent stitches at the female parts. Vulva very sore to the touch.

Neck and Back: Conium is an important remedy in indurated swelling of cervical lymph nodes.

'Crawling in the spine, as from falling asleep'. Permanent sensation of numbness in the region of the shoulder blades.

Tensive pains in back, especially in the muscles below the scapulae, aggravated by raising the arms. Pains as if sprained in the left side of back, also in the neck.

Stitches in small of back, with a drawing pain through the lumbar vertebrae, when standing.

Pain in small of back, especially drawing or dragging downward, in connection with the menses, prolapsus of the uterus or something like that.

Bad effects from spinal injury. There is a case report about a young man who had fallen from the second story onto the stone pavement of the street. More than a year later he still suffered from very annoying pain in the lumbar region (on which he had fallen), especially when laughing, sneezing or taking a quick breath. Conium brought about a great, rapid and permanent amelioration of the pain.

Extremities: Weakness, powerlessness, prostration, lame feelings and paralysis of the extremities are symptoms of Conium.

'Loss of power on awaking from siesta, arms and legs as if separated from the body'. The limbs are stiff, heavy, almost useless, moving them provokes a 'disagreeable feeling', can hardly walk.

Paralysis first of the lower, then of the upper extremities.

Trembling of all limbs. Sensations of numbness and coldness, especially in fingers and toes, sometimes spreading from there towards the body.

Bruised feeling in all the joints, especially during rest; much better or disappearing during motion.

Shoulders feel sore, as if pressed on. The clothes seem to lie on them like a load. Swelling and induration of the axillar lymph nodes, also when there are tumours of the mammae.

Cramp-like pain in the muscles of the forearms, especially when leaning on arms. Cracking in the wrist, especially in the evening.

Perspiration of the palms. Yellow spots on fingers; yellow finger nails. Gait is faltering, vacillating, staggering as if drunk, dragging his legs after him.

When he closes his eyes, he is able to walk straight and steady, but when they are open he begins to stagger.

Pain going from hypogastric region down legs, in dysmenorrhoea. Feeling of weakness, even to trembling, in the right thigh, while walking.

Or else: on walking in the open air, cramp-like pain in the anterior muscles of the right thigh. Tiredness and 'fatigue pain' in knees. Cracking of the knees on becoming erect. Cramps in calves; tensive, stiff pains in the calves.

'Painful reddish spots on the calves, later turning yellow or green like from contusions, and preventing the mobility of the foot which is bent like from shortening of the tendons'.

Coldness of one foot, with distension of abdomen. Sensation as if the bone pierced the skin at the heel.

Numbness and insensibility of the feet; they tend to become cold, with liability to catch a cold.

Sleep: *Insomnia and late falling asleep, only after midnight. Restless sleep, nightmares, anxious dreams and frightful dreams, interrupting the sleep.*

Dreams of dead people and corpses; of people who are alive in reality but dead in the dream.

Or else: sleep too deep, like stupefied, unrefreshing; headache aggravated after sleep. Especially after waking from siesta symptoms like 'insensibility', confusion, powerlessness etc. will occur.

Irresistible sleepiness during the day. 'He could not refrain from sleep with all his will power; had to lie down and sleep'.

Fever: Great internal and external heat, with great nervousness. Burning heat through the whole body. Sensation of internal and external heat after sleep. A fever symptom from the Chronic Diseases; 'Sensation of heat in whole body, also increased warmth of skin which can be felt externally, with dry and sticky lips, without thirst, even with aversion to drinks, and with an insipid saliva in the mouth; noise and shining objects affect him, as well as any motion; he wants to sit lonesome with closed eyes'. Chilliness, shivering and coldness, especially early in the morning and in the afternoon; at 5 am; from 3 to 5 pm.

'Chill with trembling in all limbs, so he always has to stay in the warmth of the sun'.

The Conium perspiration has one striking and very important modality: 'Sweat as soon as she closes the eyes, only in the beginning of the sleep; even by day, when sleeping in sitting position'.

Skin: Itching of the skin, especially of the backs of the fingers. 'Itching stitches, as from fleas, one directly after the other, here and there on the body, but always single stitches, never two at the same time'.

Yellow discolouration of the skin, also of the finger nails and the whites of eyes. Brown spots on the body. Urticaria after violent bodily exercise.

Obstinate herpetic eruptions in different places, e.g. around the neck, behind the ears, in the crook of the knee, on hands and forearms; usually moist and burning, worse by warmth.

An example by Hartlaub: 'Sudden herpetic eruption on forearm, beginning as a small spot and gradually spreading over arm;

skin became porous, very red and raw, with furrows and depressions. Sore, broken places formed here and there in the skin, viscid lymph or blood oozing from them, lymph drying and forming white crusts under which the exudation still continues; intense itching in affected parts, with irresistible desire to scratch, particularly in evening; surrounding lymphatics swollen and involved...' Burning nodules on the skin during the menses, disappearing with the end of the bleeding. Petechia, especially in old people. Tendency to necrotic ulcers. (Vithoulkas)

CONVALARIA MAJALIS
(Lily of the Valley)

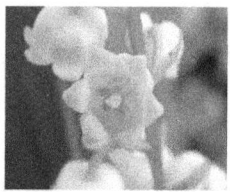

Heart ailments with sleepiness. Edema. Time seems to pass too slowly. Pain in the sacro-illiac joints. Has to sit up to sleep.

Feeling as if his heart beat through the chest. *Sensation as if the heart stopped beating then starting very suddenly.*

Palpitation from least exertion. Angina from tobacco smoking. Irregular heart beating. Better open air (Carbo-veg) worse in a warm room.

Nash says of this remedy: *I have used it with much satisfaction in women who complained of great SORENESS IN THE UTERINE REGION AND SYMPATHETIC PALPITATION OF THE HEART. It has also served me well in dropsies of cardiac origin, especially in women who have at the same time the above- mentioned soreness in uterine region. I once checked the progress of a very bad case of cardiac dropsy after the effusion in the chest had so increased that the patient could not breathe when lying down, and there was much bloody expectoration. I used the 30th potency in this case, though many times very fine results follow the use of the remedy in much lower preparations. The dropsy all disappeared and she was able to be around and enjoy life very well, though the organic heart trouble was not removed.*

BOVISTA has been of use to me in only one affection, but in that it is invaluable—menorrhagia. The FLOW IS ALWAYS WORSE, or sometimes FLOWS ONLY IN THE NIGHT IN BED. I do not know of a more-reliable symptom. It has helped and cured many cases, both acute and chronic.

It has also sometimes a flow BETWEEN the periods like, AMBRA GRISEA, but the latter remedy has more nervous or hysterical symptoms.

USTILAGO MAYDIS is also a remedy that is very useful in menorrhagia or metrorrhagia, and I think I have observed that it is best adapted to those cases where the flow is of a passive nature. (THLASPI BURSA PASTORIS.) There is apt to be more or less pain and irritation, at the same time, in one or both ovaries. It is especially useful in these cases at the climacteric. I have cured some very bad cases, and always use both this remedy and BOVISTA in the 200th potency.

CRATAEGUS
(Hawthorn Berries)

This remedy is indicated for people who have an **extreme sensitivity to the opinion of others and extreme sensitivity to unfairness – they react to this by withdrawing**. This leads them to suppress their emotions and thus we can see a connection to a reason for the high blood pressure as they hold everything inside and they can't express what is bothering them.

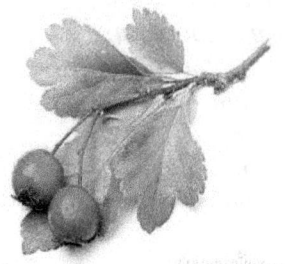

"I have to be fair and everyone else has to be fair or I will withdraw".

Avoids others if feels there will be conflict or criticism.

(Proving Boucher Institute)

They want others to treat them fairly and they also do their best to treat others fairly and not hurt others in any way. We see this same trait in Natrum muriaticum. If the person who needs Crataegus feels there will be conflict they won't answer the phone for example.

This is a remedy that can be used for headaches, stomach aches and nausea. In later stages they get high blood pressure and heart ailments.

Boericke says of this remedy: *Heart.--Cardiac dropsy. Fatty degeneration. Aortic disease. Extreme dyspnœa on least exertion, without much increase of pulse. Pain in region of heart and under left clavicle. Heart muscles seem flabby, worn out. Cough. Heart dilated; first sound weak. Pulse accelerated, irregular, feeble, intermittent. Valvular murmurs, angina pectoris. Cutaneous chilliness, blueness of fingers and toes; all aggravated by exertion or excitement. Sustains the heart in infectious diseases.* (Boericke)

CUBEBA
(Cubebs)

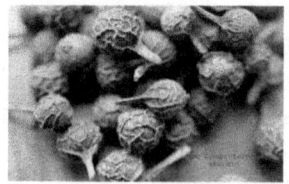

Study Guide

*Head has a fine tremor. **SUDDEN ANGER**. Bladder infections.*

Case 1: 18 y.o. She had a chronic trembling of the head with a chronic ear and chronic bladder infections. Angry and intolerant of others so she feels better when alone. Sudden anger lashing out at others. After Cubeb 30c once a week, she was better in all respects and her mother was very happy as well.

Boericke: *Urine.--Urethritis, with much mucus, especially in women. Cutting after urination, with constriction. Hæmaturia. Prostatitis, with thick yellow discharge. Cystitis.*

Nash: *This remedy, also fallen into disrepute from its empirical use in the old school, has an important place in the therapeutics of gonorrhoea, if after the first or inflammatory stage is passed under the usual remedies for that stage there still remains burning in the urethra after urination and the discharge remains thick, yellow or pus-like. Notwithstanding MERCURIUS or PULSATILLA, we may find our remedy in CUBEBA. I have made some fine cures myself in such cases. With PULSATILLA the discharge, while thick, or yellow, or green, is more likely to be BLAND, as it is on mucous membranes elsewhere.*

MERCURY has a similar discharge, but all the symptoms are WORSE AT NIGHT. When the discharge becomes thin (gleety) neither of these remedies are, as a rule, appropriate. (Nash)

CUPRUM METALLICUM
(Copper)

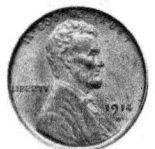

Materia Medica

Cramps, spasms, remorse and guilt.

Case 1: Teen with very severe menstrual cramps. She feels very bad about being sexually active and at times she won't let herself have sexual feelings and breaks off her relationship with her boyfriend. Her *toes would cramp painfully.* After Cuprum 30c the guilt and cramps are better.

From Hpathy.com: *Essence: maintaining control: cramp. These are serious people who work hard. They want to get on with their work, to carry on and expand. They are not allowed to ease up, whatever has been built up should be maintained. They are serious, hard working, responsible, sometimes even extremely ambitious or fanatical.*

They don't want to lose control and this tendency to hold on can cause cramps, either on the emotional or on the physical level. They have to be kind and keep their emotions under control, but it is rather a forced sort of smile. They won't let go of their own ideas and thoughts, which are often very conservative. They are rigid and precise. The physical signs of this rigidity are usually symptoms of cramp, often cramp in the calves, as if they are always having to stand on tip toes. But they can also be cramps anywhere else in the body; in the thighs, back, stomach, heart etc.

Maintaining order: telling tales Rules are there to be obeyed. As long as they follow the rules nothing can go wrong. Or if something does go wrong they won't be blamed, because they have always obeyed the rules. They love rules, it gives them a sense of security. And it is very important to them that nobody steps out of line. If someone doesn't follow the rules they will report them. These are the children who tell tales.

Detaining people who make mistakes: guard: Their desire to control can be quite obsessive. Everything has to be checked, everything has to be perfect. They consider it their task to maintain order and can get very angry if other people step out of line.

Maintaining order: ritual: Another way of maintaining order is through ritual. Ritual is a key word for Cuprum. Their rigid desire to follow the rules can lead to ritualistic behavior, a seemingly meaningless set of actions that are constantly repeated in the same order. This remedy could be very useful for people who are frequently involved in rituals, people such as priests or judges. There is often also a sort of superstitious element in these rituals, 'touch wood', 'cross your fingers' etc.

Protection against criticism: They are very sensitive to criticism, especially when someone tells them they haven't stuck to the rules. They don't want others to interfere with their affairs. They can get extremely angry when someone criticizes them, or touches them, or even looks at them. Cuprum children don't want to be touched, looked at, carried or driven. Hence their desire to hide or to escape. They want to avoid criticism and the pressure and restrictions of having to fulfill their task. Pressure of work can aggravate their complaints and if it gets too heavy they don't want to carry on any longer.

Their own criticism of other people is always about not obeying the rules or not doing their duty. (Hpathy.com)

Lippe's redline symptoms and keynotes: Contact renews and aggravates the ailment (Nux-V.) Giddiness accompanying almost all ailments, the head falling forward and on the chest. Metastasis to the brain from the other organs. Constant protrusion and retraction of the tongue like snake (Lach.) CONVULSIONS WITH BLUE FACE AND CLENCHED THUMBS. Spasm of the glottis (Brom., Chlor., Lach., Phos, Samb.)

There is blueness of the face and lips (Carb-V., Lach., Verat.) Delirium in attacks, with incessant, disconnected talking. VIOLENT CONVULSIONS, WITH PIERCING CRIES (Apis, Bell., Glon., Hyos., Plb., Stram., Verat-V.).

Spasms or convulsions beginning in fingers and toes and spreading from thence.

Affections arising from repressed eruptions, brain affections, convulsions, etc.

Convulsions during pregnancy (Apis, Cedr., Cham., Cic, Hyos., Lyc.) Puerperal convulsions (Bell., Cic., Hyos., Stram.) SEVERE SPASMODIC PAIN IN THE ABDOMEN WITH CONVULSIONS (Plb.).

ICY-COLDNESS OF THE WHOLE BODY (Camph., Carb-V., Kali-P., Laur., Phos., Sec., Verat.).

Metallic taste in the mouth (Cocc., Merc., Nat-C., Rhus-T., Seneg.) CRAMPS OF THE MUSCLES, THOSE OF THE CALVES AND THIGHS ARE DRAWN UP INTO KNOTS.

Cough relieved by a drink of cold water. (Amm-Caust., Caust., Coc-C., Iod., Kali-C., Op., Sulph., Verat.) Cold water also relieves vomiting (Phos., Puls.)

Whooping cough: the attacks come on in quick succession, accompanies perhaps by spasms, threatening suffocation (Ipec.) Mental or bodily exhaustion from over-exertion of mind, or loss of sleep (Nux-V.)

Vomiting before menses.

It is to be thought of in laryngismus stridulous and in spasmodic asthma, with thumbs clenched in the palms, blueness of the face, constriction of the throat and dyspnoea so intense that even a handkerchief cannot be tolerated near the face.

In whooping cough it is of great value, especially when the spasmodic character of the cough is very prominent; there is vomiting, the face becomes purple and the child seems to almost suffocate. The paroxysms are better from drinking water.

Study Guide

CYCLAMEN

Terrors of conscience (Ruta, Carc, Cuprum, Aids nosode).
Grieves over duty neglected. Depression, with weeping desire to
be alone. Aching in morning, with *flickering before eyes*;
sneezing with itching in ear. Vertigo; things turn in a circle;
better in the room; worse, open air. One-sided headache.
Frequent sneezing with itching in ears.

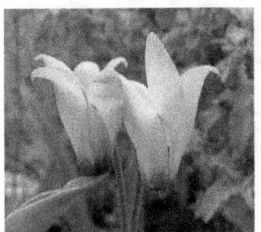

Case 1: This was a young women who was a typist. She could
no longer work because of the pain in her fingers and hands. She
had guilt about everything. From Boericke we find: Terrors of
conscience, grieves over duty neglected. After taking this
remedy her hand pains were relieved and she was able to go back
to work.

Flickering before eyes, fiery sparks, as of various colors,
glittering needles, dim vision of fog or smoke. Saliva and all
food has a salty taste; pork disagrees. Menses: too early, too
profuse, black and clotted; membranous (too late, pale, scanty,
Puls.), better during the flow (worse: Act-rac, Puls).

Burning sore pain in heels, when sitting, standing or walking in
open air (Agar. , Caust. , Val. , Phyt.).

CYPRIPEDIUM
(Yellow Lady's Slipper – Orchidaceae)

The child wants to play at night. ***Child wakes up in the middle of the night and wants to play.*** The child is over-stimulated from video games. Ailments from excitement. They scream if you try to put them back to bed. Convulsions from teething.

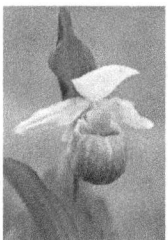

Compare to Coffea; overstimulated. Boericke: *The skin symptoms correspond to those of poisoning by Rhus, for which it has been found an efficient antidote.*

Nervousness in children; from teething and intestinal troubles.

SLEEPLESSNESS. Cerebral hyperasthesia in young children often the result of overstimulation of brain.

Child cries out at night; is wakeful and begins to laugh and play. Headaches of elderly people and during climacteric.

DROSERA
(Sundew)

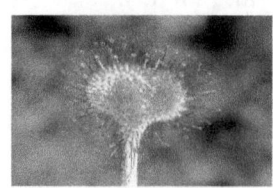

Study Guide

Suspicious of others, chronic cough. This remedy can be used for a variety of respiratory illnesses such as whooping-cough, laryngitis and bronchitis. Barking cough or spasmodic dry irritative cough. One cough comes after the other very rapidly. Choking cough; retching cough. Could have a sensation of crumbs in the throat or a feather on the larynx.

History of betrayal resulting in lack of trust.

Cough starts when the head touches the pillow i.e. cough worse from lying down. Chills with shivering. Hot face and cold hands. Feels suspicious of others.

Deep voice and horse.

Case 1: Female, smoker for many years with COPD. The cough was coninuous and exhausting. She hated everyone and had no friends. She did not trust anyone and was mean and hard on those around her. History of betrayal from family as a result no trust in anyone. After Drosera 30c the cough was better in a few days.

DULCAMARA
(Bittersweet)

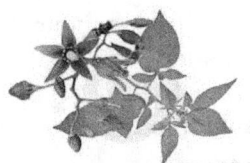

Worse from COLD DAMP weather. Joint pains, colds and allergies.
Dulcamara is another remedy that can be used for colds, flu, bronchitis and ear aches. It is very similar to Rhus tox as both remedies have the following similar symptoms: WORSE WHEN THE PERSON IS EXPOSED TO THE COLD, DAMP WEATHER – LEADING TO COLDS AND OR ***RHEUMATIC STIFFNESS.***

For Dulcamara, look for:
- Cough that is worse from cold weather
- Whooping cough
- Loose rattling coughs

- Must cough a long time to expel the mucous
- Flu with stiffness of the back and across the shoulders
- Worse after getting cold and wet
- Headache from sinusitis, worse from cold drafts or getting a chill
- Pains in the face
- Sinuses filled with yellow mucous
- Stuffy nose
- Neuralgias (a sharp pain, from an inflammation of or pressure to, the nerves) of the face
- Asthma from cold weather
- Chills beginning in the back
- Stiff and painful joints that are worse in wet cold weather
- Rheumatism alternates with diarrhea
- Warts on the hands or the face
- Herpes on the lips
- A general feeling of icy coldness

ANXIETY FOR OTHERS SUCH AS HER CHILDREN.

SHE WANTS TO SET STRICT LIMITS ON THEIR BEHAVIOR AND SCHEDULE.

SHE IS CONTROLLING AND DICTATORIAL. (BORAGE)

Take one dose then wait six to ten hours to see if there is some improvement of symptoms. As long as the patient is getting better there is no need to repeat the dose. If there is any relapse then repeat the remedy before trying a different remedy.

ELAPS CORALLINUS
(Brazilian Coral Snake)

They can have high ideals for themselves and high moral standard yet they have a tendency to betray those standards resulting in feelings of *guilt and remorse. Chilly and most often they are sensitive to cold.*

Study Guide

Generally they feel an aggravation from cold wet weather, including sadness and depression from rainy weather. They are perhaps the snake remedy that is most bothered by the cold, including *worse from cold drinks*.

A strong tendency to hemorrhage of black blood.

Desire for salads.

Case 1: *Angela, 33 year-old female*

During the initial interview Angela was crying with grief. She reported having a deep sense of loss and depression since she left her husband over a year ago.

'I can't let go of him – I still love him (2). (Obsession like other snake remedies) He didn't treat me right, but I should have stayed and made it work.'

'I feel guilty for having an affair on him (3). I let myself down, and I blame myself since I lost my integrity. I am angry he did not do enough to help me out while we were married.'

'I vomit every morning after I brush my teeth.'

Headaches on the left side with a sensation the back of the head was swollen; it felt bruised, worse from touch.

Herpes simplex. Pain in hands, forearms (2). Tingling in the arms. Shooting nerve pain in the hands and wrists worse from cold weather (2). Sensation as if her arms were swollen and painful (2). 'I wake up with enlarged hands.' Skin moles with spontaneous bleeding.

'I am very close to my father. I am an optimist. I love horses. I am afraid to have a baby; that I might die from childbirth.' (suspicious).

She did not seem especially jealous or loquacious, but there was an intensity about her. 'I am outgoing and confident, not afraid of anything.'

She owned a business and ran it well.

'I want to move to a sunny climate since I become depressed in the rainy weather (2). If my chest is touched, I will throw up and become depressed – like what is the point of life, and I want to give up. I feel my body is tight and constricted; I can't relax. I find myself gripping the steering wheel of the car.'

She was allergic to metal touching her skin. Generally chilly (2).

Grinding of teeth in sleep. Shin splints when running. Dreams of her head being swollen. She was worse from collars about the neck.

'I like ice-cold water, but I can get gum pain from drinking cold water. I binge on salads and crave cottage cheese and orange juice.'

She had a fear of bees.

Analysis: She had many symptoms characteristic of many of the snake remedies; such as, the choking, aggravation from collars, ailments from passion, and she was in general a very intense person. What made me choose *Elaps* rather than one of the other snake remedies? I have found this remedy to be unique in that it can be used when *the person has set high moral standards yet has a tendency to betray those standards*.

As a result, the patient feels a deep sense of guilt. *Elaps* can also be thought of when there is a *theme of unwanted attachment*. This patient would have liked to be free of her love for her ex-husband, but she couldn't let go. *Lachesis* and *Naja* also can display this trait. *Naja* can especially be obsessed with or brood over someone whom they know they dislike or cannot get along with. Confirming this prescription of *Elaps,* we note that she was depressed in the rainy weather, enough to want to move to a place with a lot more sun. Also, she craved salads, a known desire for *Elaps*, and was worse from cold drinks. She was sensitive to the cold as well.

Prescription: *Elaps* 30C, one dose.

Study Guide

<u>One week later</u>: She was much better in all ways. 'I feel back to my old self and happy again. The grief is much improved. I think my passions were too strong; now I can let go of my ex-husband. In the past, when a teenager, I got hives from grief over a lost boyfriend. I am good at business, driven by passion to do well, creative in the marketing department. I still want to move to a more-sunny climate.' She noted less gagging from brushing her teeth. Her sense of guilt was better by 60%. There was less pain in the jaw on waking. Sleep was better.

<u>One month later</u>: Still doing well.

<u>Over one year later</u>: She is still doing well. She moved to a sunny climate. There has been no return of the depression. She is now excited by rain; it no longer causes sadness. There are no more muscular pains, bleeding moles, or an aggravation from cold drinks. She no longer craves salad, nor is she as chilly. She is still allergic to metal. New symptom: menstrual cramps.

<u>Elaps:</u> Named because of the shape of the scales on its back resembling coral. Affects the auditory, nasal and throat passages.
Many aspect of coldness in the patient.
Black, near death, AIDS.
Feels threatened.
Unprotected (fear of being beaten).
Hemorrhagic Qualities.
Elaps is distinguished from the other snakes by the per-eminent blackness of its discharges and hemorrhages.
Black ear wax.
Hemorrhage from lungs black as ink and watery, especially from the right lung.
Stitches in apex of right lung.
Black and frothy diarrhea.

Other Characteristic Symptoms
- fruit and cold drinks lie like ice in the stomach and cause a cold feeling in the chest.

- internal coldness of same parts of body esp. of the stomach.
- spasm in esophagus so food and liquid can't pass down easily.
- affects the auditory, nasal and the throat passages.
- deafness with chronic otorrhea and a buzzing as if a fly were in the auditor canal.
- nose with a foul smelling discharge (ozena).
- inflammation with fissures of the pharynx and difficult swallowing.
- right side paralysis

Guiding symptoms of Elaps Similar to other snake poisons (passionate, loquacity, sensitive to a collars, choke easily, fear snakes, deep sleep) but unique in the following ways: *Chilly* easily and *aggravated from cold drinks*. Cold feeling in the chest or stomach from drinking cold drinks or fruit. Headache or pain in the gums or abdomen from cold drinks. May also be aggravated from heat or have heat alternating with chill. Depression from cold, wet weather. *Craving for salad*, ice, oranges, yogurt, sweet buttermilk. Aversion to bananas, meat and bread. Worse from eating fruit and bread. *Hemorrhage of dark or black blood*. Passion leading to obsession.

Emotional Profile: The patient in need of *Elaps* is often animated, passionate and driven. They reach for high moral standards, but fear of falling from grace. They want to do what is correct thing, to be respected. They can be held back because of timidity. More withdrawn than *Lachesis*, they are usually not as loquacious.

Suppression of emotions, beaten down. They desire and work hard to be the best, but they also can feel defeated, in a pit of despair, a fallen angel. Intense emotions of passion leading to strong attachments; then they can't let go, even if the person is not right for them (*Naja*); protracted grief or disappointments (*Ignatia*). Strong ambition for business success (*Nux-v*). High moral principles, and they can feel very guilty from betraying these ideals. Feels abused, lack of confidence, suppressed anger, desire to kill (*Staph*). Feels violated; fear of rape. Fearful, suspicious and apprehensive of some fatal disease, that something bad will happen. Fear or anxiety about malignant disease; "fear of death" in other words, of dying of something that was very terrible.

TF Allen proving: "Imagines he is being beaten. Irresistible desire to scream at the top of her voice. Fearfulness, dread of being alone, as though something would happen, or as though rowdies would break in. Excessive horror of rain (tenth day)."

I have had no cases to confirm a fear of rain, but I have seen two cases where there was a definite depression from rainy weather (see also case eleven below by C Hering in which the patient "never felt happy in wet weather.") C Hering: "Fear of being left alone, as if something horrible might happen. Angry about one's self, does not wish to be spoken to. At the least contradiction, body shudders, blood boils, with prickling." Difficult to listen to others, hears what they say but cannot understand (PN).

General symptoms, general modalities, confirming symptoms: Abdominal pains are ameliorated from lying on the abdomen.

Proving by HC Allen: Worse at night. Coldness aggravated by drinking cold water (*Caps.*); after a drink, shivering from head to foot with chattering of the teeth. Flushes of heat, with redness of the face and ears. Heat, with thirst, alternating with chilliness. Can be thirsty - unquenchable thirst. Bread does not digest. Fruit lies in the stomach like ice. Weight in the stomach after eating. Periodicity is marked. Great sensitiveness to cold: draft, wind, wet weather agg.

Main areas of pathology qualified by modalities: Vertigo, with tendency to fall forward.

Headaches. Violent headache, when the desire for food is not immediately satisfied, ameliorated after eating; severe pain in the vertex as if the brain were shaking, with nausea, which prevents her from keeping the head quiet; lancinating pains, first in one side, then in the other; occipital headache after mental exertion; sleeplessness.

Violent headaches which are felt first in the left, then in the right eye, and extend from the forehead to the occiput (A.L. Blackwood).

Pain at root of hairs on head. Falling of hair.

Eyeballs feel sticky under lids and as if rough. Sensation of sand in the eyes. Burning in lids. Burning and dryness in both eyes on waking. Aversion to light, desire to close eyes. Eyes red and inflamed; watery; glassy look. Violent itching in left eye. Stye on left eye, and lancinating pain.

Deafness. Cracking in the ears on swallowing. Buzzing, whistling or ringing in the ear. Ear wax black and hard. Chronic otorrhoea when accompanied with deafness.

Bad smell from the nose. Stoppage of the nose. Snuffles from the least current of air; child must breathe through the mouth; foul smell from nose; bright blood gushes from nose and ears; white and watery mucous discharge from nose; wakes up gasping. Nose bleeds. Bad smell (like putrid herring pickle) from the nose.

Red face. Its other symptoms which I have repeatedly confirmed are: Burning pain in the esophagus and stomach, commonly described by the patient as "acidity," which is ameliorated by cold drinks.

Cough, with expectoration of black blood, and a tearing sensation in the cardiac region; almost constant cough, with frightful pains throughout the lungs, as if they were torn out, especially in the upper portion of the right chest.

The passage of liquids is arrested as by a spasmodic contraction of the esophagus. Food turns spirally when going down the esophagus, or, sometimes, each morsel falls heavily, as through a metallic tube, into the stomach, which trembles violently. Liquids pass down the esophagus with a gurgling noise.

Abdominal pains ameliorated by lying on the abdomen. The intestines feel twisted, as if by a cord, and strung together in a knot, with strangulating sensation.

Bloody dysentery. Urine full of uric acid crystals. Diabetes. Hypertension. Ulcers. Allergic rhinitis. Asthma.

Hemorrhagic fibroids. Itching of vulva and vagina. Dysmenorrhea with a flow of black blood. Sensation as if something burst in the womb, then continuous stream of dark colored blood, better when urinating. Discharge of black blood between menses. Great weight at the uterus, on rising, aggravated by walking. Weakness of the genitals; impotence. Violent beating of the heart. Very stiff neck.

Cyanosis of the extremities, with reddish spots on them. The blood becomes congested in the hand, which is blue and as if paralyzed; it has to be kept held up to prevent this effect. The left foot is blue and swollen, with red spots. The right side is numb and as if paralyzed, from the shoulder to the knee.

Rheumatic pain - sticking, intermittent, ceasing for several minutes, in the whole left side; commencing in the limbs, at 4 pm; the pain disappeared about 6 pm, with mental exhaustion and great indifference. Painful peeling off of the skin of the fingertips. Itching of the soles of the feet, the skin of which peels off. Pricking, as with thousands of pins. Glands of axillae, itching with "tetter" (scaly, eczematous eruption). Boils. Carbuncles. Gangrene (*Sec*). Ailments from bites of insects and snakes (*Led*); from poisonous plants.

Case 2: The patient had spring hay fever with a lot of itching of the nose and sneezing. The striking aspect was that when she experienced the symptoms she would become very angry. She would scream for the next remedy, scream to be "fixed" and to get better. This is a very intense reaction to the itching of the nose! It just drove her crazy. This patient had a history of bad relationships with men; she could never find a man to stay with her. As in my rhinitis case, she did not have the menstrual difficulties we have been taught to associate with *Elaps*. The emotional intensity was similar to *Lachesis* and more in line with what we have

Materia Medica

been taught about *Elaps*. *Elaps* has worked for this woman for four years now. (ES)

Case 3: Mrs. T.S., consulted me on 3.30.94 for very intense headaches, from which she had been suffering for the last three years. She was accompanied by her husband, and was dressed in brightly colored clothes and bright make up.

P: 'I hated her (her mother-in-law). I hated her like poison. I used to wish her dead so many times. If I could, I would have killed her myself and tried to get away with it on grounds of insanity. But I knew I could not do that. I wanted to kill her so many times. I was on the edge, on the point of it so many times. My husband never understood that; he was so madly in love with his mother. And that was the cause of my headaches. And I reached such a pitch that if I used to touch my head, it used to ache. The tension, doctor, the tension . . . of having an old lady in the house who, if I would reach for the salt, would say: "Do not put too much salt." If I reached for the oil, she would say, "Do not put too much oil." If I reached for this, she would say, "Do not do this." And she used to call me "mad." "You are mad; you are mad," she would always say. I have led a very rough life, very unhappy life mainly due to my mother-in-law. And she...wherever she is, she will suffer for it. I believe in that. She will not go straight to heaven, as we Catholics believe, but she will be wandering somewhere because she made me suffer; she made me go through hell. She used to shout and scream all the time.

She used to call me a prostitute. She could see that there was not a single man coming to my door, not a single man, yet she would call me a prostitute. I do not know why. My husband used to ask her if there was any man coming, and she would say that there was not. He used to then ask her why she was calling me a prostitute. She used to call me such filth- the bitch! She used to call me filthy names that I could not understand. My neighbors would understand and they used to say that if they told me what all those meant, I would feel very bad. They used to all say that she did not treat me like a daughter-in-law, but like a servant.

They used to all say that I fight with everyone. I call them names; I abuse them. I have a big fight. Once in every two or three years, I let off steam. It takes me a long time to get angry; I simmer and simmer, and then suddenly I blow my top and get angry.'

Case analysis: In this case, she has dreams of falling and flying. Her autobiography is entitled, 'The Great Abyss and the Glory Beyond It.' This is how she sees her life - falling down into an abyss and then rising up from that fall. Her talk is very egoistic; she is boasting, showing off. She feels she is very great, divine, and has always to be on the top. And her fear is of falling off from that place at the top where she sees herself. Of the snake remedies, *Elaps* has dreams of falling into an abyss. The miasm in the case is cancer. This need to do everything on her own, to look after her son on her own even if it adversely affects her health, and to do everything to perfection, to cook, to play the piano, to write, etc., are features of the cancer miasm. She was the best student in her school. She takes too many things upon herself and believes that she has to do them all perfectly. She feels desperate and wants to kill. She talks in the superlative; things appear extreme for her. Her perspective of life is very bleak; she feels she has been living in hell, in an abyss. One can see how the miasm is close to syphilis.

Rubrics: Delusion, falling forward, she is. Dream: falling, abyss, into. Company, desire for. Delusion, is being injured. She was given one dose of *Elaps* 1M on 3.30.94.

Follow up 4.05.94: She had felt some relief in her headache for half a day, but then again her headaches were the same. Over the next year-and-a-half the remedy was repeated only four times. There was a marked improvement in her headaches and in her moods, and she was able to reduce the antidepressants. She moved out of Bombay and continued to follow up through letters and over the next one year there was still further improvement.

On 22nd March 1997, she sent me a letter asking for further medication.

P: 'The headaches are bearable. I have reduced my medication to half of what it used to be.' "9.03.97: She is feeling much better. Her headaches are much better. She is happy and relaxed, but occasionally loses her temper with her son when he does not keep things in order. Her husband says that she is much better. Although she does have mood swings, she is much calmer. Her headaches are miraculously cured; earlier she used to scream with pain. She says of her mother-in-law: 'She was good woman despite everything.' She speaks about her in normal tones and does not harbor bad feelings towards her anymore, has made peace with her. Remedy not repeated." (R. Sankaran)

Case 4: Ulceration of throat, aggravation on the left side, difficulty of swallowing liquids, occurring five or six times a year, lasting two or three weeks at a time; attacks brought on by exposure to rain or wind; dislikes wet weather apart from the throat affection, never feels happy in wet weather. (C Hering)

Case 5: Pain in right lung for eight days; cannot turn to either side nor sit up without assistance; sleeplessness; sibilant rales with crepitation in both lungs; right lung sounds dull under mamma and near armpit to percussion; each inspiration causes a crackling sound; respiration very difficult, almost agonizing; vomiting all forenoon; diarrhœa all day; constant cough; urine like blood. Pneumonia. (C Hering)

Case 6: 1993 IFH Case Conference, by Eric Sommermann, PhD.

This case is still in progress. It cannot be presented yet as a cured case, but *Elaps* has had a definite positive action after many other remedies had failed. It is a case of a female with hemorrhagic fibroids who has been treated for about four years by a skilled homeopath. She received *Ignatia, Lachesis, Medorrhinum, Staphysagria, Lycopodium, Sulphur, Natrum muriaticum, Aurum muriaticum natronatum, Calcarea fluorica,* and *Phosphorus*. The *Phosphorus* seemed to work acutely to stop the bleeding, but then the bleeding would return. The fibroids had continued to grow, and a hysterectomy seemed imminent.

Initial Visit: January 6, 1993. Female, Age 50

Study Guide

This woman looks 35 and is attractively dressed in bright colors. She has an interesting but troubled history. It is an effort to get the case because she has a lot of trouble keeping her conversation focused. She is a talented but starving artist with a large portfolio. She grew up in a family of artists. Alcohol is a big problem in the family. All the men in her family have risen in the profession and have made good money. Her brothers were treated as budding artists and were helped on their way by her father.

She says that her father and brothers treat women like dogs. Her father was mean. He was the boss in the family and was very strict. She and her mother were his prisoners. She was afraid during her whole childhood, but she was the caretaker for the family. Her father was physically violent with her mother. Her mother was too easy and sweet. Her mother finally divorced her father, started drinking, and then died of a heart attack at 53.

Her father and brothers continued to use the patient and hold her down as an adult. She says her family has 'ripped her off' all her life. She feels they control the art scene and have prevented her from advancing. She began drinking. They then stole her material and made money from it, but never gave her any of the money. She eventually sobered up and sued them, but lost the suit. She says they bought off her lawyer, who also sexually harassed her. Yet, she still maintains a relationship with them. They call her all the time and won't leave her alone.

She has trouble expressing her anger toward these men. They don't take her seriously; they treat her like a little girl. She says her father doesn't know how she feels.

She is very angry with the attorney. She feels that she's been violated and that the law hasn't served her.

"For the last three months everything has been upside down. She has had a lot more stress during the holidays because her father was around again. She was really depressed. She gives presents to family members she doesn't like. She wants to fight but she's tired.

She is single and has had a lot of trouble in relationships. Men want to run her life. 'They start out nice and sweet. Then they want you to follow them and give up your own life. They think you want to be in their life.' She is trying to avoid the man in her most current relationship, but he doesn't leave her alone.

She does a lot of walking when she's angry. She tries to confront these men over the telephone, but they're not interested in it. She wants to scream.

She has a lot of menstrual bleeding (2), with big clots the last few days. She uses five or six pads a day for two weeks. She gets cramps in her uterus with the bleeding (2). Doctors have diagnosed fibroids with an enlarged uterus. They want to take the uterus out.

Fears high places (2). Fears snakes (3). She can't even see them on television or a picture of them. Fears someone will take control of her life.

She has recurring insomnia (2). She used to be a night owl. She has been taking Vasotec for high blood pressure for several years.

Case Analysis: I didn't feel I had many chances to prescribe for the case, because a hysterectomy appeared imminent. I gave *Phosphorus* 10M right away to stop the bleeding while I thought about the case. The *Phosphorus* didn't work.

Besides the emotional pathology and history, there were very few symptoms to use in this case. The main pathology contained only common symptoms, and there were few keynotes. All the main polychrest remedies had been tried and had failed.

I actually found the remedy by noting the similarities to the case of rhinitis I just described (*given earlier in Dr. Sommerman's IFH presentation*). Here is a woman who has a history of abusive relationships with men. She feels like a prisoner who can't escape or confront or regain power in the relationship. In both cases, they try to break off relationships by simply avoiding the person, which is ineffective on the whole. There seems to be no power to resist the men they attract, even though their sex drive is not excessive. They look younger than their age, and there is a certain vulnerability about them. They get treated like 'little girls' who don't know what's good for them.

There is a lot of suppressed anger, which manifests as a desire for revenge (in this case, the lawsuit). And there is a strong fear of snakes.

Apart from that, there are no other keynotes or guiding characteristics.

Elaps can be found under metrorrhagia, uterine fibroid, and clots. But these are common symptoms, and there is no characteristic black discharge as you would expect. I was far from certain in this case, but felt it was the best prescription I could make.

Plan: *Elaps* 200C, single dose.

First Follow-up: February 9, 1993

The bleeding stopped within a day of taking *Elaps*. She feels as if the remedy 'tightened her up.' She has had one menstrual cycle since the remedy. It was a normal five-day flow. This was her best cycle in a long time. Before, she couldn't get out of bed the first two days.

She was very mean with her boyfriend before her last menstrual cycle. He isn't what she wants. He has been saying that she is moody. Her father is still very hard to talk to, and she can't trust him. She can't stand where she lives, and he doesn't help out. They don't know how it hurts. They're the kind of men like the Anita Hill thing.

Her insomnia persists. It could be due to the Vasotec.

Assessment: She is experiencing a definite improvement. The family dynamics are difficult.

Plan: Wait.

Second Follow-up: March 22, 1993. Telephone consultation.

She has been bleeding excessively with clots for two days (2). It is coming out like water. Her energy is not great. She's in a fairly good mood. She recently changed blood pressure medication to a diazide derivative through an HMO doctor. She is going back on Vasotec.

Assessment: The remedy may have been antidoted.

Plan: *Elaps* 200C, single dose.

Third Follow-up: April 29, 1993

Her menses have been good. She is not sleeping much (2), probably due to Vasotec. Her mind doesn't stop. She thinks about how 'lousy' her family is. She gets wrapped up in the world's problems. She does a lot of creative work at night.

She is on Augmentin for a sinus infection and bronchitis.

"She has sidestepped her family in the art industry and has made financial arrangements for showing her work with promoters. She never thought she could do this before.

Assessment: She is doing fairly well.

Plan: 1. *Sulphur* 30C, twice a day for two days. (*No explanation here provided*)

EUPATORIUM PERFOLIATUM
(Thoroughwort)

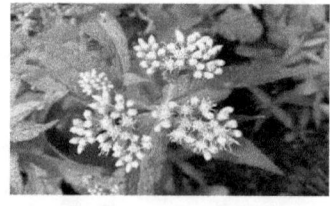

*Flu with a sensation that the **BONES** are **BROKEN**.*

Study Guide

Thirsty for cold drinks. Nausea from the smell of food.

Eupatorium is one of the most important remedies that can be used for influenza. A person that needs it will have all the typical symptoms of influenza, such as chills, fever, sore throat, headache, cough etc.

This remedy is indicated when the following additional and specific symptoms are present:
- *thirsty for cold drinks*
- Achy muscles and a SENSATION THAT THE BONES ARE BROKEN
- pain and achy feeling in the muscles and joints and especially *pain in the bones*
- very thirsty for cold drinks, drinks by the glassful
- aching pains in the back
- pain in the arms, legs and the wrists
- *nausea worse from the smell of food*
- *Headache worse from lying down*

If the patient is thirstless, then this remedy is not indicated and it would be better to try Rhus tox, Gelsemium or Arnica.

Case 1: Chest pain, cough, fever, weakness, sore throat. Feel as if the bones in my wrist had been broken in two. Thirsty. After Eupatorium I felt almost all better the next day.

EUPHRASIA
(Eyebright)

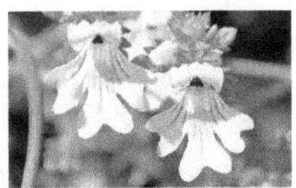

Hay fever with burning discharges from the eyes. Acrid lacrimation; it burns the cheeks. Cough with lacrimation (All-c, Puls, Nat-m, Squilla). Can't stop blinking. I once gave this remedy successfully to a person who was very allergic to her cat. Her tears would burn her cheeks.

The eyes water all the time and are agglutinated in the morning. The margins of the lids are red, swollen and burning. Fluent coryza in the morning with cough; worse from warmth and cold.

FERRUM METALLICUM
(Iron)

Flushing from slight exertion. Obesity with a red face. These people get angry from contradiction, they are very domineering, never give up and always want to get their own way. Of all of our remedies they have the the greatest determination and strong convictions. They tend to be overweight, red in the face, even bright red from slight exertion. Often noise can make

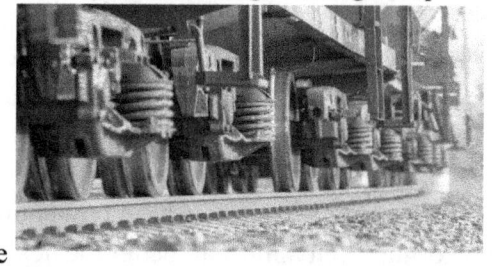

them angry. Think of a strong iron locomotive, nothing can stop it.

If they have itchy skin with Ferrum symptoms think of Ferrum sulphur.

FERRUM PHOSPHORICUM
(Phosphate of Iron)

Ferrum phosphoricum is indicated in the first stages of an *acute inflammation; such as a sore throat.*

A PALE FACE with CIRCUMSCRIBED RED FLUSHES OF THE CHEEKS. Tendency to be overweight and very difficult to loose weight.

Study Guide

For example, at the beginning of a cold, a sore ear, or a sore throat. Usually at this stage there are no unusual symptoms and there are very few core symptoms that need to be present in order to give it. But these may include: A PALE FACE with CIRCUMSCRIBED RED FLUSHES OF THE CHEEKS, *or a pale face alternating with flushing. Think of the complexion of Santa Clause.*

Mentally the person is *frustrated from the challenges of daily life - she is sympathetic, fair and persistent, but this daily grind is wearing her down.* So one can see this symptom could fit almost any person and that is why it is in fact a very common remedy.

Typically to one degree or another all Ferrum patients show very strong determination, they can be stubborrn and show anger from contradiction. Thier parents of these patients become easily exasperated as the Ferrum child no matter how small and sweet looking often do not comply to disapline, they will argue and seem to never give in.

Other symptoms that indicate Ferrum phosphoricum are:
- coughing up pure blood, with pneumonia
- congestion in the head and face, red face
- thirst for large quantities of water
- cough with a red face
- bronchitis in young children
- otitis media (*ear ache*) first stage
- hot palms of the hands
- difficult dentition (irritation of the gums from new teeth) in infants and young children
- pain in the forehead
- headache with a hot red face
- diarrhea with blood

Recommendation: give this remedy when the person has vague symptoms, the face is pale, some flushing and no other remedy fits better. Prescribe some vitamin C (500 mg a day) and cod liver oil, (one teaspoon a day) to help the immune system, rose hip tea with lemon and honey and plenty of bed rest.

Often the body is sick because it is in need of a break from the toils and tensions of life.

Ferrum phosphoricum will help strengthen the immune system and speed up the inevitable recovery. If the infection progresses the symptoms may become clear enough to give Belladonna, Chamomile or another remedy. Ferrum phosphoricum would be a good constitutional remedy to consider for a person who experiences anger from contradiction or frustration from an injustice. If this remedy is for the acute illness and chronic illness then they will often be obese as remedies with iron (Ferrum) in them are for people who gain weight easily and can't loose weight no matter how hard they try. Often these peole who are in need of this remedy for chronic ailments are very empathetic to others, social but also stubborn. They don't give up easily.

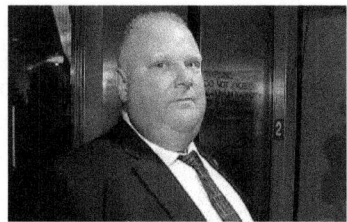

This person above has the typical complexion and body type for the Ferrum patient. It is mostly genetic, they would find it extremely difficult to loose weight no matter how much they exercise but this does not mean they do no benefit from the exercise. .

Note the red face but pale skin under the redness. These people can communicate easily have charisma (Phoshorus). ***Anger from contradiction;*** this anger is typical of all Ferrum patients. Ferrum patiens are usaully honest and well meaning but one can't easily get them to change their mind.

It is thought that Margaret Thatcher had one of the Ferrum constitutions. - they called her the 'iron lady' as she would not bend her opinions easily. Perhaps Kali-ferrum - Conservative and rigid.

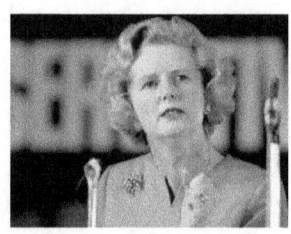

Study Guide

For most acute ailments it is recommended to give one dose of the 30c and wait at three hours to see if there is a reaction. If the patient is improving the remedy does not have to be repeated. If the symptoms start to return or stop improving; then repeat the remedy. If there is no improvement after twelve to eighteen hours then search for a better remedy. The more severe the symptoms the faster the patient should improve if the remedy is correct.

GELSEMIUM
(Yellow Jasmine)

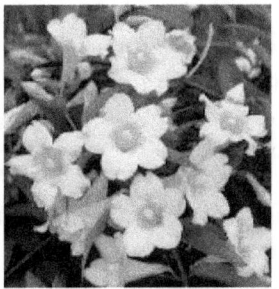

Shock - FEAR: *trembling, can't think, weakness.* **RUNS AWAY, wants to escape.**

Compare with Aconite: both go into shock from fear. Gelsemium has more weakness Aconite more palpitation and hyperventilation.

The fear that is generated in the Gelsemium person is depicted in this famous painting by Francisco Goya's (1746-1826). Goya has massed his figures in four distinct groups...those already dead, those about to be

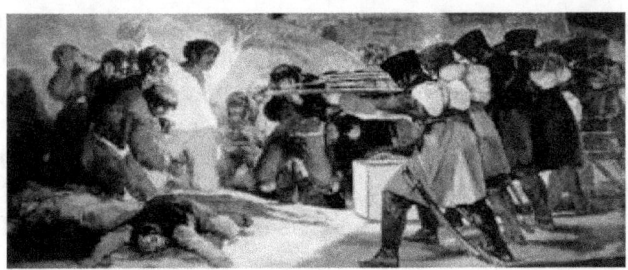

Materia Medica

shot, those waiting to be placed before the rifles, and the firing squad itself. In these real life situations the helpless victim is pleaing for mercy, **they tremble, loose control of their bladder and bowel and become paralyzed with fear.**

If a patient were to survives this type of fright such as war or attack from an enemy the nervous system can be severely damadged, resulting in a loss of muscle strength, PTSD, chronic anxiety etc.

More common examples include fear before a piano recital, fear after a confrontation or near car accident, fear from a job interview. The police officer went into shock after being shot at. Fear affected her in such a way that she lost her memory during the math exam. FEAR TO FAIL.

Cowardice, trembleing: he feels trapped in a relationship; wnts to run away. He feels that at work too much is expected of him so he stays home and gives up his profession.

At the stoplight his car was hijacked at gunpoint; she lost control of her bowel and could not stop trembleing.

Gelsemium is also one of the first remedies to think of for influenza.

There are specific symptoms that indicate its use, which are.
- *dull thinking*
- *drowsiness*
- *THIRSTLESS*
- *desire to be alone*
- *INDIFFERENCE TOWARD EVERYTHING*

A general feeling of profound <u>weakness and lack of stamina on all levels</u>. For example the muscles become weak, the person only wants to lie and rest. There is weakness of the emotions as they do not want to face the challenges of life any longer. The responsibilities of life seem to get too overwhelming and the person develops *a lack of self confidence.*

This desire to avoid everything further makes them retreat to their room and avoid visitors. *Fear of commitment in a relationship.* Nervous breakdwon from work; wants to stay at home, wants to avoid people completely; *cowardly.*

Study Guide

Gelsemium will build confidence when there are no physical symptoms and can therefore be used for situations such as: <u>stage fright, before an examination, or before a job interview</u>. In these situations, as well as the influenza, there may be diarrhea that is triggered by the anxiety.

In the later stages of the flu there can develop:
- *mental dullness and weakness* of memory
- a desire to be left alone
- timidity
- apathy
- aversion to confrontations (Magnesiums, Silicas)
- *fear of responsibility*
- complaints, from fear and anticipation
- trembling from exertion
- chill alternate with flushes of heat
- heaviness of the head
- *drooping and falling of the lids of the eyes*
- headache in the occiput, (back of the head) which radiates to the forehead (Opposite: Viola which has a frontal headache that radiates to the occiput).

Also, may experience:
- sore throat with difficulty in swallowing
- tonsillitis
- swallowing causes pain in the ear
- heaviness in the chest
- the heart feels it will stop beating, better if he moves about
- sleepless from anxiety
- shaking chills

On needing Gelsemium for the flu the patient will have almost <u>*no thirst*</u>. The patient will not drink very much, only one or two drinks a day. This is what distinguishes it from Eupatorium perfoliatum, the next closest remedy. The Eupatorium patients desire large quantities of cold drinks; while the Gelsemium patient does not want to drink. A few times I have seen this remedy work very well for anticipation anxiety when there was a lot of thirst for small sips as the mouth was so dry.

Compare with: Lycopodium; both have lack of conficence and want to run away from responsibility. Lycopodium is more selffish, they seek out superficial gratification and can try to dominate others. Gelsemium is more mild, yielding and averse to confrontation.

GINSENG

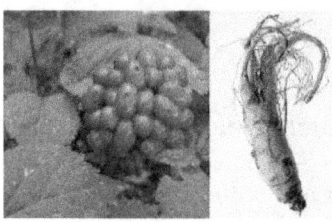

Love of work. Endurance for work ----------> burnout.

Desire to and enjoy to work 14 to 16 hours per day. Similar to other stimulants such as Coca, Coffea and Kola. Ginseng gets hiccup easily. *They feel tranquil and courageous in dangerous situations such as a car accident or house fire.* They have a clear head in these situation and seem to know just what is the right thing to do. Sciatica, lumbago. Tonsillitis. Menstrual cramps.

Stomach ulcers with vomiting after eating. Not as irritable as Coffea. Not as easily offended as Kola. Kola can also work for many hours or even a double shift but they like to do two things at once which annoys their partner. For example when their partner talks to them they want to read a book or play a video games all at the dame time. Ginseng has the most even vitality to work over many hours.

Coca is also a remedy for people who love to work but they want to work at things that are very challenging such as build a rocket to mars or try to find a cure for cancer.

Study Guide

GLONOIN
(Nitroglycerin)

C3H5N3O9

THROBBING pains worse heat. (Bell, Com).

Glonoin is the first remedy to consider for the symptoms of <u>sunstroke.</u> **Headache with mental confusion.**

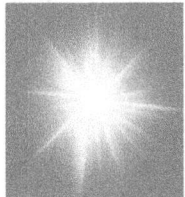

Example: In the cases which I have treated, the person usually experienced a *severe throbbing headache, the blood seemed to rise to the head causing flushing* and a sensation as if the head would blow off or explode.

Case 1: In one case the headache was so severe the patient could hardly speak. She was given a dose of Glonoin 30c, went to sleep and awakened to feel much improved. Typically, the person needing Glonoin has a surging of blood to the head, which gives a feeling that the head has become enormously large, accompanied with a violent headache. Other symptoms include, ***pulsating pain, a hot, pale face, dizzy feelings, fainting spells, and nausea and vomiting.***

Chronic: Migraine headaches, surging of blood to the head. ***Gets lost*** in well known streets. Supressed anger.

Case 2: She has blinding headaches. She gets lost trying to drive home with the headache. Her mother is trying to force her into a marriage, she feels she can's disobey yer mother. Suppressed anger. After Glonoin the headaches are all better. She marries a different man she loves and her mother is also happy about this.

GRAPHITES
(Carbon)

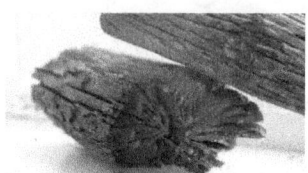

Can't loose weight, STOCKY build. This is the build where no amount of exercise or diet can affect a change in weight. The exercise is still of great benefit though. Many Carbon remedies have this same problem: Adamas, Carbo-veg, Calc-c, Kali-c, etc).

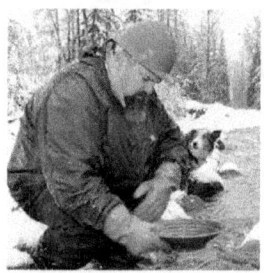

Typical build of Graphites.

Callosites on the hands or feet. Eruptions behind the ears.
This is another remedy that can be used for ear infections. The main symptom to look for is that when there is pain and obstruction in the ear the person has a *strong desire to swallow often*. Usually the left ear is worse. Puss exudes from the ears.

Other symptoms are:
- Impaired hearing. Noises in the ears
- Moist eczema of the ear or behind the ear with itching
- Like Belladonna there is a strong sensitivity to light
- *Aversion to sweets and salt*

Case 1: I had a patient who had various chronic physical and emotional symptoms, skin cancer being one of them. He said: "I have never liked salt, I never use it because of that." Based on this symptom alone I gave him Graphites and over the next few months all his complaints were cured. I caled him a few years later to see how he was doing and he reported that none of his symptoms had ever returned.

Sometimes there are many general symptoms in a case that do not especially indicate one remedy above another. Then one has to find at least one unusual symptom and give the remedy based on that peculiarity.

Graphites has been known to cure the following symptoms: Obesity. But I have also seen it work in people who were of normal weight. Unhealthy skin, rough, hard, thick, dryness, cracking, inability to perspire, dandruff. Eczema with a sticky, honey like discharge. Thick calluses on the hands or feet.

Emotionally may be:
- *Irresolute*
- Weeping especially from music

Physically may have:
- Constipation, with large stool
- Agglutinated (sticky) eyelids in the morning
- Eczema of the eye lids
- Cracking in the corners of the mouth
- Cramping pains in the stomach, which are better from hot drinks especially hot milk.
- Chilliness and a sensitivity to cold

Newborn babies blow bubbles when crying, have eczema of the face. With teenage girls, the menses are suppressed or delayed.

HEPAR SULPHUR
(Burned Calcium Sulphide)

Chily, LACK OF VITAL HEAT, feels insecure - dependent on others.

Hepar Sulph is a powerful and deep acting medicine. It is indicated for some of the most *severe and chronic* infections possible, such as:

- colds
- influenza
- bronchitis
- pharyngitis
- otitis media
- tonsillitis
- sinusitis
- croup, abscesses, boils and
- pneumonia, appendicitis, peritonitis, nephritis, enodcarditis.

In order to use it with accuracy the following 'picture' of symptoms needs to be present.

CHILLY AND AGGRAVATION FROM COLD, INTOLERANT TO BECOMING COLD and even when one part of the body becomes cold or exposed there is a _shiver_ of _coldness felt throughout the rest of the body._ This can happen for example when someone is in bed and puts one hand out of the covers. Immediately the rest of the body gets a chill from this.

So the Hepar person will be _worse_ from _uncovering and intolerant to drafts._ Ears sensitive and painful to the wind and open air. Better from heat, warm wraps, warm room and a hot bath.

If you ask the question, 'So are you more sensitive to cold or heat?' and the person says: 'I am not really sure, as I am sometimes bothered by the heat and a little worse from the cold.' This response indicates that Hepar can't be the correct medicine. They must be able to spontaneously say, 'I am so chilly since I got sick, my body is so difficult to keep warm, if I uncover I get cold all over again, even if I put one foot out of the covers my whole body gets cold.' With this answer there is a strong possibility that Hepar will be the correct medicine.

There are very few other remedies that have this degree of sensitivity to coldness and so it becomes the *most reliable general symptom* on which to base the prescription of Hepar. Lack of vital heat can't stay warm. Gen; heat, lack of vital: (Camph, Hep, Verat. etc).

The next most important symptoms are as follows: Swelling and hardening of the cervical glands which can be felt by palpation.

Study Guide

A tendency toward *suppuration* and discharges of mucous from any mucous membrane. This could, for example, be pus in the middle ear leading to a bulging ear drum, pains in the ear, or eventually an ear drum that bursts spontaneously from the pressure of the puss. Catarrh (a runny nose) or a collection the pus in the eustachian tube that causes a pain in the ear. Difficulty in hearing, caused by the above conditions.

Tonsillar abscess, boils, acne, cysts, all are very sensitive to touch. These are all examples of the same process of suppuration and can occur in any part of the body; the gums, the roots of the teeth, beside the nails, at the base of the spine, in the ovaries, and on the back.

Pus gives off an offensive, sour odour. Stitching or splinter-like pains, especially felt in the throat. Intense sensitivity to pain. Complains intensely, as seen in someone needing Chamomile.

Desire to eat fatty foods, sour foods, vinegar, pickles and hot spicy foods. A tendency toward allergic type reactions to chemicals, pollen, dust. Typical they have hay fever symptoms, such as sneezing, watery eyes, itching. Various types of chronic coughs. May have a fear of bees.

The emotional disposition of Hepar in not always present in the person who needs this medicine. If it is present, then the certainty of it working is much greater and not only will the symptoms of inflammation get better but the temperament will also improve.

In general the Hepar person is in a state of extreme sensitivity to the external environment. So this becomes true on the emotional level as well, experienced as a type of hypersensitivity to any negative stimulus.

<u>There is a type of insecurity that only improves when there is a guaranteed comfort.</u> Small stresses, such as being left alone in the house, can be intolerable for the Hepar child or adult patient. A child may not want to be in their room alone. They feel they need protection because of this great sensitivity. They feel traumatized by watching or hearing about anything cruel.

There may have been some kind of trauma that led to this insecurity and sensitivity but the fact that it remains, is the reason to consider the use of Hepar. It is often difficult for a person to admit to these feeling of overdependence, sensitivity to unfairness, timidity, lack of confidence and they will not be so apparent unless one gently and respectively asks in a non-judgemental way such as; How do you feel when alone? What things have you done that have been totally independent of what other people wanted or expected of you? If you don't like your situation why don't you leave? This type of inquiry may reveal to you the state of vulnerability that is found in a person that needs Hepar.

For example I had a patient with a large golf ball sized boil on her knee. It had been there for a few years. The abscess was so deeply rooted into the tissues of the knee that surgery was not an option. She told me the story of how she was adopted into a large family and expected to do all the work. A kind of Cinderella story.

While the other children were given elaborate birthday partieses hers was often forgotten or in later years she was not invited to family events. She felt extreemely vulnerable, first of her he birth parents had forsaken her and now this new family was also neglecting her.

She was very hurt, but also angry but could not show the anger or else she could suffer more rejection, become homeless or suffer exposure to the harsh elements. After Hepar the boil and abscess totally resolved. She became a lot more outspoken but in a way that allowed her family to realize the pain they had caused her. As a sesult she was treated with more respect and felt closer to them all.

The next clue to the emotional state can be found in the symptom of swelling, pus, and allergic tendency. These are processes in the body that are *hyperactive* reactions. Those reactions that are excessive and more than is necessary. On the emotional level the expression of this same hyperactive process ranges from mild irritability, to a feeling of **constant inner anger and indignation, suppressed anger, temper tantrums, fits of anger, and even violent anger.**

In countries where we see people suppressed there is always the possibility of violence.

Racism, sexism etc are all examples where discrimation can lead to suppression and eventual violence.

Study Guide

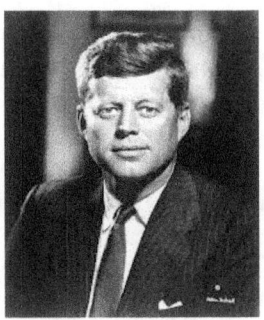

"Those who make peaceful revolution impossible will make violent revolution inevitable"- John F. Kennedy.

Festering anger and festering abscess are different branches on the same tree as are exploding boils and the exploding anger. Those needing Heper can become impatient, abusive and quarrelsome from the least cause. He may even be so angry that he has the impulse to kill.

Chronic infections and ***chronic unforgiveness,*** sensitivity to cold, sensitivity to lack of emotional warmth are two more examples. The root cause of all these examples is the same and that is what the body cures when Hepar is given.

I like this image of Geronimo because you can see the grief, vulnerability, fear, disbelief, hurt, anger, defiance and lonliness all together. These traits a typical in Hepar and Causticum.

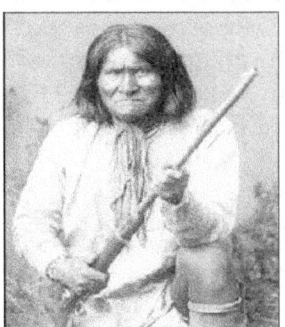

Those who fight against injustice are often beaten down, given no voice and so they resort to violence.

These people often get infections but to give antibiotics does nothing to heal the source of the infection which is the immune system that is not working as it should. The antibiotics at best only temporarily take away the bacteria just as one can try and kill the flies that come to live at the garbage dump. Once the antibiotics run out the infections will usually return because the internal constitutional environment is prone to an infection, just like those flies are attracted to the smell of rotting garbage. If the cells of the body are strong, fed with healthy food and given a remedy like Hepar then the inner environment will be changed and the cells of the body will no longer attract but rather become immune to any virus or bacteria.

The person needing Hepar sulphar commonly has suffered *an emotional injury or a situation of abuse,* and subsequently are not strong enough to react and overcome the situation. Perhaps they are too young or the stress was too much for them. The trauma is therefore internalized and the cycle of shame and insecurity begins. But within the deepest parts of the person's identity, there is the conviction that what happened to them was an injustice and so over time this sense of indignation gets stronger until it finally erupts as physical symptoms or emotional anger. The rage can become intense, leading to homocidal tendencies, radical ideas, revolutionary and destructive. There is often an impulse to kill those who have offened them (Lach, Scorp, Hyos, Stram). Severe anger from injustice can also be found in Causticum and Halialeetus.

As was mentioned earlier someone can need Hepar and not have all these emotional dilemmas because the emotional level may be healthy and the expression of the imbalance is therefore only expressed as frequent colds or an acute ear infection. The modalities of physical symptoms - such as the cough being very sensitive to cold air; and the general symptoms will still indicate the use of Hepar if in fact it is the simillimum.

Hepar is made from sulphur heated with calcium. Hahnemann did the proving of this medicine about 200 years ago. I have seen it make order out of chaos, bring a sense of peace to people with tortured lives and heal where nothing else would. In the end people have to be healed with the remedy that is a catalyst. It is better to treat the person as a whole. When they are healed, then they can cure whatever illness they many have.

Study Guide

HYDRASTIS
(Golden Seal)

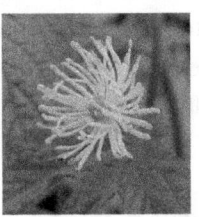

<u>Mucous in strings from any portal</u>. Sinusitis. Thick ropy secretions from sinuses, stomach, uterus or bladder. Ropy vomiting. Headaches especially when related to constipation. Tongue white, swollen and show the imprint of the teeth (Merc). Liver is tender with gallstones. Weak digestion.

All gone sensation not better from eating. Fissure of edges of tongue and rectum. Chest inflammation with thick tenacious expectoration. Ulcers and cancer. Weakness, cold sweats, Weak memory, can't remember what he is reading or talking about. Vindictive, angry, spiteful, ready to snub anyone. Aversion to go out or do anything. Compare to Kali-bichromicum.

HYOSCYAMUS
(Henbane)

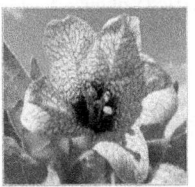

<u>Jealousy</u>, suspicion, anger violence. UNCONTROLLED EMOTIONS, leading to fights, lots of screaming and accusations. For example the husband is late getting home; his wife does not believe that he was in a meeting at work, she starts

an argument and accuses him of having an affair. They fight about it for hours; eventually she wants to kill him. This is typical for Hyoscyamus; they love their partner so much that it makes them feel too vulnerable to being abandoned. They become jealous and suspicious for almost no reason. They often have a high sexual desire or act in a shameless manner. Muscle spasms or twitchings.

Case 1: She would take off her clothes at work for anyone who asked. (Repertory: Mind, Naked, wants to be. And Mind, Shameless).

Case 2: Often he would beat up on his girlfriend when she was late coming home as he thought she was going to leave him.

Case 3: She had epilepsy, and wanted to kill her husband because he was not being faithful. After Hyos her anger, suspicion and seizures all abated.

In many cases the sexuality is suppressed and there are more subtle expressions of this remedy; like we see here:

Case 4: Very severe acne, as a teen he fell in love, was then rejected and it almost 'killed him' as his emotions were so tied to her. Since then for 20 years he would not let himself have a girlfriend or even any friends at all. (Vithoulkas seminar 1989)

Hpathy.com: *One common etiology of the Hyoscyamus state is emotional neglect in childhood (delusion, deserted, forsaken). This stress leads to adaptation in the will to have one's emotional needs met. The Hyoscyamus person can gain attention by shocking, annoying or provocative speech and behavior (inciting others, mocking, mania to ridicule, disposition to contradict, desire to fight). Hyoscyamus individuals may tell risqué jokes or act like 'clowns' (jesting), and although not listed in the books, some Hyoscyamus individuals describe an attraction to, dislike or fear of clowns. The desire for attention leads some to behave like chameleons when in company, but these multiple persona undermine a truer sense of self-identity, as the desire for attention distracts them (and those in their company!). The sense of self-esteem or self-worth is often very low, and Hyoscyamus individuals may feel a strong sense of guilt (anxiety of conscience, delusion that he is a criminal, self-reproach).*

They can experience great difficulties learning to be vulnerable in a relationship. The Hyoscyamus adult has not been taught to trust, or if they did trust in the past, the trust was broken. So to have someone really 'see' them, with all their fears and defenses exposed, can be very threatening. They may expend a great effort to maintain defenses against this possibility (deceitful, sly).

Hyoscyamus characteristics can be found in such positive rubrics as precocity, intellectual, introspection, inquisitive, and clairvoyance. Hyoscyamus may be compared to Pulsatilla (complementary–Hyoscyamus demonstrates a more extreme need for attention), magnesiums (fears of abandonment), Lachesis and other animal remedies (loquacity, themes of attractiveness), Veratrum (themes of persecution), thuja (chameleon personality, reproaches oneself) and Belladonna and Stramonium (other members of the solanaceae family). The reader may read the proving and examine other rubrics for Hyoscyamus in order to fill out the above description.

In summary (with apologies to Shakespeare!), the Hyoscyamus state can be respectfully characterized as: 'To be exposed or not to be exposed, that is the question.'

Nervous system: Hyoscyamus is full of convulsions, contractions, trembling, quivering and jerkings of the muscles. Convulsions in vigorous people, coming on with great violence. Convulsions that involve the whole economy, with unconsciousness, coming on in the night. Convulsions in women at the menstrual period; and then the lesser convulsions of single muscles, and contractions of single muscles.

Little jerkings and twitchings. In low forms of the disease it takes on the latter, jerkings and twitchings of muscles. In low typhoid states where there is great prostration with twitching. He feels it himself if conscious, enough to realize it, but others see it. An evidence of great prostration of the nervous system. Sliding down in bed, twitching of the muscles.

Suspicion runs through acute sickness; it runs through the mania in insanity. Suspicion that his wife is going to poison him; that his wife is untrue to him. Suspicious of everybody. Wants to kill everyone.

"Refuses to take medicine because it is poisoned."

"Imagines, that he is pursued, that the people have all turned against him, that his friends are no longer his friends.

He carries on conversations with imaginary people."

Lying there picking the bedclothes, and muttering. Even when he is in a stupor and realizes nothing apparently, that is going on, he makes passive motions, mutters, talks to himself, and once in a while utters a shrill scream. Picking his fingers, just as if he had something in his fingers when there is nothing there. He picks at the bedclothes the same way. Picking at his nightshirt, or picking anything he get his fingers on. Or, picking in the air, grasping as if he were grasping at flies. (Hpathy.com)

IODUM
(Iodine)

Hyperthyroid, restless, worse from heat, emaciation and hypogycemia.

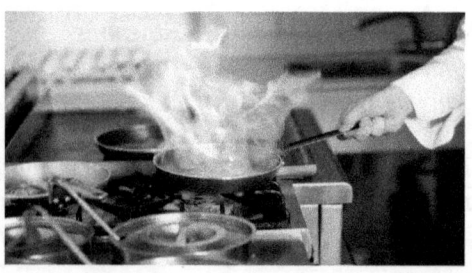

The burners (mitochondria) are turned on high and as a result there is too much energy with restlessness.

Study Guide

Everything is done in a *hurry. These people need open cool air and are worse from a warm room.* The thyroid gland produces too much T3, they are loosing weight and have to eat often. *Many symptoms from missing a meal.*

Here is what H C Allen has to say about this remedy: *Persons of scrofulous diathesis, with dark or black hair and eyes; a low cachectic condition, with profound debility and great <u>emaciation</u> (Abrot.).*

Great weakness and loss of breath on going upstairs (Calc.); during menses (Alum , Carbo an. , Coc.).

Ravenous hunger; eats freely and well, yet loses flesh all the time (Abrot. , Nat. m. , Sanic. , Tub.).

Empty eructations from morning to nigh, as if every particle of food was turned into air (Kali c.).

Suffers from hunger, must eat every few hours; anxious and worried if he does not eat (Cina , Sulph.); feels > while eating or after eating, when stomach is full.

Itching: low down in the lungs, behind the sternum, causing cough; extends through bronchi to nasal cavity (Coc. c., Con. , Phos.).

Hypertrophy and induration of glandular tissue – thyroid, mammae, ovaries, testes, uterus, prostate or other glands – breasts may dwindle and become flabby.

Hard goiter, in dark haired persons (light haired, Brom.); feels > after eating.

Palpitation, worse from least exertion (compare, Dig. – from least mental exertion, Cal. ars.).

Sensation as if the heart was squeezed together; as if grasped with an iron hand (Cact. , Sulph.).

Leucorrhoea: acrid, corrosive, staining and corroding the linen; most abundant at time of menses.

Cancerous degeneration of the cervix; cutting pains in abdomen and hemorrhage at every stool.

Constipation, with ineffectual urging > by drinking cold milk.

Croup: membranous, hoarse, dry cough, worse in warm, wet weather; with wheezing and sawing respiration (Spong.).

Child grasps at larynx (Cepa); face pale and cold, especially in fleshy children.

Relations. – Complementary: to, Lycopodium.

Compare: Kali-iod, Calc-iod, Ferrum-iod, Nat-iod, Mag-iod, Bar-iod, Acet-ac., Brom., Con., Kali-bi., Spong. in membranous croup and croupy affections; especially in overgrown boys with scrofulous diathesis. (Allen)

Case 1: Child of three. Very thin, restless, never wants to wear any clothing. Her body is like a furnace. She is very irritable if gets hungry so often will take food without asking every two hours. After Iodum 30c much better in all respects.

IPECACUANHA
(Ipecac root)

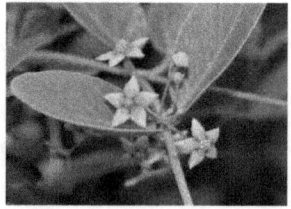

Cough with gagging and almost vomiting. Anger and disdain.

Chronic nausea when <u>there is anger or disgust at something.</u> He <u>holds everything in contempt.</u> The feeling of disgust is so strong they have to remove themselves from the situation.

Study Guide

Discontented, capricious (Ant-c, Cham, Cina).

Case 1: He hated the idea that people were making money from selling things at Christmas so he would no participate in any aspect of the holiday with his family of friends. He had chronic nausea as his chief complaint. After Ipecac his nausea is all better and he feels more accepting.

2: He hates society so goes and lives in the mountains alone and off the grid. He has a chronic cough with gagging at the end of the coughing spell.

3: She hates men after being raped and has chronic nausea since the trauma. All of these patients benefited from Ipecac.

Here is what the genius Kent had to say about this remedy:
Ipecac. has a wide sphere of action among acute sickness. Most of its acute complaints commence with nausea, vomiting.

The febrile conditions commence with pain in the back between the shoulders, extending down the back, as if it would break, with or without rigors, much fever, vomiting of bile and seldom any thirst. This is the general aspect of the beginning of an Ipecac fever or gastric. trouble or chill in intermittent or bilious attacks.

The stomach is disordered. There is a sense of fullness in the stomach, cutting pains in the stomach and below the stomach, going from left to right. The cutting pain in colic goes from left to right. The patient is unable to stir or breathe until that pain passes off. It holds him transfixed in one position, coming like the stabbing of a knife in the region of the stomach, or above the navel, going from left to right, and is attended with prostration and nausea.

Nausea: All the complaints in Ipecac. are attended more or less with nausea; every little pain and distress is attended with nausea. The sufferings seem to center about the stomach, bringing on nausea.

There is continuous nausea, and gagging. The cough causes nausea and vomiting. It is a dry, hacking, teasing, suffocative cough, accompanied by nausea and vomiting. He coughs until his face grows red, and then there is choking and gagging. With every little gush of blood from any part of the body there is nausea, fainting and sinking.

Hence its value in uterine hemorrhages; bright, red blood with nausea; a little blood is attended with fainting or syncope, but the great overwhelming nausea runs through the complaints of this remedy. Though there is sometimes thirst, it is usually absent. When Ipecac. does its best work, there is thirstlessness.

With the Ipecac. fever, or with the chill, there is likely to be pain in the back of the head, a bruised pain through the head and back of the neck and sometimes down the back, and drawing in the muscles of the back of the neck. A congestive fullness in the head, a crushed feeling in the head and back of the head; the whole head aches and is full of pain.

Ipecac. is sometimes as restless as Arsenic., but the Ipecac prostration comes by spells, whereas the Arsenic prostration is continuous. You will see Ipecac patients tossing over the bed as much as they do when they need Rhus, turning and tossing, and moving the hands and feet, with restlessness.

This is especially the case when the spine is somewhat involved. Ipecac has symptoms that look like tetanus it has opisthotonos, and it has been a useful remedy in cerebro-spinal meningitis with vomiting of bile, with pain in the back of the head and neck, and drawing of the muscles of the back, retracting the head.

Study Guide

Stomach: When cerebro-spinal meningitis has gone on until the patient is emaciated, when remedies have seemed but to palliate momentarily, and the whole body is inclined backwards, and there is vomiting of everything, even the simplest article taken into the stomach, the tongue is red and raw, and there is constant nausea and vomiting of bile, Ipecac will cure.

Ipecac cures inveterate cases of gastritis when even a drop of water will not stay down; everything put in the stomach is vomited, continuous gagging, sharp pain in the stomach, pain in the back, below the shoulder blades, as if it would break, vomiting of bile, continuous nausea and great prostration. Irritable stomach. It also cures when the abdomen is distended, and sensitive, a tympanic state, when there is vomiting of bile.

Ipecac has proved a useful remedy in epidemic dysentery, when the patient is compelled to sit almost constantly upon the stool and passes a little slime, or a little bright red blood; inflammation of the lower portion of the bowel, the rectum and the colon. The tenesmus is awful, burning, and continuous urging with the passage of only a little mucus, and blood. With this there is constant nausea; while straining at stool, the pain is so great that nausea comes on, and he vomits bile. At times, whole families are down with it. It runs through a whole valley and may be epidemic, but it commonly relates to endemics.

In infants, it is indicated when a cholera-like diarrhea has been present and it ends in a dysenteric state, with continued tenesmus, and the expulsion of a little bloody mucus, the child vomiting everything it takes into the stomach; nausea, vomiting, prostration and great pallor. It is also useful in such conditions when the stool is more or less copious, and is green, and the child passes, frequently, copious quantities of green slime. Much crying when at stool, much straining, with passages of green slime, vomiting of green slime, and vomiting of green curds; milk turns green and is vomited.

Chest: The chest complaints of Ipecac. are interesting. Ipecac is especially the infant's friend and is commonly indicated in the bronchitis of infancy. The usual bad cold that ends in chest trouble in infants is a bronchitis.

It is very seldom that an infant gets a true pneumonia, it is generally a bronchitis with coarse rattling. The child coughs, gags and suffocates, and there is coarse rattling which can be heard throughout the room, and the trouble has come on pretty rapidly. The child is pale, looks dreadfully sick, and sometimes looks very anxious. The nose is drawn in as if dangerously ill, and the breathing is such as appears in a dangerous case. Ipecac. will sometimes modify this into a very simple case, break up the cold, and cure the child.

In the old books, the pneumonia of infancy had a distinct and separate description, and the typical symptoms were those of Ipecac. You will see a great similarity of symptoms when you study Ipecac. and Ant. tart. together in chest troubles. If you have been studying them together, you will say,

"How do you distinguish them; they both have rattling cough and breathing, and both have the vomiting?"

Well, the Ipecac. symptoms correspond to the stage of irritation, while the Tartar emetic symptoms appear in the stage of relaxation. That is, the Ipecac symptoms come on hurriedly, come on as the acute symptoms, whereas the Tartar emetic complaints come on slowly. The latter is seldom suited to symptoms that arise within twenty-four hours, or at least the symptoms of Tartar emetic (Antimonium tart) that arise in twenty-four hours are not of this class. (Antimonium tart is also full of contempt).

This group comes on many days later, comes on at the close of a bronchitis when there is threatened paralysis of the lungs; not in *the state of irritation, not the dyspnoea from irritation, not the suffocation of that sort, but the suffocation from exudation, and from threatened paralysis of the lungs.*

When the lungs are too weak to expel the mucus the coarse rattling comes on. Then there is the great exhaustion, deathly pallor of the face and sooty nostrils.

We see now that these two remedies do not look alike. If we observe the pace of the two remedies, we see that the complaints differ. It is not so much that they belong to stages, although they do, but rather that Ipecac brings on its symptoms rapidly and effects a crisis speedily, and that Ant. tart. brings on its symptoms slowly and effects a crisis after many days.

You can readily see the value of Ipecac in whooping cough, for it has the paroxysmal character, the red face, and vomiting and gagging with the cough. The red face, thirstlessness, violent whooping, with convulsions, with gagging and vomiting of all that he eats are the symptoms that you will generally find.

Hemorrhages: I have hinted at the hemorrhages, and these open out a great field for Ipecac I could not practice medicine without ipecac, because of its importance in hemorrhages. When I say hemorrhages, I do not mean those from cut arteries, I do not mean hemorrhages where surgery must come in; I mean such as uterine hemorrhages, hemorrhages from the kidneys, from the bowels, from the stomach, from the lungs.

You must know your remedies in hemorrhages; if you do not, you will be forced to use mechanical means; but the homeopathist who is well instructed is able to do without them. In the severest form of uterine hemorrhages, the homeopathic physician is able to do without mechanical means, except when mechanical means are causing the hemorrhage.

This does not relate to hourglass contractions, it does not relate to conditions when the after birth is retained, or when the uterus has a foreign substance in it, because under such circumstances manipulation is necessary.

A distinction must be made. But when we have simply the pure dynamic element to consider, simply and purely a relaxed surface that is bleeding, the remedy is the only thing that will do the work properly. When the uterus is continuously oozing, but every little while the flow increases to a gush, and with every little gush of bright red blood the woman thinks she is going to faint, or there is gasping, and the quantity of the flow is not sufficient to account for such prostration, nausea, syncope, pallor, Ipecac is the remedy.

When with the gushing of bright red blood there is an overwhelming fear of death, Aconite. If your patient while going through the confinement has had a hot head, an uncontrollable thirst for ice cold water, and after the confinement, everything has gone on in an orderly way, and the placenta has been delivered, and although you have no reason to expect such hemorrhage it comes on, Phosphorus will nearly always be the remedy.

In those withered women, lean and slender, who are always suffering from the heat, who want the covers off and want to be cool, who have had a tendency to ooze blood from the uterus, and now have a hemorrhage that is alarming either with clots, or only an oozing of dark liquid blood, you can hardly do without Secale. A single dose of any one of these medicines on the tongue will check a hemorrhage more quickly than large doses of strong medicine.

The hemorrhage will be checked so speedily that in your earlier experiences you will be surprised. You will wonder if it is not possible that it stopped itself. In copious menstruation Ipecac. is

Study Guide

often indicated When the woman has taken cold, or has a shock. In cases where she is not especially subject to copious uterine flow at the menstrual period, she is naturally alarmed, for it is something she has never had before, and the flow is likely to continue for many days, attended with this weakness. All her power seems to go with a little gush of blood. Ipecac. will cure and end the menstrual flow normally. A fortunate thing in nature is the tendency to check hemorrhage, which is always good.

There are a large number of medicines that control hemorrhage, and these you must keep at your finger's ends. They belong to emergencies. You must know the remedies that correspond to violent symptoms and violent attacks. Ipecac is full of hemorrhage. Vomiting of great clots of blood, continuous vomiting of blood in connection with ulceration. In persons who are subject to violent attacks of bleeding, who bleed easily, who have a hemorrhagic tendency, Ipecac will control temporarily the hemorrhage when the symptoms agree.

Urines: Severe pain in the back in the region of the kidneys, shooting pains, frequent urging to urinate, and the urine contains blood and little clots of blood. The urine is extremely red with blood, which settles to the bottom of the vessel, and lines the whole commode with a layer of blood the thickness of a knife blade. Every pint of urine that it contains will have that coating of blood in the vessel; every attack of pain in the kidney is attended with that condition of the urine. Ipecacuanha will stop that bleeding. It is true that when patients have bled until they have become anemic, and are subject to dropsy, Ipecac ceases to be the remedy; its natural follower then is China, which will bring the patient in a position to need an antipsoric remedy.

Colds: Then there are the "colds."

Simple, common coryzas among the children. When a cold

settles in the nose, and the nose is stuffed up at night or when the adult has a coryza, with much stuffing up of the nose, blowing of mucus and blood from the nose, much sneezing, and the cold goes further down and is followed by hoarseness, extending into the trachea with rawness, and finally into the bronchial tubes with suffocation and settling in the chest, think of ipecac.

The Ipecac. colds often begin in the nose and spread very rapidly into the chest. With these colds in the nose there is copious bleeding of bright red blood. Every time he takes cold in the nose he has copious bleeding; a tendency to nosebleed with the colds. The inflammation that comes upon the mucous membrane in Ipecac. is violent.

The irritation comes on suddenly, and the mucous membrane inflames so rapidly that the parts become purple, turgescent, and bleeding seems to be the only natural relief. Stoppage of the nose and loss of smell; the nose becomes so stuffed up that he cannot breathe through it.

With the head symptoms, with the colds, with the whooping cough, with the chill, and with many of the inflammatory complaints, the face becomes flushed, bright red, or bluish red, and the lips blue; with the chill the lips and the finger nails are blue. The chill is violent, sometimes congestive in character and often a rigor. The whole frame shakes, and the teeth chatter.

There are old incurable cases of asthma that are palliated by Ipecac. and carry around a bottle of it from which they say they get much relief. It is useful in cases of humid asthma, in cases of asthmatic bronchitis, when they suffer from the damp weather and from sudden weather changes; every little cold rouses up this bronchial attack, and he suffocates and gags when he coughs, or spits up a little blood.

He has to sit up nights to breathe, and the attacks are common and frequent. These patients say they get relief front Ipecac., and it is not surprising that Ipecac relieves that state of asthmatic breathing, because it has such symptoms. Some of these cases are incurable, they are people advanced in life.

This remedy, more wisely administered, will give more relief. A powder of Ipecac. will break up the attack, so that the patient is comfortable, and then will go on in an ordinary sort of asthmatic way, until catching another cold. The cough is rattling and asthmatic.

Convulsions: As a convulsive medicine Ipecac is not well enough known.

Convulsions in pregnancy. Convulsions in whooping cough; frightful spasms, affecting the whole of the left side, followed by paralysis; clonic and tonic spasms of children and hysterical women. Tetanus, rigidity of the body, with flushed redness of the face.

These are strong features of Ipecac, and they have not been sufficiently dwelt upon, and the remedy is not sufficiently known as having these states so prominently. Medicines like Belladonna are more frequently spoken of in the books and in treatises of spasms, yet Ipecac. is just as important a remedy to be studied in relation to spasms, and its action upon the spine.

Skin: In suppressed eruptions, the symptoms will very commonly point to Ipecac.

When the eruption does not come out, or an eruption has been driven back by cold, sometimes acute manifestations of stomach and bowels follow and colds settle in the chest from suppressed eruptions, Ipecac will also cure erysipelas, when there is the vomiting, the chill, the pain in the back, the thirstlessness and the overwhelming nausea.

Ipecac. is often sufficient for the nausea and vomiting when the scarlet fever rash is slow to come out. Instead of the rash coming out as it should, Ipecac symptoms come on in the stomach with nausea and vomiting. Ipecac. will check the nausea and vomiting, will bring out the eruption, and the disease will run a milder course. (Kent)

KALI BICHROMICUM
(Potassium Bicarbonate)

Stringy discharges, sinusitis. (Hydrastis).

Kali Bichromicum will treat certain colds when the main symptom is sinusitis with THICK STRINGY DISCHARGE. Chronic sinusitis.

Post nasal catarrh, pressure and fullness in the sinuses.

Dry cough, constriction in the airways, asthma, tightness in the chest. Loss of sense of smell. Throat dry and rough, profuse yellow sticky tenacious discharge.

Pains felt in one small spot. Headaches in one spot, sinus pains in one spot, rheumatic pains in one spot. Generally sensitive to cold.

Symptoms are often worse from drinking beer or they feel they are allergic to beer.

This remedy is indicated for people *who like a routine and display a conservative type of lifestyle.* They are compliant, middle of the road and family oriented. They like things to be done well, have high standards and can feel strongly about *things being done a certain way* – they feel they know the best way. They may have a job that is very repetitive, with no challenge, but don't mind it much as it provides security for their family.

All the remedies that contain potassium have this general emotional disposition (routine oriented, controlling their environment) with a tendency to wake up between 2 and 4 am. Such as Kali-carbonicum, Kali-sulphuricum, Kali-muriaticum and Kali-phosphoricum. Kali-carb is the generic example of this remedy. They have a

Study Guide

strong sensitivity to cold, swelling of the eye lids – lower or upper and wake up between to 2 to 4 a.m.

They often have a lack of empathy and understanding for those who are different.

Kali-sulp is more warm blooded and may put their feet out of the covers at night or have some skin irritation or itchy skin.

Kali-mur is more sentimental and can feel emotionally vulnerable. They can feel worse from sitting in the sun. See the description below.

Kali-phos is useful when the kali symptoms are present but the patient is more sympathetic and social in their nature. They like to start well organized programs that can help others. Such as a support group for those who have lost a child. They suffer from very severe fatigue, even too tired to read or study.

All of these Kaki remedies like order, hold stong principles, they are conservative, like things done properly by the rules but often this becomes a rigidity, too black and white, too proper and too detailed.

KALI CARBONICA
(Potassium carbonate)

Bag-like swellings of upper eyelids. Or swelling under the eyes or lower lids. See below:

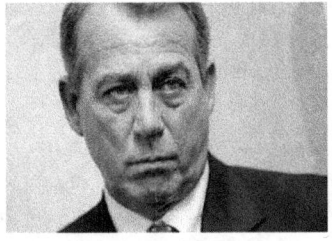

Waking at 2 to 3 am; then difficult to sleep.

Pains in the lower spine with stiffness.

Conservative outlook on life. Likes rules and things have to be done a certain way. Rigid outlook on life. Too proper. See things in terms of black and white. Fear of change and new things.

This idea of having a strict approach to others can be found in the following rubrics: Mind, Proper. Mind, dictatorial. Mind, duty – too much sense of.

Worse from cold. Sinus problems. Asthma, relieved when sitting up or bending forward or by rocking; worse from 2 to 4 a. m.

Kent says of this remedy: *The patient is whimsical, irascible, IRRITABLE TO THE VERY HIGHEST DEGREE, quarrels with his family and with his bread and butter. He never wants to be alone, is FULL OF FEAR and imaginations when alone, "fear of the future, fear of death, fear of ghosts." If compelled to remain alone in the house he is wakeful, sleepless, or his sleep is full of horrible dreams. He is never at peace, is full of imaginations and fear. "What if the house should burn up!" "What if I should do this or that!" and "What if this and the other thing should happen!"*

He is oversensitive to everything, SENSITIVE TO EVERY ATMOSPHERIC CHANGE; he can never get the room at just exactly the right temperature; he is sensitive to every draft of air and to the circulation of air in the room. He cannot have the windows open, even in a distant part of the house. He will get up at night in bed and look around to see where that draft of air comes from. His complaints are worse in wet weather, and in cold weather.

He is SENSITIVE TO THE COLD and is always shivering. His nerves feel the cold; they are all painful when it is cold. The neuralgias shoot here and there when it is cold, and if the part affected be kept warm the pain goes to some other place. All his pains change place and go into the cold part; if he covers up one part, the pain goes to the part uncovered.

Study Guide

This remedy is full of sticking, burning, tearing pains, and these fly around from place to place. Of course Kali carb. has pains that remain in one place, but usually THE PAINS FLY AROUND in every direction. Pains cutting like knives. Pains like hot needles, sticking, stinging and burning. These pains are felt in internal parts and dry passages. Burning in the anus and rectum, described as if a hot poker were forced into that passage; burning as with fire. The haemorrhoids burn like coals of fire. The burning of Kali carb. is like that of ARSENICUM.

Again from studying the text it will be seen that it is a common feature of this medicine to have its symptoms come on at 2, 3 OR 5 O'CLOCK IN THE MORNING. In Kali carb. the cough will come or have its greatest < at three or four or five o'clock in the morning. The febrile state will occur from 3-5 in the morning.

The patient, who is subject to asthmatic dyspnoea, will have an attack at 3 o'clock in the morning, waking him out of sleep. He will wake up with various symptoms and remain awake until 5 o'clock in the morning, and after that to a great extent they are relieved. Of course, there are plenty of sufferings at any time in the twenty-four hours, but this is the worst time. He wakes up at 3 o'clock in the morning with fear, fear of death, fear of the future, worries about everything and is kept awake for 2-3 hours, and then goes to sleep and sleeps soundly. (Kent)

KALI MURIATICUM
(Potassium Chloride)

This remedy is made from potassium chloride. It has the ability to stimulate the immune system in such a way as to cure infections that are associated with *THICK, TENACIOUS, GLUEY EXUDATION* (mucous). (Caust, Hydrastis, Kali-bi, Senega)

In the ear this is called a serious otitis media. The tympanic membrane is retracted, there is difficulty in hearing, often a blocked eustachian tube and swelling of the cervical glands. Snapping noises in the ears. A sense of fullness in the ears. Painless, or nearly pain free ear infections.

After Kali muriaticum the 'clot'of fibrous mucous will be dissolved, absorbed back into the body or discharged out through the eustachian tube.

A few years ago I was at a conference and a medical doctor found that if this remedy was used after a stroke or heart attack as the result of an embolus, (a fatty deposit from the arteries that breaks off and becomes lodged in a small artery blocking it) the recovery time was significantly shortened. He found the speech and paralysis after a stroke was not as severe as those persons who he had previously treated without this remedy. Again it seems that Kali muriaticum has the ability to dissolve clots and fibrous tissue.

This would be a remedy to use after many antibiotics have been used and although the ear is sterile the body does not seem to be able to rid itself of the fibrous mucous.

In chronic cases you may see a patient who is a bit like Natrum muriaticum and Kali carb: Rigid, strong principles but also romantic, sentimental and full of grief.

KALI NITRICUM

These patients often resemble Nitric Acid – **holding a grudge, anxiety about health and craving fat.** The Nitrate in many remedies creates anxiety as found in this remedy. Often it is an anxiety about health.

Too strict about some aspect in their life. Rigid and proper which makes others feel too controlled.

- Irritable, short-tempered, may hold a grudge (Nit-ac)
- Hard-working, responsible, strong sense of duty.
- Anxiety about health (Nit-ac).
- Craving for fat (Nit-ac).
- Sinusitis, polyps, nasal obstruction, discharges may be watery.
- Colitis, diarrhea.

- Primary use is in respiratory conditions – asthma, bronchitis, tuberculosis, pneumonia, allergic rhinitis, etc.

- Asthma worse at 3 a.m. (Kali).

- Back pain, sciatica, left-sided (Kali).

- Spiritual death (Nit-ac). They feel there is no meaning in life or very strict about rules regarding religion.

- Heart problems.

- Sleeplessness at 3 a.m. (Kali).

- Aggravation, such as asthma at 3 a.m. (Kali).

KALI PHOHORICUM

Desire to create a structure for the benefit of others. All the Kalium remedies like to do what is correct, best, most safe, most proper. If Phosphorus is added then the patient can display a strong empathy

Case 1: Her child died in an accident. Chronic fatigue syndrome since then. Her reaction was to *organize a grief support group for others*. After Kali-phos her vitality and strength returned in full measure.

We think of Kali-phos in cases of *mental and physical exhaustion,* especially after periods of stress or over-exertion, or a long period of study. Often needed by students and intellectuals who have made some enormous effort and have a type of mental breakdown. Especially needed when great exhaustion and mental dullness is associated with nervousness and over-sensitivity (Asar).

- Example of breakdown state: overly sensitive, frazzled nerves, flinch at least sound, tired, mind doesn't work, can't sleep at night, irritable over trifles, restless, feel unable to cope.

Materia Medica

- Great depletion, weakness, fatigue, muscular weakness – chronic fatigue syndrome

- Mental exhaustion – mental breakdown from over-work (Lecethin)

- Irritable – with breakdown

- Nervous excitability, anxiety – with breakdown

- Nervous restlessness – with breakdown

- Hypersensitivity to all stimuli, starting from noise – with breakdown

- Feeling unable to cope – despondency, nervous dread, depression

- Insomnia – from frayed nerves, nervous excitability (often given for insomnia only)

- Also for multiple sclerosis, neurasthenia (Alum-phos)

- Diarrhea, vaginitis, headache, indigestion

- Children: hyperactive, nervous, excitable, nightmares, crave sugar

- Chilly, < cold, > warmth and rest

- Right-sided

- Chilly, < cold

- Sensitive to thunderstorms

- Aggravation at 3 a.m. and 9 p.m

- Desires: cold drinks

- Aversion: salt, fish

- Hemorrhages of bright red blood

- Bone problems, growing pains, osteoporosis

Study Guide

- Neurological problems
- Migraines
- Tuberculosis, lung complaints, bronchitis, asthma
- Back pain, sciatica

Mind:

- The patient is often more extroverted than other Kali's because of the Phosphorus influence
- Easily upset from hearing bad news or hearing of world catastrophes (Phos)
- Tend to be very open in homeopathic consultations (Phos)
- Children can be very homesick if they move, lose contact with friends
- Easily frightened. Fears being alone, disease, death, something bad will happen (Phos)

KALI SULPHURICUM

Rigid in some aspect of the personality with Sulphur symptoms such as feeling worse from heat . Wakes 4 or 5 a.m. Sinus problems. Itchy skin.

Similar to Pulsatilla but mental/emotional symptoms differ – often called "the irritable or chronic Pulsatilla" – if Pulsatilla is indicated but doesn't work, consider Kali-s. (Potassium sulphate is found abundantly in the flower of Pulsatilla)

- Warm-blooded, < warmth, warm rooms > fresh air, > walk in fresh air (Sulph, Puls)
- Yellow discharges and yellow coated tongue (Puls)

Materia Medica

- Colds from temperature changes in spring-time (Puls)
- Chronic otitis, catarrh of the ears (Puls)
- Chronic sinus with obstruction, yellow mucous (Puls)
- Respiratory conditions, bronchitis, etc. (Puls)
- Asthma, > open air (Puls). Allergic hay fever. Arthritis (Puls)
- Back pains and sciatica (Kali)
- Cold hands and feet (opp to Sulph)
- Skin conditions, inflammations with yellow pus
- Aversion: eggs (Sulph)
- Aggravation 3 to 5 a.m. (kali)

Mind:

- Feels anxious when stuck inside, better for a walk in fresh air (Puls)
- Timid (2) (Puls). Lacking in confidence (2) (Puls)
- Busy, hurried, restless. Discontented, irritable (3), angry (3), and critical. (Puls is not so critical or angry)
- Aggravated by consolation (opp to Puls – Puls tends to be more demanding, to need more attention
- Irresolution (2) (Puls). Desire for company (Puls)
- Kali: Principle of duty; Closed; Optimism; Work, task; Family
- Sulphuricum: Clothing; Beauty, grace, harmony; Joy; Love and relationships; Jealousy. Egotism, desire for compliments

Study Guide

LAC CANINUM
(Dogs milk)

Feels unfortunate – INFERIOR and less than others – *feels he is always looked down upon or that he is looking up at others i.e. others seem more important.*

DESIRE TO PLEASE OTHERS to be included again. The child is rejected, she is not included, she is forsaken and feels alone.

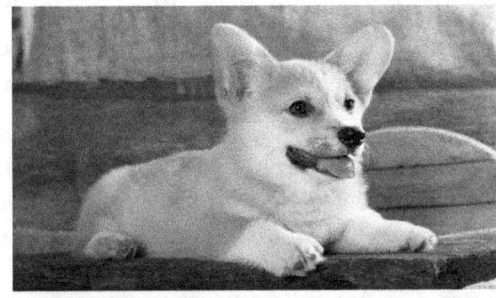

Fear to be abandoned so will try and do good deeds to help other people; that way they are wanted and loved by others. The worst thing they fear is to be alone. Appeasement at almost any cost (Magnesiums, Car, Aids nosode). Yielding to others. Feels dependent on others but less important.

Keynotes: **Salivation on the pillow at night.** Feels as if walking on air, or not touching the bed when lying down, floating. Fear of snakes.

Pains are better from cold. ***Erratic pains, alternating sides.***

Kent says of this remedy: *The fingers were not aggravated from hard pressure, but she would scream if they touched. This state is difficult to cure "outside of Lac can. and LACHESIS. LACH. has produced a similar condition. The sensitiveness of the abdomen so that the sheet cannot be permitted to touch the skin belongs to both.*

Another strange state is a peculiar vertigo, a condition, when walking, in which she seems to be floating in mid-air, or, when lying, as if she were not on the bed. Other remedies have this. The sensation as if floating, or not touching the bed, or sinking down, belongs to LACH. The sensation of gliding while walking is strong under ASARUM EUROPEUM.

The complaints, almost regardless of kind or quality, CHANGE SIDES.

The rheumatism is first found in one ankle and then in the other, and then back again to the original site. If in the knee or hip or shoulder the RHEUMATISM ALTERNATES SIDES. The headaches and neuralgias do the same thing. The ambulating erysipelas first attacks one side, then the other. In inflammation and neuralgia of the ovaries the same alternation is observed. Sore throats affect alternately the sides of the throat or tonsils. Many cases of this sort have been cured by this remedy. The trouble commenced on the right and went to the left and LYCOPODIUM failed, but when it returned to the right the alternation was noticed and the remedy revealed. Only a limited number of remedies have alternating sides.

One or two provers had many symptoms, and so not all are reliable; but this remedy SO INTENSIFIES THE IMAGINATION AND SENSES that it would be easy for them to imagine symptoms, and that itself is suggestive. Full of imaginations and harassing, tormenting/thoughts. Wandering features in the mental sphere, wandering and alternating states. Cannot collect the thoughts.

She wants to leave everything as soon as it is commenced, a condition of irresolution common to quite a number of remedies. She is impressed with the idea that all she says is not so, thinks everything she says is a lie, as if there is no reality in the things that be. In this it is somewhat analogous to ALUMINA, in which the patient feels as if someone else and not himself were saying everything, a lack of consciousness of the reality of things.

Every time a symptom appears she thinks it is a settled disease; fear and anxiety that some horrible disease has come upon her, a delusion that she was suppurating and in a loathsome state; infested with snakes.

Horrible sights are presented to the mental vision, not always snakes, and she fears the objects will take form and present themselves to her eyes. This is analogous to LACH., which has the feeling that the atmosphere is full of hovering spirits, although he never sees them. Imagines he wears someone else's nose. Imagines she is not herself and her properties not her own. Imagines she sees spiders, snakes, vermin. She cannot bear to be alone.

Study Guide

LAC HUMANUM
(Human Milk)

Detachment and Isolation: Estranged from family, no connection or bond.

Can't trust new people. Feels deeply empty. NUMB to life.

Completely cut off from life leading to suicidal thoughts.

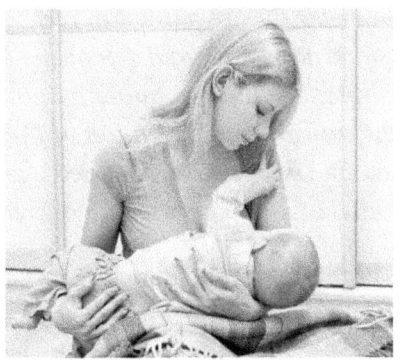

Situation if which the child was not wanted or not understood: Adopted children, emotionally abandoned children, divorce of parents, both parents going to work. When the parents did not bother or want to know their child. No bond between parent and child.

Breast feeding failures: This can be the beginning of the feeling of rejection and loss in bonding. Loss of ambition: *gives up, no use in trying any longer.* Aversion to lift the head up.

Indifference: Can't feel any longer, lack of feelings for anything or anyone. Indifferent to family, can't make new friends. What is the point in trying (Calc-nit, Nit-ac).

Feels unworthy: Not good enough to be loved. Loathing of self and life. To feel worthy may be into compulsive washing and cleaning. A desire to be perfect.

Depression: a wall of pain around the patient, the person feels totally isolated and can no longer make contact with others. No positive emotions can flow into the patient. Hopeless, cut off, estranged from family, giving up to die, suicidal. Consolation is not helpful; turn away from affection.

Depersonalization: Feels a loss of identity. Feel like an outsider. No sense of purpose in life.

Compensate with control, a lot of structure, may be fastidious. May learn that duty can hold them together but don't know who they are.

In order for the patient to feel 'okay' he or she may insist on continuous and total symbiosis (sense of oneness) with their parent or caretaker. Such as holding hands all day, being held all day or having the unwaivering attention of the parent 24/7. This is a desire to go back into the womb to be nurtured again without having to individualize. Can't individualize. Can't separate from their childhood doll.

May have many feelings of insecurity and fears. Fear of others. Fear something will go wrong or that something bad will happen. Fear of criticism, aversion to conflict or confrontation.

Later in life can't bond with others, feels isolation, can't maintain a relationship with others. Always feels isolated and alone. May go and live on the street as this reflects most closely what they feel the world is like or may go to the other extreme and join a group with extreme beliefs in order to feel a part of something.

Breakdown state of the personality, catatonia, psychotic break: No confidence, feel they are nothing and worthless. Helpless. Crave love and symbiosis. Become extremely dependent or give up and want to live on the street. May only have one way to communicate with the world, such as dancing, sex, work, sport etc; then isolated the rest of the time and no connection. Feel life is a dream and not real. Depersonalization, wish to be a baby again. No identity, shallow personality, fake person (Thuja).

Dreams of death of mother, father or baby. Alcoholism, drug addiction. Feels empty and depressed on waking. Forgetful, makes mistakes. Sexuality increased or decreased.

Study Guide

Can't sleep: feels too alone. Has to sleep with TV on.

Suck thumb – needs extra nurturing to feel okay.

Allergies and eczema. Early tooth decay.

Swelling of breast before menses. Other PMS symptoms. Post partum depression – can't bond with their child. Menses dark brown or black.

Nausea better eating. Gestational diabetes, craving sugar. Eating disorder to feel emotionally nurtured. Crave milk, aversion to milk or allergy to milk. Weakness of muscles.

Headache, migraine, dizziness, vertigo, an empty feeling, flushes, loss of hair, coldness of the extremities, weak libido, lack of feeling, awkwardness, general chilliness, eczema, psoriasis, molluscae.

Lac humanum: Source: human milk, one donor
Proving: by J.Houston and E.Halahan 1993 (Great Britain)

Lac maternum
Source: mixture of human milk from nine donors at different stages of lactation, including colostrum.
Proving: Tinus Smits (Links 2000)
No classical proving.

Case 1: Three year old female spayed Corgi dog. Hemorrhagic cystitis. Frequent urination (4). Bright red blood in urine, no clots. Wants to be alone, won't look up, will not come when called. Wall of sadness. Isolation, lost, numb, depressed. No appetite. Normal thirst. Plan: Lac humanum 30c once a day for three days. After one day 50% better. After three days 90% better. One year later no relapse, bladder is now strong like a tank. (Sulph, Canth, Aurum sulph, Sarsap, Uva ursi, no help until Lac hum given.)

Compare:
Psorinum: both can have bad smelling eczema, depression, hopeless feeling.
Abrotanum: Child can't breast feed and looses weight. Failure to thrive.

Camphora: Forsaken, isolation, no friends.
Sepia: Indifference, aversion to affection, low sexual desire.
Nitric acid: Life has no meaning.
Aurum: Suicidal depression, feels unworthy, loathing of self.
Lac-caninum: feels rejected, isolated. But Lac-caninum will try to please others which is a feeling of optimism that Lac human does not have.
Pulsatilla: Forsaken, alone feeling. But Pulsatilla is better from consolation while Lac humanum is not better from consolation.

Bibliography: The Homoeopathic Proving of Lac Humanum Jacqueline Houghton and Elisabeth Halahan

LACHESIS
(Bushmaster Snake)

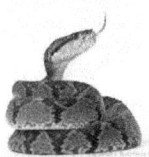

Loquacity, want to control others, jealousy, too passionate. Better onset of menses. **WORSE FROM TIGHT COLLARS** **or any tight clothing.** This is a good remedy for sore throats, ear aches and or sinusitis.

Typically, the person needing Lachesis will be:
- Loquacious (very talkative)
- Jealous, A FORCEFUL PERSONALITY
- DOMINEERING
- *Envious, suspicious, mistrustful, possessive*
- Overly passionate
- Aggressive
- Malicious
- Full of hatred

Study Guide

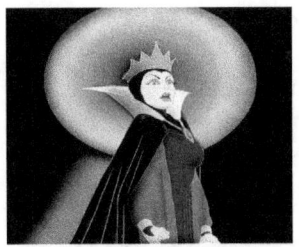
(Disney)

The evil queen in story of Snow White is a typical Lachesis. She is proud, domineering, insanely jealous, passionate to a fault, her ego is too strong, vengeful, homicidal, sexually powerful but also completely unfulfilled, lonely and tragic.

They feel a need to control others.

Fear of snakes.

Worse from tight shirt collars or constriction on the throat or abdomen. Many different symptoms such as headaches and irritability are worse before menses but great relief when the menses begin.

Ailments during menopause such as hot flushes and hot perspiration. Plethoric, swollen, mottled or purple face.

<u>Sensitive to heat and headaches from exposure to the heat of the sun</u>, or other sources of heat. The head especially is worse from being overheated leading to headaches. Feel faint in a hot room.
Easily feels full of anger, hypertensive, suffocating or under pressure and needs an outlet such as talking, sexual expression, eczema, flushes, discharges or haemorrhage. Analogy: a pot boiling over, a pressure cooker ready to burst.

Symptoms worse on the left side. Diseases begin on the left and spread to the right side. Great sensitiveness to touch.

All symptoms, especially the mental ones, are worse from oversleeping. Aggravated feeling, such as a feeling of suffocation, sudden starting or choking upon falling asleep, or waking in the morning with a headache.

Symptoms are worse:

Materia Medica

- In the spring, such as hay fever
- From hot drinks
- When swallowing liquids
- From suppression of discharges
- From suppression of skin eruptions or
- From the suppression of sexuality

Rushes of blood (blood is pushed by the heart to one area of the body in an intense way).

Hypertension, asthma, migraine headaches. Sore throats, ear aches, asthma, cough, fever, chest infections. Sciatica on the right side. Briefly stops breathing during sleep.

Case 1: In one case I had there was an acne rosacea only on the left side of her face. She was angry before her menses with a great relief in mood once the menses would start. The acne and PMS were bettter after Lachesis 30c once a week for a month.

Case 2: In another case a 35 year old man came to see me for headaches. He was quite the character. He would run down people that cut him off in traffic and smash in their winshield with a bassball bat and then drag them trrough this broken window and then beat them. After Lachesis he became a much calmer person, even sent nice Christmas cards to his relatives. I asked him what happened to his ruthless anger and he said he did not know, he did not have it any longer and just could not get himself worked up.

Case 3: In another case I saw a man in his 20's about to be married but he was impotent. After Lachesis he was able to remember being sexually molested by a nieghbor and so wanted to go back to that country, find him and kill him. In this case we can see how when the anger is suppressed it can lead to physical ailments. I talked him out of this violent revenge and said that he had his whole life ahead of him plus he no longer had the impotence. A few months later he reported that the anger was no longer controlling him and so the molestation was becoming a memory that no longer affected his life.

Case 4: In another case a woman in her 30's came to see me with her main symptom being a fear of being poisoned. She was afraid to even eat food she had prepared as perhaps they had poisoned the food at the grocery store or from where it was grown or made. The panic was so severe she could barely work or funciton with everyday affairs. After Lachesis this all calmed down and she looked back on this behaviour with puzzlement, not really understanding how she had acquired this fear.

In all of these cases the following symptoms were present, suspicion, anger, intollerance of tight clothing about the neck, worse from heat and the sun.

LECITHINUM
(Phosphatidylcholine)

This remedy has the social aspect of phosphorus: excitable, friendly, easy connection to others, but they burn out more easily like we see in Phosphoric acid and Kali-phos.

Their mind is tired, can't think or read a book as it makes them feel totally exhausted - (Kali-phos).

It is also one of the main remedies for scleroderma, the tissues become hard and tight. The best keynote is: *dry face, it feels cracked after washing or as if there was a dry egg on it.* It is a good remedy for students who burn out because they are often very empathetic people. Phosphatidylcholine chemical structure:

Case 1: Female 25 years old, x-ray technician. Frequent colds, (every two to three weeks has a cold/flu) with weakness, can't think when has a cold, has to stay home and does nothing. She is very social, friendly, open and full of empathy for others. Close bonds to family. Lives with her boyfriend and says they are

Materia Medica

aways joking around and every night is like a giggle fest. *Very dry skin especially on the face where after washing the face feels it will crack.* Wakes tired like as if not slept. Father had *scleroderma* and died from it. Aversion to fish and vegetables. After the remedy no more colds, vitality much better, no more weakness, face not so dry. Ten months now since taking this remedy and still doing well.

Case 2: Female in 50's multiple joint and muscle pains, lots of shooting pains, muscles contract, *tight, stiffness all over, muscles feel sclerosed.* Heartburn (Phos), esophagus *full of scarr tissue,* lots of acid reflux, very dry face – *feels it will crack after washing it.* Worries about her children and granchildren all the time (Phos), 'I put myself in their shoes, I can't help it, they are such dears, I love them so much.' She starts to cry. Ulcers in the stomach (Phos). Osteopenia (Phos). *She is my most friendly patient,* very exciteable, acts as if we are best friends, she asks me over for dinner with her husband, tells all her friends about me, makes me feel like I am *magnetized in her presence.* X-ray shows bone s*purrs in the spine* and degenerative joint disease. Weak all over.

Kali phos helps some but nine days after Lecithinum the joint pains are 70% better in the arms and 100% in the lower limbs. This was in 2004 with Lecithinum 30c and then 200c. It is now 2014, ten years later and she never relapsed, exercises at swimming laps three times a week and doing very well. She still is *very exciteable* but able to let go of many of the problems which her grandchildren are suffering from.

In some patients who need this remedy there will be *total mental exhaustion* like we see in Kali-phos, Picric acid and Phosphoric acid. There is an aversion to think, *incapacity to read one page,* sleepy but can't sleep, the mind wanders and feels slow.

Like Tuberculinum we can use this remedy for exhaustion from burning the candle at both ends. This is because *they can be the most outgoing, social and excietable types of people* like Tub, Med, Arg-nit and Phosphorus.

Can't read a book as the mind won't work or be able to understand what they are reading (Taxus).

Think of this remedy when you see many phosphorus symptoms but the thirst is normal. Then ask about the dry skin. :-)

LYCOPODIUM
(Club Moss)

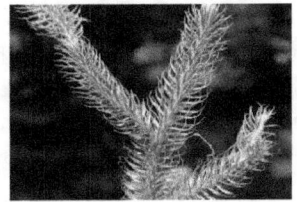

Lack of confidence. Cowardice. Fear of new things. Tries to create a persona of power over others. Act confident but underneath he feels like a failure.

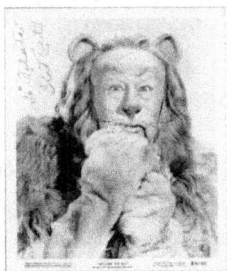

The cowardly lion from The Wizard of Oz is a good example of Lycopodium. His bravado is very superficial; he is lion with no courage.

These people try to impress by being flamboyant or dictatorial but deeper down they feel inadequate and fear failure. If he is relied upon too much he wants to run away from responsibility (Anac, Ethy, Gels). Fear of new things, of public speaking, ailments from too much responsibility. Fear to be alone and of large social gatherings. Apprehensive.

Case 1: After getting married and having a child the responsibility seemed too much so he left his family and found himself a younger new girlfriend.

Case 2. She immigrated to a new country, her stomach always felt bloated, she felt inferior to others, she tried to act strong, competent and confident as a compensation. She was afraid others would find out how she really felt about herself.

Case 3. He was a bully at school but at home acted well in front of his parents especially his father who would discipline him for every mistake. He felt a failure in his father's eyes and could not please him.

Case 4. He hides from confrontation. Before playing baseball he gets an upset stomach and wants to stay home. All of these cases did well on Lycopodium.

Digestive problems, bloating (China, Carbo-veg) and easily filled up from a little bit of food.

Tired on waking, and tired from 4 p.m. to 8 p.m. Diarrhea from anxiety. Symptoms worse on the right side. Better from warm food and drinks.

Cold hands and feet. This remedy treats many different chronic ailments.

Nash: *The patient sits down to the table VERY HUNGRY, but the first few mouthfuls fill him right up and he feels DISTRESSINGLY full; in a Pickwickian sense "too full for utterance." This alternation of hunger and satiety is not markedly found under any other remedy.*

Constipation predominates under LYCOPODIUM, and like NUX VOMICA there may be frequent and ineffectual desire for stool, but while that of NUX VOMICA is caused by irregular peristaltic action that of LYCOPODIUNT seems to be caused by a spasmodic contraction of the anus, which prevents the stool and causes great pain.

Many liver troubles.

LYCOPODIUM is also one of our best remedies for impotence. (AGNUS CASTUS.) An old man marries his second or third wife and finds himself not "equal to the occasion." It is very embarrassing for the whole family. A dose of LYCOPODIUM sets the thing all right and makes the doctor a warm friend on both sides of the house.

Young men from onanism or sexual excess become impotent. The penis becomes small, cold and relaxed. The desire is as strong as ever, and perhaps more so, but he can't perform. (SELENIUM, CALADIUM.) I have known apparently hopeless cases of this kind cured by the use of this remedy, high single doses at intervals of a week or more. Give it low, however, if you want to, but do not blame me if you don't succeed.

LYCOPODIUM affects the right side most, or at least the troubles begin on the right side. Swelling and suppuration of the tonsils I have aborted more than once in old quinsy subjects by an early dose of this remedy. In fact, I have had such success with LACHESIS, LYCOPODIUM, LAC CANINUM and PHYTOLACCA that some who employ me for nothing else come for those powders that "BREAK UP QUINSY" so quick. In diphtheria, if the disease begins in the nose or right tonsil and extends to the left, you will think of LYCOPODIUM, but remember that MERCURIUS PROTOIODIDE also begins on the right side, but there is no difficulty in choosing between the two. (BROMINE diphtheria begins below and comes upward, just the reverse of LYCOPODIUM.) Pains in the abdomen, ovarian and uterine regions also begin in right side, RUNNING FROM RIGHT to left; right foot gets cold while the other remains warm, eruptions begin on right and travel across to left side. Sciatica the same; any complaint that begins on right and goes to left makes me think of LYCOPODIUM. The "sides of the body" subject is of more account than some imagine. Drugs have an affinity for particular parts, organs and even sides of the body.

Upon the respiratory organs this remedy also has a strong influence. It is one of our best remedies for chronic dry catarrh of the nose, which becomes completely closed, so that the patient has to breathe through the open mouth, especially at night. Here the choice often lies between this remedy, AMMONIUM CARB. and HEPAR SULPHUR., other symptoms, of course, deciding the choice. In infants SAMBUCUS comes in for a share of attention.

LYCOPODIUM has often saved neglected, MALTREATED OR IMPERFECTLY CURED CASES OF PNEUMONIA from running into consumption. It may even come into the later stages of the acute attack itself, and here as usual the disease is apt to be in the right lung, and especially if liver complications arise. The disease has passed the first or congestive stage, and generally the stage of hepatization, or is in the last part of this stage, and is trying hard to take a favorable turn into the breaking-up or third stage, the stage of resolution. Just here is where many cases die, neither free expectoration, nor perfect absorption of the disease product taking place. There is extreme dyspnoea, the cough sounds as if the entire parenchyma of the lung were softened; even raising whole mouthfuls of mucus does not afford relief, the breath is short and the wings of the nose expand to their utmost with a fan-like motion. Now is the time when LYCOPODIUM does wonders. Again, even when this stage is imperfectly passed, and the patient still coughs and expectorates much thick, yellow, purulent or greyish-yellow, purulent (sometimes foetid) matter, tasting salty, with much rattling in the chest, LYCOPODIUM is indispensable. Here the choice may have to be made between this remedy and SULPHUR, KALI HYDROIOD. or SILICEA. The characteristic aggravation as to time, of this remedy, is from 4 TO 8 O'CLOCK p. M. COLOCYNTH has 4 to 9 aggravation of abdominal pains, and HELLEBORUS NIGER, of the headache, with coryza; but the 4 to 8 aggravations of LYCOPODIUM are general, not confined to any one, or one SET of symptoms.

LYCOPODIUM profoundly impresses the sensorium. We see by studying its pathogenesis that it DEPRESSES. This is found particularly in typhoid. The patient lies stupid, eyes do not react to light; lower jaw drops; apparent impending paralysis of the brain.

This condition may also be found in the advanced stage of many different acute diseases, such as cerebro-spinal meningitis, typhoid fever, pneumonia, etc. Now if you get the 4 to 8 p. M. aggravation this remedy surely comes in. But this depression of the sensorium is also found in chronic form. You remember what was said of this remedy in the impotence of old men. If you find corresponding failure in the sensorium of old men, the memory fails, they use wrong words to express themselves, mix things up generally in writing, spelling, and are, in short, unable to do ordinary mental work on account of failing brain power, remember LYCOPODIUM. Here again ANACARDIUM, PHOSPHORUS, BARYTA or OPIUM may come in for comparison. Also PICRIC ACID and AGNUS CASTUS. (Nash)

MAGNESIA CARBONICA
(Magnesium carbonate hydroxide)

All the Magnesium remedies have the following symptoms in common: *Worse from conflict, worse from any argument especially for a child when their parents argue.*

They always try to make peace. Fear of abandonment or never well since being forsaken.

Cramps in any part of the body but especially legs.

Wakes up tired, sleep is unrefreshing. Feels awful in the morning.

Forsaken, alone; will do almost anything to not be abandoned. Mild and yielding. The orphan child.

Difficult to digest milk.

Examples: After his parents separated he could not recover as there was too much conflict that he was exposed to. After being a foster child she could not feel secure or wanted. After being a soldier in Iraq he was full of anxiety and PTSD. He wakes up tired, the conflict cut him up inside and he can't recover from this stress. In fact he never was a soldier, he was a Magnesium and they should never be put into conflict; rather they are the ones who have the skills to negotiate and find peaceful solutions to political conflicts. Ginseng is the perfect soldier, nothing scares them.

Kent says of this remedy: *Like other MAGNESIAS it has most violent neuralgic pains, pains along the course of nerves, pains so violent that he cannot keep still, and he moves about and IS RELIEVED BY MOTION. The provers felt these pains mostly in the head and face, but clinical experience has demonstrated that it has violent neuralgia everywhere. We are justified, from the proving, in considering it as especially related to the LEFT SIDE OF THE FACE; NEURALGIA IN THE NIGHT; DRIVING HIM OUT OF BED, keeping him in constant motion. As soon as he stops moving the pain becomes very severe, shooting, tearing and cutting.*

It has varied eruptions upon the skin; dry, scaly, dandruff-like eruptions upon the skin, very unhealthy hair and nails. Particularly does it affect the teeth and roots of the teeth. In every change of the weather the roots of the teeth become violently painful, burn, shoot and ache continuously. Toothache before and during menstruation. During pregnancy she suffers all the time with toothache, tearing pains in the left side of the face, although the roots of the teeth are perfectly sound. The hollow teeth are unusually sensitive, and painful. The teeth are so sensitive that they cannot be manipulated by the dentist. This is like ANT. CRUD., but Magnesia carb. especially affects the roots of the teeth, while ANT. CRUD. affects the dentine more particularly. Sensitiveness of the teeth, so that he cannot bite upon the teeth, and the teeth feel too long. Magnesia carb. and CHINA, when no other symptoms are present, are prominent remedies among the affections of the teeth during pregnancy.

There is a kind of marasmus that you will puzzle over if you do not know this remedy. If we analyze the remedy in general, we will see that it produces a state of the body like that prior to tuberculosis. He does not undergo repair, he loses flesh, and the muscles become flabby as if some serious disease were coming. In children of tuberculous parents there is that tendency to go into marasmus. The child's muscles are flabby, the child will not thrive in spite of feeding and medicines. It seems to be laying the foundations for some serious trouble. Finally, it emaciates and the back of the head begins to sink in, as if from atrophy of the cerebellum.

The appetite increases for milk and meat and animal broths, and yet they are not digested, and when the milk is taken it continually passes the bowel in the form of white potter's clay, or like putty. The stool is soft and of the consistency of putty. If you go through a china factory where the men are forming with their hands, in such wonderful manner, all sorts of beautiful dishes, and moulds, you will see that the original clay, as they are manipulating it, is white. It is a perfect picture of the Mag. carb. stool, composed of putty-like undigested milk.

I have observed, especially among illegitimate infants, those that have been conceived by clandestine coition, that they have a tendency to sinking in the back of the head. The occipital bone will sink in, and the parietal bones jut out over it, and there will be a depression. That is not an uncommon thing in children that go into marasmus. They are very likely to have a potter's clay stool. It does not run, and it is not hard. The white, hard stool is quite another symptom, and the soft, semi-fluid white stool leads to another class of remedies, but this pasty stool, looking as if it could be moulded into any kind of shape, is a Magnesia carb. stool.

I once had in charge an orphanage, where we had sixty to one hundred babies on hand all the time. The puzzle of my life was to find remedies for the cases that were going into marasmus. A large number of them were clandestine babies. It was a sort of Sheltering Arms for these little ones. The whole year elapsed, and we were losing babies every week from this gradual decline, until I saw the image of these babies in Magnesia carb., and after that many of them were cured.

The Mag. carb. baby SMELLS SOUR LIKE THE HEPAR BABY. Wash it as you will and it smells sour; the perspiration is sour, and the whole baby smells sour. It is not especially the stool. The stool smells strong and pungent, putrid, and very often the whole child has a pungent odor, like an unclean baby, though it be well washed.

The MAGNESIAS produce inactivity of the rectum and anus—a paresis. The stool is large and hard, requiring great straining to expel. It is dry, hard and crumbling. The stool will remain partly expelled and then crumble, breaking up in many pieces. Another stool that is laid down in the books as a most striking condition of Magnesia carb. is green; it is the diarrhoeic stool, and the green part floats upon the watery portion of the stool.

"Stools green, like scum on a frog pond; sour, frothy; with white floating lumps like tallow, bloody, mucous." Floating like lumps of tallow, is more characteristic of PHOSPHORUS, and many a time has DULCAMARA cured it.

The face of the chronic adult case is pale, waxy, sickly and sallow, and you wonder why this patient will not right up, and will not thrive. She has a sickly countenance, HER MUSCLES ARE LAX, she becomes so tired and sweats upon little exertion.

She is disturbed in every change of the weather, and is worse at the beginning of menstruation. She seems to take cold whenever menstruation is coming on. She says: "I know my menstrual period is coming on, because I have a cold in my head."

Magnesia carb. has coryza every month before the monthly period. These patients take on an appearance as if going into decline, and yet they go on year after year unable to do anything, not able even to keep house, have a violent craving for meat and an aversion to vegetable food, grow thin and increasingly flabby, muscles relaxed, and with tendency to prolapsus.

The walls of the abdomen have a tendency to fall down and to be relaxed, and the rings favor the formation of hernia. That is the kind of relaxation. The nerves are painful, and the muscles are tired.

When you have such a case and have prescribed, and they persist in spite of every remedy, you know that the case does not well indicate a remedy, that the conditions are latent and there is a tendency to some grave internal disorder.

The organs are threatening to break down; the kidneys, the heart, the lungs, or the brain are about to undergo organic change. (Kent)

MAGNESIUM MURIATICUM
(Magnesium chloride)

Like Magnesia carbonica the people who need this remedy are also severely *aggravated by quarrels or disharmony in their family.* They just want everyone to get along. Mag mur is more isolated and hurt more easily than Mag carb. They may have resentment, grief and deep emotions that they can't express.

Deep down they feel disappointment. They suppress what they feel and try to help others or do their duty so that peace is maintained. They can feel that the world is unjust to them, that too much is demanded of them but they are too yielding to assert what they want from others. The resentment can create a sour temperament or even bitterness.

Like Mag carb they can't digest milk very well and like all other Magnesias *they wake up feeling tired in the morning.*

Like Nat mur they do not like to talk about their feelings. They like to have things quiet and are quite sensitive to noise.

It is a good liver remedy. Pressing pain in liver; worse lying on right side. *Liver enlarged with bloating of abdomen*; yellow tongue.

MAGNESIA PHOSPHORICUM

Similar to other Magnesia remedies but more empathy and more friendly to others.

Wakes tired but not as much as the other Magnesias.

Mild, worse from being alone.

Neuralgic pains that are better from the application of warmth. Headaches and menstrual colic better from warmth.

Cramping of muscles with radiating pains. Pains such as menstrual cramps, are better from warm applications.

Worse from conflict like other Magnesiums. Wake tired. More empathy and like to be social like Phosphorus. CRAMPS in the back or legs. This remedy is most easily confused with Carcinosin.

Study Guide

MAGNESIA SULPHURICA
(Epsom Salt)

Magnesia plus Suphur symptoms. Feel controlled by others but don't really mind it. Difficult to be assertive. *Give in rather than get into an argument.*

Yielding, want to make peace with everyone.

Case 1: 35 year old married man. Itchy eczema and hay fever. Red lips. Mild character, lets his wife make most of the decisions. Goes along with what the rest of the family wants to do. No egotism. Likes to get along with others, aversion to conflict. Warm-blooded, wakes tired.

Worse from heat like Mag-iod. Mag iod more restless with hypoglycemia.

MERCURIUS
(Quicksilver)

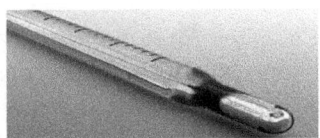

SENSITIVITY TO HOT AND COLD. Salivation. Suspicious.
The patient will find it difficult to find a comfortable temperature. The person seems to take on the character of mercury itself; when it is hot, they feel too hot; when it is cold, they feel too cold. The patient can't maintain their resistance to hot or cold. For example when the bed gets hot she perspires and has to throw off the covers. Then she feels a chill so turns up the heat. Then gets cold again and has to open the window. Not many remedies have this symptom so when it is present it becomes a super keynote for Mercury.

SWOLLEN TONGUE. IT SHOWS THE IMPRINT OF THE TEETH.

Materia Medica

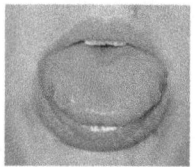

SALIVATION ON THE PILLOW WHEN SLEEPING. Wakes up in the morning with wet spots on the pillow.

Swollen cervical glands. The lymphatic glands of the neck are puffy and hardened. This is a common symptom in chronic infections of the upper respiratory tract, bronchi, throat, and nasal passages.

Perspiration at night which aggravates. Often a cold and clammy sweat all over the body. It can be a profuse, heavy sweat. It does not bring relief of any symptoms and the person will say that they feel worse from it.

Pale and sickly looking. The face can be swollen, moist white and pale with sunken dark eyes, and dry lips. The tongue is swollen, coated white and showing the imprint of the teeth.

Symptoms are worse at night. Bone pains, fever, ear pains, sleeplessness, cough and sore throat all can be worse at night.

Effects of infection such as: pus formation, abscesses, and ulcerations. Thick mucous from the sinuses, thick yellow discharge from the ears. Boils in the ear canals. Swollen tonsils with pus and bad breath. Bronchitis and pneumonia with heavy tough mucous which is difficult to cough up. Ulcers of the mouth and throat. Deformaties as a result of syphilis inheritance.

These key symptoms if followed will lead to many successful outcomes for the average acute case who needs Mercury. In most of the cases over the past twenty years of practice, I have not seen any definite mental state that accompanies the physical acute symptoms of Mercury. They are a little irritable from the pains, they want to be taken care of and may be a little worried about how sick they are but most often they do not display the mental sympstoms such as suspicion andparanoia which we often see in the chronic cases.

In Chronic cases we can see the flollowing: They can be very conservative people, extremely shy and introverted. There are a variety of other emotions that can be present such as sudden anger, violent impulses, suspicion, paranoia, anxiety, or depression. It is not common to find a mercury person with an acute illness that has any of these mental symptoms. Perhaps when the acute symptoms have been suppressed over many years with antibiotics, then the defence mechanism breaks down on deeper levels, leaving the person unable to deal with the emotional stresses of life. The result is then an expression of one of the many severe mental pathologies of Mercury such as feeling surrounded by enemies. In these cases we can find more severe physical pathology such as ulcerative colitis, cancer and or autoimmune diseases.

Usually, in the acute stages of gastoenteritis the person has extreme fatigue, food is not assimilated, there can be vomiting and diarrhea and they lose weight.

Case 1: Diarrhea with blood, salivation while sleeping, senstive to hot and cold. One dose of Mercure 30c. Next day all better.

The infections of the ear, that Mercury will heal; can be in the first stage of the ear infection or for the chronic, continuous ear infection. Even when every antibiotic has been tried and nothing works any longer Mercury can take up the task and accomplish wonders. In either case the first acute or very chronic it can be a Mercury case, if the concommitant symptoms fit – they are all listed above in italics and bold.

Often the infections start in the throat. The throat gets swollen, bluish red, stitching, burning, raw pains or severe pains. Pains into the ear on swallowing. Complete loss of voice. Ulcers and swelling of the tonsils.

The nose is stuffy, congested sinuses, sneezing, acrid burning discharge, worse in a warm room. Can have profuse and fluent coryza (nasal discharge). They feel worse in general from damp weather.

Other conditions that Mercury can treat: Spongy bleeding gums, gum abscesses, mononucleosis, hepatitis, whooping cough and trembling limbs.

There is no question that Mercury used in large material doses is potentially harmful and there is every reason why we should avoid it where-ever and when-ever possible. For example many people have chosen to replace the mercury amalgam silver filings in there teeth cavities with a composite, gold or porcelain filling. We also need to make laws stricter so that less mercury gets into the environment where it can affect wildlife and has the potential to also get into the food chain. These steps will in time mean less risk of Mercury poisoning.

With all this concern over safety why has homeopathy chosen to use it as a medicine? Mercury has some unique and positive features and characteristics that can be retained when diluted beyond the point where any atoms are present.

This fact must be emphasized, that when these medicines are made in a homeopathic pharmacy at each dilution one part of the solution is added to 99 parts of water. If after 12 dilutions this solution was put under the most sensitive analysis not one molecule or atom of Mercury would be found. At 30 dilutions, the homeopathic 30c dose, it is even more dilute but stronger in its ability to heal than a 12c dilution.

MEDORRHINUM
(Gonorrhea Nosode)

Aversion to rules.

Confident in being a rule breaker. Anything goes.

Creativity with no boundaries.

Through history there have been many times where these people inspire others to start a revolution of new ideas and want to break many of the old norms of society. For example, Henry Miller in 1928 best captures this era in his writing and in the movie about him called <u>Henry and June.</u> Watching this movie will give one the main perspective of this remedy.

A quote from Henry Miller:

> *"Do anything, but let it produce joy. Do anything, but let it yield ecstasy."* Henry Miller, <u>*Tropic of Cancer*</u>

Note how he says: "Do anything" that is the rallying call of an iconoclast.

> *"What is a fanatic? One who believes passionately and acts desperately upon what he believes. I was always believing in something and so getting into trouble. The more my hands were slapped the more firmly I believed."* Henry Miller, <u>*Tropic of Capricorn*</u>

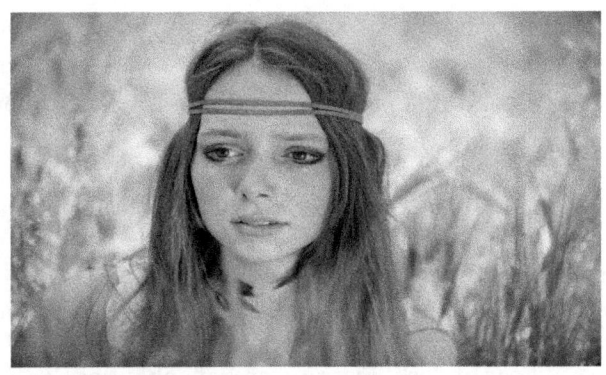

He does not mind getting into trouble as long as he believes in what he is doing out of passion and ones personal belief.

Extremes – does things to excess, goes to extremes in many things (partying, drugs, sex, emotions, violence, etc.) – can be maniacal, aggressive, forceful, wild, impulse, overexcited (GV).

Another era when this influence was strong was in the 1960's. Freedom, rebellion from authority, breaking rules, sexual revolution, mind expanding drugs, new music etc.

The Medorrhinum person is often the passionate adventurer – tries new things for the experience; wants to break the norms of society. Somewhat fearless. Iconoclastic.

- *Very sexual, sensual, passionate, even promiscuous.*

- Can be obsessed with sex, always thinking about it.

- Doesn't believe in rules – loves the forbidden, finds it stimulating to cheat or do illegal things, have affairs, etc.

They are the people who start and sustain a sexual revolution: 1920's and 1960's.

- Aggression – often an inner hardness, can be aggressive and violent, even cruel – although the opposite state of great sensitivity may also be present at other times.

- Body can't keep up with their excesses – becomes depleted, even psychotic.

- Spaced-out states after excessive partying, etc.

- Wild, scattered, out-of-control feelings – chaotic mind. "The mind develops a kind of internal wildness. There is a sensation as if a storm were occurring inside the mind. It is a wild, scattered, out-of-control feeling that is felt inside." (G.Vithoulkas)

- Cruelty to animals. Excessive love of animals, especially in children.

- Keynote: Fear or sensation of someone beside or behind him.

- Fear of dark, insanity, anxiety about health, claustrophobia.

- Seems vague or scattered in conversation (Alum, Arg-n, Cann-I).

- Loses thread of conversation – begins a sentence and forgets what he was about to say.

- Can be vague, confused, absent-minded, forgetful, losing words or threat of conversation.

Study Guide

- Misjudges time – feels a recent event happened a long time ago, or that time moves too slowly.

- Hurried, restless. Sensation - time goes too slowly.

- Night people – like to stay up late, feel better at night.

- Perpetually planning or looking ahead – essence is "what comes next?".

Two types (Vithoulkas): State of excess/profusion: extroverted, aggressive, impulsive, over-excited, passionate, sexual, wild.

State of inversion: Very sensitive type, introverted, shy, even to the point of being unable to speak in the interview, suppressed, reserved.

- Often thought to be hard types who are not very likable and need a lot of distraction.

- But some Medorrhinums "express from the heart" – you can feel the intensity and sensitivity as they describe their symptoms – they seem like Phosphorus but more intense.

- Central idea – "intensity of all sensations and great hypersensitivity".

- Anticipation fears – as strong as Lyc, Arg-n.

Physicals:

- Easily susceptible to gonorrhea – may have had gonorrhea, or may be an inherited miasm.

- History of early heart disease in parents.

- Tendency to have all kinds of warts, tumors, fibroids.

- Tendency to have chest inflammations, chronic colds, coughs, sinusitis, rhinitis.

- Tendency to have heart problems.

- Tendency to have rheumatic pains, esp. after gonorrhea.

- Extremely profuse discharges from all mucous. membranes, and vaginal discharges.

- Bites fingernails (keynote).

- Sleeps on abdomen or in knee-chest position (keynote) (i.e. children sleep on knees).

- Hot feet, uncovers feet at night.

- Great sensitivity of the soles of feet – can't walk on rocks (keynote).

- Loves fruit, esp. oranges, and even unripe fruit. Also craves: ice, meat, fat.

- > by the sea, from sea bathing.

- > evening and night.

Children: Diaper rash.
- Restless, hyperactive, into everything.

    Huge amounts of energy.

- Sexuality develops very early – age 10 or 11.

- Sleeps on knees (knee-chest position) or on abdomen.

- Fear of dark, of monsters in the dark or in the closet.

- Very thirsty.

- Ravenous appetite soon after eating.

- Desires ice, fruit, unripe fruit.

- Chronic cystitis or leukorrhea in young girls.

Study Guide

- Hot feet in children – love to take off their shoes and walk barefoot on a cold floor.

Children (from Philip Bailey):

- Adventurous, fearless. Precocious, quick developers.

- Very inquisitive, always wanting more information about the world around him.

- Not shy, love to talk to strangers.

- Boundless energy. ADD, or ADHD.

- Can be cruel – with insects and animals – but generally grow out of it.

- Very early sexual interests (even at ages 3 to 5) – fascinated by sexual games, and their genitals.

- Puberty – early sexual energies and experiences, very strong sex drive.

- Puberty – can become vain.

From Philip Bailey: Essence is "the passionate adventurer."

- Breadth of character can cause it to be mistaken for many other types.

- Confident, self-possessed, optimistic.

- Not possessive, not attached to things and people, more detached.

- Individuality, independence, flexibility, detachment (like Merc).

- Gets on well with people and enjoys company, good social skills.

- Extremes of temperament from introverted to extroverted, from kind to cruel, from intellectual and detached to highly emotional and intuitive.

- Enormous appetite for life and for experiences of all kinds, just to see what they are like – always hungry for more.

- Adventurers, exploring the world, or emotions and relationships, or intellectual, philosophical, mystical exploration.

- Can be hedonistic, given to sensual excess – especially in youth, usually mature out of it.

- High sex drive and need for new experiences – may try bisexuality or homosexuality in youth.

- May indulge a lot in daydreams, or slip away into a vague state where everything seems unreal, separated, detached. (Can-ind).

- Sense of detachment and expansion is very characteristic, esp. under stress – a kind of spaced-out feeling (Alum, Cann-I) .

- Whenever a patient seems vague or scattered consider Med, Alum, Arg-n, Cann-i.

- Mental wildness – sense of being out of control, sense of chaos in the mind during stress.

- Hurried, panicky when anxious (Alum, Lach).

- At their best in the evening and at night – lyrical, poetic, spontaneous, etc.

NATRUM CARBONICUM
(Sodium Carbonate)

Sensitive people, hurt easily but more composed than Natrum muriaticum. **GRIEF with DIGNITY. Noble gestures. Like to serve others.**

For sore throats and other respiratory infections.

Study Guide

SENSITIVE TO THE SUN: HEADACHES FROM THE SUN, TIRED AND WEAK FROM SITTING IN THE SUN.

Aversion to the taste of milk: she or he will never drink milk.
In order for this remedy to be correct both of the above symptoms need to be present: *worse from the sun and aversion to milk.*

If Natrum muriaticum does not work then consider this remedy.

Refined, responsible and diplomatic. Desire to please others, composed, introverted, well mannered, strong dignity, loyal and long suffering. Avoid those who hurt them.

I do not know the remedy which would have best fit Nelson Mandella (perhaps none), but he displayed the traits of dignity, politeness, diplomacy and grace which we can associte with this remedy.

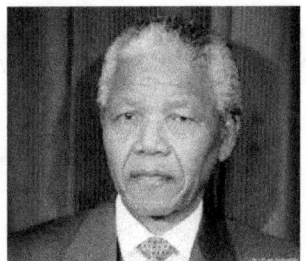

He could feel the suffering of others and his own suffering but he could reach beyond that and not sucumb to revenge and hatred (Lach). When you are the guest of a Narurum crbonica you will always feel you are treated with diplomacy.

Tragic life, withdraw but do their best to act happy. They want to be open and cooperate but down deep they are closed and don't want to discuss their grief.

Polite; won't intrude or impose on others.

Worse before a storm or any change of weather. Dry cough, dry skin, stomach-aches, rheumatism. Old sprains. Kyphosis. Stomach problems. Joint pains. Etc.

NATRUM MURIATICUM
(Table Salt)

OVERSENSITIVE,

HELD IN EMOTIONS,

GRIEF.

WITH THE GRIEF THEY DO NOT WANT CONSOLATION.

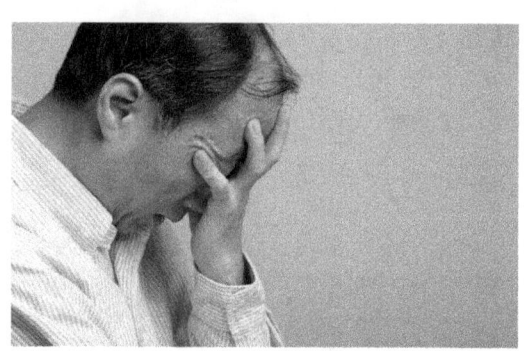

A wall of invulnerability[2] (G. Vithoulkas). They are too easily attached to others and then can't disattach – as it causes pain and heartbreak. *Very deeply felt emotions.*

Oversensitive to the slightest criticism or rejection. Worries about the opinions of others. Silent grief. After a criticism he will isolate himself and feel resentful.

Responsible, hard working, punctual, serious about life, looks to others for approval, introverted.
Falls in love too easily with the wrong person, infatuated but does not reveal what they feel to others. She falls in lover with her bus driver who is already married! Too romantic, too sincere, too infatuated without really knowing the person. Imagine if a Natrum muriaticum would fall in love with a Medorrhinum person – one heart is broken the other thinks nothing of it.

Bitterness and anger from being hurt, difficulty in forgiving, but will not reveal this emotion to others.

Resentment if others try to intrude into their personal space or try to make them open up their feelings. *They try to stay composed.*

This sensitivity will manifest itself emotionally in the person, whose goal in life is "not to hurt, or to be hurt."

---

[2] Homeopathy Medicine of the New Man, Vithoulkas p. 130.

Reactions to minor insults are exaggerated. Grief and depression often follow the insult.

Thoughts of "How could they say that to me?" Compare Staphasagria to this as they feel the same emotion to an insult.

Consolation aggravates. Prefers to suffer in silence.

Worse with sun (especially headaches), (Bell, Glon, Nar-carb, Lach)

Ailments of grief and sorrow. Seem to never recover from a grief – can't let go of old memories. Sensitive emotionally. Feelings are easily hurt. *The person dwells on insults or criticisms.*

Introversion may be a result of such insults, criticism, or grievances of the past. Weeping may be involuntary or uncontrolled. Cries when alone.

Herpetic eruptions (cold sores) of lips and mouth. Dry eruptions especially on the edge of the scalp. Drying and itching of flexor surfaces (Chlorum). Cracking of lips (esp. corners), fingers and nails. Hangnails. Headache which feels like hammers in the head and are worse with the sun. Hay fever. Thirsty. Back pain, which is better with firm support. *Craves salt, chips, olives.* Worse at 10 am.

Dreams of robbers in the house and can't sleep until they search the whole house.

Averse to consolation. They do not like to open up and talk about themselves in the interview. It is painful for them to say how they feel. They can resent your prying into their personal life. *Sad yet unable to weep. Wants to be alone to cry. When they do cry it can be overwhelming.*

Aversion to fats, cuts the fat off of meat. Sore throats, cough, ear aches, bronchitis and allergies.

Take one dose of 30c and wait overnight to see if there is a reaction to the remedy. As long as there is improvement then wait and do not repeat the dose. When there is a relapse or the improvement stops then take another dose.

Materia Medica

Case One: Hay fever, cold sores on lips. Never got over love for boyfrined when a teen. She feels like her heart is still aching. Likes to listen to sad sentimental music alone. Worse from direct sun it makes her very tired. Reserved and very sensitive to what others think and say. After Nat-mur: hay fever better, more cheerful and outgoing, able to let go of the past.

NATRUM PHOSPHORICA
(Sodium Phosphate)

Closed with self expression, desire for others to be open.

Likes others to be open and expressive but with their own feelings they are closed and secretive. Many strong feelings well up inside of them too painful to talk about. Resent anyone who tries to get too close to them. Want others to be happy and feels sympathy for others. Generous.

Mouth blisters especially on the tongue. Acid stomach. Heartburn.

NATRUM SULPHURICUM
(Sodium Sulphate)

Romantic but sad and depressed. Discontented, tearful; lively music makes her sad. Must use all self-control to prevent shooting himself. He may feel: *I deserve more from this world.*

Irritable, < mornings; dislikes to speak or to be spoken to. Spirits low, extremely timid and anxious; mind enfeebled. Jaundice after anger.

Mental troubles arising from a fall or other injuries to head (Arn, Cic, Cocc, Hell). Melancholy with periodical attacks of mania.

Aversion to conflict. A strong liver remedy. Worse from cold and damp. Warts. Itching worse from undressing. Better after stool.

Natrum and Sulphur symptoms in the same patient. Itchy skin, worse from heat and sun.

NICCOLUM

He or she wants to correct others.

Dictatorial. The police state; and tries to impose these standards that are too strict on his family or at work.

Very strong sense of duty. Hard working, do not want much for themselves. Wants to correct others (Kali, Borage). Children who correct their siblings and parents. Struggle and fight against injustice. Intolerant to contradiction. Hunger in middle of night.

NUX MOSCHATA
(Nutmeg)

Sleepy in daytime, irresistible drowsiness (Op). Dreamy, thoughtless, disconnected. Can't recognize well known streets. Vertigo when walking in the open air. Very dry mouth during sleep so that the tongue sticks to the roof of the mouth. Bloating abdomen.

May have the flu or mononucleosis with these symptoms. I had a cancer patient once with these symptoms; he could not stay awake in the daytime. His mouth was very dry at night. This remedy definitely helped him for a time.

NUX VOMICA
(Poison nut)

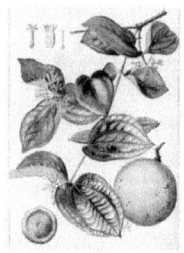

Fastidious, impatient, ambitious and irritable. Anger when things not in their place. Wants to be successful at any cost.

Type A personality.

Hahnemann said of Nux: "*Nux vomica is chiefly successful with persons of an ardent character; of an irritable, impatient temperament, disposed to anger, spite or deception.*" Nux vomica is best adapted to the thin, spare patient with an irritable and nervous temperament who is prone to indigestion and hemorrhoids.

William Boericke says of this remedy: *The Nux vomica individual is very **impatient**, competitive and ambitious. The major focus of his life is his work and achievement. This person is compulsive with his work. People of such temperament have a focused nature and often have strong, aggressive personalities.*

*This **anger** is very characteristic of Nux vomica. The patient can be irritable, at first only sporadically, but as he becomes more pathological the irritability becomes anger, then rage, then frank violence. He becomes infuriated at the slowness and insufficiency of his co-workers. Even an inanimate object can anger the patient: he may tear his shirt if the button doesn't come out easily.*

*Nux vomica patient is very **competitive** in all aspects of his life.*

*He must win even at the cost of his own health. A Nux vomica patient finds it difficult to accept the limitations of anything and he cannot resign himself to circumstances. To keep up with work pressures, he uses various stimulants like coffee, cigarettes, drugs, alcohol, or even sex. From all this come the **bad effects of stimulants** as initially they may help him to cope, but later on, toxicity develops and the entire nervous system becomes overwhelmed and oversensitive.*

*Such patients are easily subject states of collapse **from over work or abuse of substances or from indulgence and excess**. The Nux patient is also very **fastidious** and becomes angry if objects are not in their proper place.*

*Nux vomica has a **characteristic peculiarity** of waking in the morning, falling back to sleep, then waking again feeling worse. He has a bitter taste in his mouth and his tongue is coated. There is a dull headache and he is constipated. All this happens because of inappropriate sleep or we can say **sleeplessness**. His mind is so wrought up that his thoughts run around and don't let him sleep. There is a typical **morning aggravation with waking at 4 a.m.***

*The Nux patient is very chilly and has a repugnance to cold and cold air. He feels cold from the least movement or from uncovering. He **must be covered in every stage of fever, chill, heat and sweat**.*

*On the physical plane, Nux vomica pathology centers largely on the **gastrointestinal tract**. There is marked craving for spicy and fatty food, alcohol, beer and stimulants.*

***Hiccough**; from overeating. **Eructations** are sour, bitter; nausea and vomiting especially in the morning and after eating. The patient feels **"I would be better, if I could vomit"**.*

*Stomach pain worse after anger; worse from tight clothing and better by warmth. Soreness of abdominal wall, worse after eating. **Peptic ulcers and gastritis in workaholic patients**. Uneasy, fitful and **fruitless urging for bowels to act**; > stool. **Constipation**, inactive peristalsis. Strains hard at stool; feels as* *if a part remains unexpelled.* (Boericke, Materia Medica with Repertory)

The nervous system seems bound up and works against itself. This is described best by Kent: *"Another state running through Nux is that actions are turned in opposite directions. When the stomach is sick, it will empty its contents with no great effort ordinarily, but in Nux there is retching and straining as if the action were going the wrong way, as if it would force the abdomen open; a reversed action; retches, gags, and strains and after a prolonged effort he finally empties the stomach."* (Kent)

Case 1: 40 year old patient with painful muscle spasms. Very ambitious, his family is ready to leave him as he never spends any time with them. He is often irritable, answers his phone in the interview in order to take care of business matter. After Nux his spasms are better and he starts to have a more balanced life.

If the muscle spasms that are even more severe; such as they bend the patient or make him completely rigid or seizures with impatience then think of *Strychninum* (Nux and Ignatia contain *Strychninum*).

Strychninum: convulsions, severe irritability, back spasms which are of the most severe type. May have anxiety that something bad will happen.

OPIUM
(Papaver Somniferum)

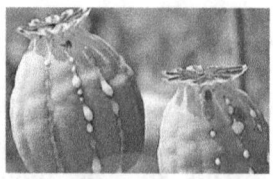

Sleepy all the time or SLEEPY IN THE DAYTIME

Study Guide

Painless in situations that one would think would be painful

Severe constipation. Can't tell the truth, spaced out.

Ailments from shock and fright. *Shock leads to dissociation and numbness.* Loss of integrity, lies and steals easily, no longer knows what is true. (Morph, Salix alba). Looks happy, but can't find the truth.

May be a charismatic person but also a charlatan. Easily lie to get what they want.

Apathy, loss of consciousness. Breathing stops on going to sleep.

Painless paralysis, twitchings of limbs, convulsions. Narcolepsy.

PETROLEUM
(Coal Oil)

Seasickness or car sick with accumulation of water in the mouth. Aversion to fats.

Head – sensation a cold breeze blowing on it.

Vertigo on rising from a seat. Moist erruption behind the ears.

Tips of fingers are dry, <u>cracked</u>, rough, fissured worse every winter or from putting the hands in water.

Dry hands which crack and bleed. Feel better in a warm place.

May have some Graphite symptoms as both are carbon remedies.

PHOSPHORUS
(Elemental Phosphorus)

THIRSTY FOR <u>COLD DRINKS</u>. May be up to ten drinks per day. Prefer ice cold drinks or better still <u>carbonated ice cold drinks – soda pop</u>. STRONG EMPATHY FOR OTHERS,

VERY SOCIAL.

Friendly people who easily make contact with others and make others feel included and cared for.

The universal symbol for Phosphorus – happy to see and connect with everyone if just for a minute:

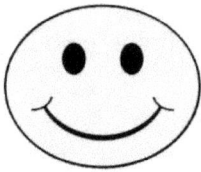

Fear:
- Of being alone
- Of the dark
- OF THUNDERSTORMS
- That something bad will happen
- May have panic attacks

Emotionally:
- A VERY OPEN, SYMPATHETIC, SOCIABLE NATURE (PULS)
- Effervescent, a bubbly affectionate personality (Arg-nit)
- Easily reassured
- The person who needs Phosphorus will usually have many friends. She can be so helpful to others that she becomes exhausted (Car, Cocculus, Kali-phos).

Desires fresh air.
Symptoms worse from lying on the left side.
Bruises easily, bleeds easily.
Other pathologies that phosphorus will treat include:

- Nausea and vomiting which are better from cold drinks. Diarrhea, with involuntary stool
- Tightness of the chest, burning in the chest, oppression of the chest
- Tickling in the larynx when speaking. Looses her voice. Hard, dry, tight hacking cough
- Symptoms better from sleep and generally refreshed by sleep
- Numbness of parts especially the fingers

This remedy affects the lungs, stomach etc.

Nash says of this remedy: *Tall, slender, narrow-chested, phthisical* (tuberculosis) *patients, delicate eyelashes, soft hair, or nervous, weak persons who like to be magnetized. Waxy, half anaemic, jaundiced persons.*

Anxious, universal restlessness, can't stand or sit still. < in dark or when left alone, before a thunder storm.

Burnings prominent in every place, as in mouth, stomach, small intestines, anus, between scapulae, intense, running up spine, palms of hands, heat begins in hands, spreads to face.

Craving for cold things, ice cream, which agrees, or cold water, which is thrown up as it gets warm in the stomach. Must eat often or he faints. Must get up at night to eat.

Sinking, faint, empty feeling in head, chest, stomach and whole abdominal cavity.

Cough, < twilight till midnight, < lying on left side, > on right side. Right lower lobe most affected.

Diarrhoea, profuse, pouring out as from a hydrant; watery with sagolike particles or dysenteric, with wide open anus.

Apathetic, unwilling to talk, answers slowly, moves sluggishly.

Constipation: faeces slender, long, dry, tough and hard like a dog's; voided with difficulty.

Hemorrhagic diathesis; slight wounds bleed profusely, haemoptysis; metrorrhagia worse; vicarious, from nose, stomach, anus, urethra in amenorrhoea.

Cannot talk, the larynx is so painful; cough, going from warm to cold air, laughing, talking, reading, eating, lying on left side (DROS., STAN.).

As a general characteristic, Burning is almost as strong under this remedy as under ARSENICUM and SULPHUR. There is no organ or tissue in which it may not be found, from the outer skin to the innermost surface of every tract or parenchyma. It may be subjective only without actual rise of temperature, or it may attend organic changes in malignant diseases, with great rise of temperature.

The sensation of BURNING in an intense degree should always place PHOSPHORUS in the front rank for consideration. Again, there is perhaps no remedy having stronger action on The Nervous System. It attacks it in its very citadel of strength, the brain and spinal cord, producing softening or atrophy with all its attendant symptoms in their order, as prostration, trembling, numbness, and complete paralysis. It does this in both acute and chronic form of disease.

It will be found in acute typhoids as well as in that slowly progressive disease, locomotor ataxia. Its causes may be sudden, like pneumonia, typhus, exanthematic diseases, croup, bronchitis, when vitality reaches its lowest ebb, or may arise in a condition undermined by grief, care, or excessive mental exertion; excess in venery or onanism.

Its action at the first may be characterized by a burning heat in various parts, and especially in the skin, with restless moving and anxiety, especially at twilight. Over-sensitiveness of all senses, such as external impressions, light, odors, noises, touch, etc., and later when organic changes have taken place the other extreme, of loss of motion, sensation, and sensitiveness obtains.

In the former state there is one very characteristic symptom, THE PATIENT MOVES CONTINUALLY, CAN'T SIT OR STAND STILL A MOMENT. Instead of fidgety feet, like ZINCUM, he is FIDGETY ALL OVER. PHOSPHORUS affects every tissue. The blood becomes broken down or impoverished. Chlorosis and pernicious anaemia obtain.

Study Guide

APIS and KALI CARB. also each have anaemia or a pale waxy or what is called bloodless appearance of the patient. They all have oedema or bloating, and there is one peculiar difference in the face between them. In KALI CARB. the upper lids bloat and hang down like a bag of water. In APIS it is more in the lower lids, while in PHOSPHORUS they bloat all around the eyes; and the whole face bloats. Under PHOSPHORUS the blood becomes so broken down that it will not clot any more, and we have purpura hsemorrhagica.

Even in apparently healthy tissues we have this strong characteristic discovered by Hahnemann, viz.: "SLIGHT WOUNDS BLEED MUCH." This is what is called the haemorrhagic diathesis, and much to be feared, as many persons having it may bleed to death from any slight abrasion; and this same tendency to bleed extends to fungoid growths like fibroids, fungoids, cancers, etc., and are very dangerous and troublesome.

Then again PHOSPHORUS attacks the bones in the form of necrosis. It is so especially of the lower jaw, but is also true of other parts, as the vertebras; and I once cured a very extensive and long standing case of caries of the tibia with it.

Fatty degeneration of heart, liver and kidneys, with the characteristic anaemic condition, should call attention to this remedy. General emaciation, rapid or slowly progressing like atrophy in children, also comes under its tissue destroying power.

And so we find it to be a remedy of wide range and great power. But it is never enough for the homeopathist to know simply the action in general upon any organ or set of organs. He must know how it acts differently from other remedies when acting upon the same tissue or organs. Now while PHOSPHORUS acts upon the mind, to cause "great anxiety and restlessness" as in other remedies, ACONITE, ARSENICUM, etc., it must be remembered that it is the anxiety and restlessness that precedes another state.

It belongs to a stage of irritation in the brain and nervous system which if not checked will go on to organic changes, which will be attended with a very different set of symptoms, such as come for instance from actual brain softening in which appears APATHY, SLUGGISHNESS; TALKS SLOWLY, IS INDIFFERENT OR WON'T TALK AT ALL.

There is one particular symptom worthy of note: THE PATIENT FEARS TO BE LEFT ALONE; is afraid; afraid of the dark, in a thunder storm, etc. This is more during the irritable stage of which we have spoken. PHOSPHORUS is a great remedy in typhoids, especially with lung complications, and here we often get stupor and low muttering delirium like LACHESIS, but while LACHESIS is worse after sleep, PHOSPHORUS is generally better, if he can get to sleep.

In the late stage of brain or nervous troubles, calling for this remedy, we find the patient losing all ambition to do anything; either mental or physical labor is shunned. There is great indifference. He cannot think with his usual clearness; cannot apply himself to study or mental operations, ideas come slowly or not at all. Again the patient is sometimes amative, or like HYOSCYAMUS shamelessly exposes himself.

There is no remedy that covers a greater variety of mind symptoms arising from brain trouble than PHOSPHORUS. No remedy produces greater vertigo, with a longer list of various connections. I have found it one of the best and oftenest indicated for VERTIGO OF THE AGED.

Chronic congestion to the head is characteristic, and the sense of burning in the brain is prominent; the heat and congestion seems to COME UP FROM THE SPINE.

HEAT RUNNING UP THE BACK is more characteristic of this than any other remedy. Deafness is prominent, and is peculiar, in that it is especially DEAFNESS TO THE HUMAN VOICE, a common symptom in the aged. The most frequent use I have made of the remedy in nose affections is in a chronic catarrh, in which the patient frequently blows SMALL QUANTITIES OF BLOOD FROM THE NOSE; the hand-kerchief is ALWAYS bloody.

As I said when writing upon the tissues, the face of PHOSPHORUS is characteristically pale and bloated around the eyes, but in pneumonia we often find circumscribed redness of the cheek upon the side of the lung inflamed. This is also true with SANGUINARIA. About the mouth and tongue I do not know anything particularly characteristic. It has a peculiar symptom of the throat. THE FOOD SWALLOWED COMES UP IMMEDIATELY AS IF IT HAD NEVER REACHED THE STOMACH. This is supposed to be due to spasmodic stricture of the oesophagus.

Study Guide

Under appetite and thirst we have some very valuable indications for this remedy.

HUNGER is one, must eat often or he faints; right after or soon after a meal, is hungry; hungry in the night; must eat. He is relieved by eating, but is soon hungry again. This calls to mind IODINE, CHELIDONIUM, PETROLEUM, ANACARDIUM, etc.

The thirst is also peculiar. He wants COLD THINGS, like PULSATILLA, but AS SOON AS THEY GET WARM IN THE STOMACH THEY ARE VOMITED.

Some people have an abnormal craving for salt, or salt food, and eat too much of it. PHOSPHORUS is a good remedy to counteract the bad effects. (NAT. MUR.)

We have many kinds of vomiting under PHOSPHORUS, but nothing characteristic except the one already mentioned.

We have already spoken of the hungry, faint feeling in the stomach. Sometimes this is described as an empty, gone feeling, and here again we think of such remedies as IGNATIA, HYDRASTIS, SEPIA and others; but PHOSPHORUS does not stop here with this sensation, but extends through the WHOLE ABDOMEN. No remedy has this feeling in the abdomen so strong as PHOSPHORUS.

Under stool and rectum occur some very characteristic symptoms also, for instance: Stools profuse, watery, POURING AWAY AS FROM A HYDRANT, with lumps of white mucus, like GRAINS OF TALLOW. Stools bloody, with small white particles like opaque frog-spawn. Stools involuntarily oozing from a CONSTANTLY OPEN ANUS, or dysenteric stools with wide-open anus and GREAT TENESMUS. Constipation; faeces slender, LONG, DRY, TOUGH LIKE DOG STOOLS. No remedy has a richer array of stool symptoms, and as we see by the above few select ones, some of them are very unique and have often been verified. It will repay any physician to carefully and frequently look them over.

This remedy powerfully excites the sexual appetite in both sexes. It is almost irresistible, and leads the patient into a mania in which he will expose himself. This is succeeded by the opposite extreme of impotence, though the desire remains after the ability to perform is gone. Of course, these sexual symptoms are accompanied with concomitant symptoms of the drug.

Upon the female sexual organs PHOSPHORUS is true to its general haemorrhagic tendencies; if the menses do not appear, there is often VICARIOUS BLEEDING from the nose or lungs instead. PHOSPHORUS is BOUND TO BLEED. It is so with cancer of the womb or breasts also. They bleed easily. Upon the RESPIRATORY ORGANS also this is one of our greatest remedies. Beginning with the voice and larynx, it causes and cures GREAT hoarseness. Patient can hardly make a loud noise, and is apt to be worse in the evening or fore-part of the night. There is PAIN IN THE LARYNX, worse by talking, or can't talk at all on account of it. In croup, it sometimes comes in after ACONITUM and SPONGIA have failed. The disease has progressed downward until it involves the bronchi and parenchyma of the lungs. It is of indispensable value here, and, also when, after the violence of the affection seems to have abated, the patient hoarses up every evening and seems to be INCLINED TO RELAPSE.

In bronchitis the cough is tight, worse from evening to midnight, also from SPEAKING, LAUGHING, READING ALOUD (ARGENTUM MET.), COLD, AND LYING ON LEFT SIDE. The patient suppresses the cough with a moan just as long as he can, because it hurts him so. The whole body TREMBLES with the cough.

It has great oppression of breathing in both acute and chronic affections of the lungs. There is HEAVINESS, AS OF A WEIGHT ON THE CHEST.

In pneumonia, for which PHOSPHORUS is one of our best remedies, it attacks by preference the LOWER HALF OF THE RIGHT LUNG. It is apt to be indicated by the symptoms, either at the beginning of the stage of hepatization, when it puts a stop to the further progress of the disease, but its more frequent application comes in where the stage of hepatization is past and we want to break it up and promote absorption or resolution. Here it has no equal, as I am fully convinced by abundant experience.

Now, do not misunderstand and give the remedy blindly on a pathological indication only. If you do you will sometimes fail, and ought to. But I repeat, this remedy will oftener be found the indicated one here than any other. After the hepatization begins to break up, other remedies like TARTAR EMETIC, SULPHUR and LYCOPODIUM will come in.

In pleuritis you will find stitches in the LEFT side increased by lying upon the left side. Remember in both affections PHOSPHORUS is characteristically increased by lying upon the left side.

In tuberculosis, it is oftenest indicated in the incipient stage with the symptom of cough, oppression and general weakness already mentioned; but I have often found it indicated in the later stages, and if given very high and in the single dose and not repeated have seen it greatly benefit even incurable cases. If given too low and repeated it will fearfully aggravate.

One of the most characteristic symptoms of this remedy is, "FEELING OF INTENSE HEAT RUNNING UP THE BACK." Again the burning may be in spots along the spine. Also it has intense heat and burning between the scapulae. (See also LYCOPODIUM.)

These, like the rest of the burnings of PHOSPHORUS, often occur in diseases of the spine and nervous system, but not necessarily so. Like ZINC, these burnings may be purely subjective, but are none the less valuable as therapeutic indications.

Another very characteristic symptom of PHOSPHORUS is BURNING OF THE HANDS. It is as strong as the burning feet of SULPHUR, and is found both in acute and chronic diseases ; cannot bear to have the hands covered. The flashes of heat all over (which PHOSPHORUS has) BEGIN in the hands and spread from there even to the face. It now remains to call attention to the Constitution of Phosphorus.

"Tall, slender persons of sanguine temperament, fair skin, blonde or red hair; quick, lively perception and sensitive nature."

"Tall, slender phthisical patients, delicate eyelashes, soft hair."

"Tall, slender women disposed to stoop. Young people who grow too rapidly and are inclined to stoop. Nervous, weak persons who like to be magnetized." (Nash - Leaders)

PHYTOLACCA
(Poke Root)

This is a remedy for SWOLLEN GLANDS, tonsillitis, sore throats, and various coughs.

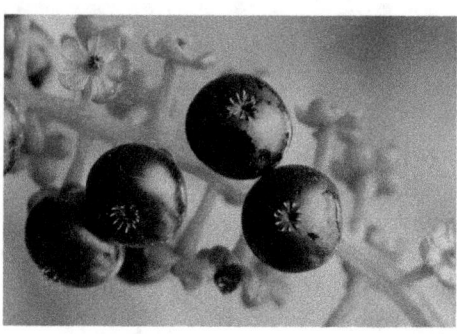

Some symptoms that indicate its use are:
- Lots of mucous from the nose
- The throat is dark, red and feels hot
- Sensation of a lump in the throat
- Shooting pains into the ears on swallowing
- Diphtheria
- Cannot swallow anything hot
- Feels better to drink cold things
- Dry, hacking, tickling cough, worse at night
- High fever, alternating with chilliness and great weakness
- Mumps
- Hard painful swelling of the cervical glands
- Back pain and stiffness
- Pains in the bones, stiff neck
- Worse from cold damp weather

Mastitis. Breast hard and very sensitive. Tumors of breast with enlarged glands. Breast abscess. Shooting pains in shoulder with stiffness and inability to raise it (Sang, Ferr)

Kent says of this remedy: *You will notice the resemblance of this drug to MERCURY, and it is an antidote to MERCURY. In those lingering mercurial bone pains, where the patient has been salivated; the pains come on at night from the warmth of the bed; the body aches; a chronic, sore, bruised state; soreness of the periosteum where the flesh is thin, over the tibia; joints; soreness of the muscles; drawing and cramping; drawing in the muscles of the back; backache, worse at night; worse from the warmth of the bed.*

Study Guide

The patient suffers from these symptoms in cold, damp weather, as in MERCURY. Tendency to ulceration, hence its usefulness in syphilis; old, chronic, syphilitic ulcers; the patient has been salivated; had MERCURY rubbed in; he became saturated with it, but it no longer helps. Ulcers in the throat; on the skin; on mucous membranes anywhere. Spasmodic conditions; drawing in the muscles; this may extend to violent spasms; opitsthotonos; sometimes the cervical region is affected and the head is drawn back; jerking and twitching of the muscles.

The symptoms are aggravation at night, on cold days, in a cold room, and from the heat of the bed; so that there is a controversy between heat and cold.

It seems that the remedy centers in the MAMMARY GLANDS. Soreness and lumps in the breasts from each cold, damp spell; becomes chilled and a sore breast results; sore breast in connection with the menses; a nursing woman is exposed to the cold, the breast inflames and the milk becomes stringy; coagulated milk. This comes out in the proving, but poke root has been extensively used by cattle raisers when the cow's milk became thick and there were lumps in the bag, and when the condition was brought on from the cow standing out in the rain. (Kent)

PLATINA
(Platinum)

***Arrogance, haughty, egotism, condescending.* PRIDE**

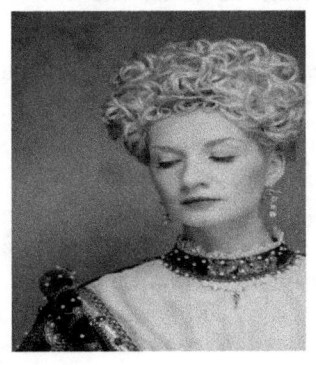

They want to appear mysterious, beautiful and superior to others.

Aristocratic. Proud. Feels taller than others. Other people seem small. Flirtatious, nymphomania.

Anesthesias of tissues. Numbness with headache.

Case 1: I had a patient with very numb lips. He could not get over the fact his girlfriend had left him. He had a strong feeling of indignation. He wanted to kill her and generally thought that everyone was less than him. After Platina he was much improved. This remedy can be used in certain cases of paralysis, multiple sclerosis. Constipation when traveling.

Burning pain in ovaries. When they walk into the room one feels they are boasting in some manner. Egotism, full of themselves.

PODOPHYLUM
(May Apple)

Explosive diarrhea. Diarrhea with gas.

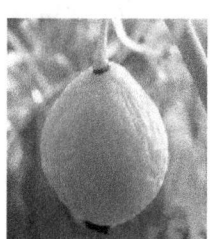 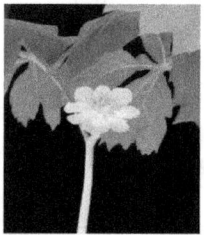

Case 1: After going to Mexico she had gas that exploded with the diarrhea. After one dose of Podophylum she is all better.

There may be loquacity during heat.

Kent says: *Everything taken into the stomach becomes sour. The glands of the stomach are as if paralyzed; there is no digestion; this goes on until we have vomiting and diarrhoea. During this there is a wonderful disturbance in the abdomen; rumbling; gurgling as if animals were floundering about; clinically, as if fish were turning and tossing in a pond, as we have seen them before a storm. Rumbling and rolling. This is attended with severe, cramping pains doubling her up.*

Abdomen is sensitive; so sore she cannot endure pressure. The soreness extends to the stomach, intestines and finally to the liver. The whole abdominal viscera are sore. sensitive to pressure.

After this comes a gurgling, watery stool, pouring out of the anus. A tremendous outpouring so that the patient wonders where all the fluid comes from, and soon it comes on again. Copious, enormous, and very frequent. (Kent)

PSORINUM
(Scabies Nosode)

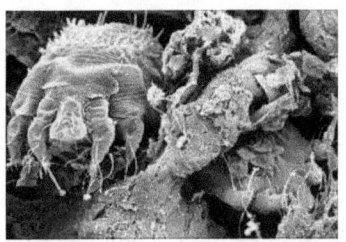

VERY CHILLY, even in summer wants to wear a hat and scarf.

Pessimism. Feels life is not worth living. Hopeless and suicidal depression (Aur, Lac-h). Street person mentality. Even if you try to help them they see no reason to work or try to get anything out of life. Giving up with depression. Bad odor to the body. They don't want to clean themselves.

Itchy skin, eczema. This is the most frequent pathology seen with this remedy.

Case 1: I treated an elderly gentleman who had depression. He felt pessimistic about life in general, that nothing was ever going to be good or prosperous. His father had suffered a lot during the depression in the 1920's. His terrible headaches came on *when-ever a storm was approaching.* Gen: Storm, approach of: PSOR. After Psorinum his headaches and pessimistic outlook were both much improved.

Case 2: Flu symptoms. Very chilly, body can't warm up. Feeling hopeless. After Psorinum 30c next day all better and positive mood restored.

Case 3: Teen with suicidal depression for eight years. At age seven she was given cortisone for eczema. This got better but then the depression came on. After Psorinum 30c one a week the depression is better then the eczema came back and finally this was taken care of with Psorinum 200c. She went to to enjoy her life and especially being involved with the theater and acting.

Case 4: Patient in 50's. He comes to see me because of pain in his rotting teeth. He lives on the street most of the time. His cloths smell terrible. He says that he does not care about his teeth just wants me to give him some pain medicine. Next time he came in his gum inflamation is much better and he is not so depressed. Also he is taking care of her person hygiene.

With this remedy the suppression of the eczema can lead to a very severe depression. In Bufo and Cicuta the suppression of eczema leads to convulsions and epilepsy. In Zinc the supression of skin ailments can lead to restlessness and encephalitis. It is not clear why and how the body has to find a new pathology from suppression.

The body seems to want to vent out its pathology. If it is blocked it will find a new way out. In Chinese medicine there is the concept of energy that has to move and complete a cycle through all the meridians. The energy can not stay in one place if it is blocked it will find a new place, new body system to effect.

Study Guide

PULSATILLA
(Wind Flower)

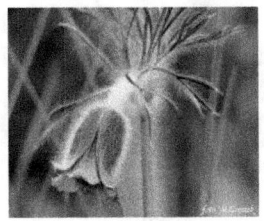

Affectionate

Feels forsaken

Clingy

Desires affection, *mild and yielding. Worse from heat. They easily create a situation where their care giver wants to give them affection. Worse from being alone, want someone there to hold their hand.*

If children are given enough affection from both parents they will be able to transition past the Pulsatilla stage. If they loose this bond too early they can need this remedy when they feel: forsaken, depressed, cry too easily and become clingy.

Pulsatilla is a very important and useful remedy for acute infections. It will often not only treat the present infection but also treat the underlying cause if there is a chronic tendency to infections.

Emotional characteristics: MILD, YIELDING, GENTLE, SOFT, TIMID AND WEEPS EASILY (Opposite to natrum muriaticum).

AN INNOCENT AND OPEN NATURE.

Materia Medica

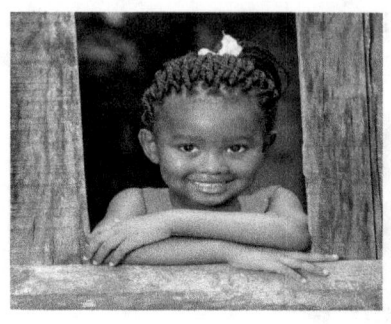

FORSAKEN FEELING.
DESIRES, AND IS BETTER FROM,
AFFECTION AND CONSOLATION.

THIRSTLESS WITH A DRY MOUTH.

Worse from a warm and stuffy room, heat and sun. **Better** from open air. *The feet feel hot at night, so they put them out of the covers.*

Aggravation from and aversion to fats. **Nausea from fats.**

Discharges are bland and thick. Many symptoms are better with gentle continued motion. Symptoms ever changing, like menses changing color every month, headaches that change their location or pains in the body rapidly shifting from one part to another.

Unlike Belladonna and Chamomile, Pulsatilla has predominantly a *mild, yielding and gentle nature.* At times when the Pulsatilla person experiences severe pain they will display some irritability and discontentedness. They often have *changeable moods,* i.e. happy affectionate and extroverted, then sad and weeping, then irritable and won't speak.

The Pulsatilla patient will try to please others, in order to receive consolation and support (Lac-can). They *crave affection and suffer* from feelings of *abandonment.* He or she will often develop *forsaken feelings* and feel alone in the world. They therefore want protection and consolation from family. *Crying easily* and *wanting* to be *held* is the most common disposition of Pulsatilla. Children will often hang on and *cling* to the parent.

In a Pulsatilla state the person will often have a lack of confidence. There will be shyness and timidity. They become easily persuaded or suppressed by others. It is hard for them to be assertive. If positive feelings are shown toward them they will open up easily, express their emotions joyfully and want a lot of personal interaction.

They need this positive interaction so much they may find ways to get attention and the love they crave by acting helpless, needy and tearful. "I am in such pain, you have to help me!" or "No one cares or understands that I am all alone. *You have to take care of me.*"

If they are abused they will become fearful, closed, extremely timid, cry easily, and search for the support of those who can help to extricate them from the situation.

In an ideal case of Pulsatilla, the emotional disposition above will be complimented by the following symptoms:
- Irritable and a general aggravation when in a warm room
- <u>Desires open air</u>
- Better from uncovering the blankets, especially their hot burning feet
- Aggravation from rich food, such as cream and <u>fat</u>
- Aversion to fatty foods and fat on meat
- <u>*Thirstless*</u> (only two to four drinks a day). Does not want to drink even though he has a dry mouth
- Desires ice cream and other cold foods

The emotional state and general symptoms may have been present for days, months or years before the following physical symptoms present themselves. Typical symptoms of an acute infection in a child leading to her crying and wanting to sleep with her parents.

Acute and chronic ear infections. Thick, bland (doesn't burn the skin) yellow green discharges. Changeable discharges. After measles the ear problems are worse. After scarlet fever there is impaired hearing.

For women and girls Pulsatilla is beneficial for the following conditions:
- Headaches in girls who are about to begin their first menses.
- Painful menses since puberty
- Irritable and weeping before menses
- Irregular menses
- Menses that are changeable in appearance
- Suppressed menses from getting the feet wet

- Violent menstrual cramps

Other symptoms and presentations include:
- Asthmatic respirations
- Coughs of variable description, which are better in the open air and worse from lying down
- Fear of the dark or being alone
- Hay fever with loss of the sense of smell
- Urinary tract infections
- Varicose veins
- Sleeps on the back, with hands on the abdomen, or hands over the head

It is very **unlikely** that Pulsatilla will have any positive effect if the patient is thirsty, likes to be heated or is aggravated by the cool open air.

From the above description, one can see that Pulsatilla can treat many different types of diseases. As long as the emotional state is present and the general symptoms fit then there is a good chance that Pulsatilla will have a good effect. Recommendation: prescribe this remedy in the 30c potency one time every seven to ten days for a month or two until the chronic tendency is permanently cured.

Case 1: A woman in her 50's with psoriasis. She could not go shopping alone and had to take her husband with her. After Pulsatilla her psoriasis got better and she was able to travel alone for the first time to see her grandchildren in another state.

SANICULA AQUA
(Mineral Springs Water Allen Park Ottawa Illinois)

This remedy is most similar to Sulphur and Calcarea carbonica: *The patient wants to uncover their feet at night* (Sulph).

Worse from heat.
Defiant, headstrong, obstinate, does not want to be touched.

Perspiration on the head and neck at night (Calc-c).

Study Guide

Fear of pain.

Fear of dark. Restless, desire to go from place to place.

Painful large stools. *Fear to have a bowel movement.* Bashful stool.

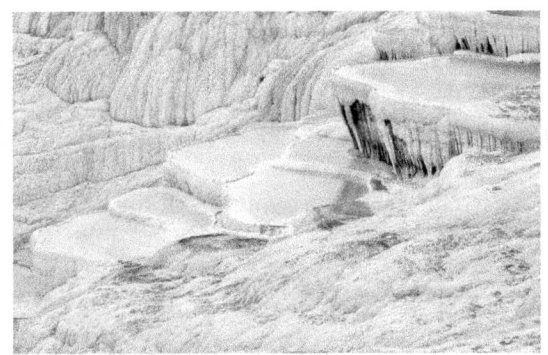

Cough excited by talking or laughing. Cracking in the skin of the hands. Pains in the shoulders. Offensive odor to feet. Car and sea sickness. Discharges smell like fish brine. Craves bacon.

Easily car sick or seasick.

The uterine symptoms remind one of Sepia and Lilium tigr - bearing down as if contents of pelvis would escape. Worse walking; jar. Must support parts by hand against the vulva. Child wants to nurse all the time, yet loses flesh. (Nat. mur., Abrot.)

Cases: three cases of children who have severe constipaton. A week between bowel movements. Very dry stool. Fear to have a bowel movement with fear of pain. After Sanicual all symptoms better.

SEPIA
(Cuttle fish ink)

Irritability with AVERSION TO FAMILY and COMPANY.

<u>Mood is better from physical exercise.</u>

Lack of warmth and affection for others. Prefer to be alone.

Chronic colds, sinusitis, sore throat.

Tired out from too many cares or too much work; become indiffernt to their family.

Materia Medica

INDIFFERENCE TO THOSE LOVED MOST.
Push their husband and children away. *Irritable from too much company. Better when alone,* unsociable. Aversion to sex. Lots of PMS symptoms.

Easily irritable from the demands of her children and husband.

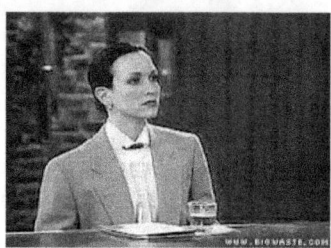

The talented actress Bebe Neuwirth plays the part of Lilith Stermin in the sitcom Frazier. She portrays a Sepia type of person: Critical, prideful, wound up like a tight spring ready to shoot out a barb of criticism, masculine, emotionally cold and independent.

Sepia can be critical of others, they often don't realize how much hurt they can inflict on others especially their children. Stasis: emotionally not caring one way or the other about those they normally love; physically, the circulation is sluggish and they have low energy. Feel worn out, and can't think clearly. Desire to be alone. This is a slightly different type of sepia i.e. indifferent from long hours of child care, no positive emotions left to give or nurture.

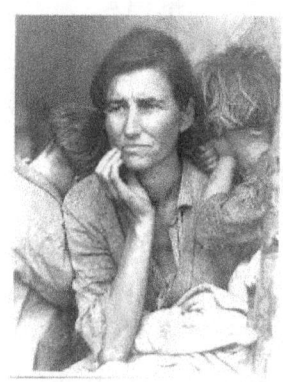

Study Guide

This famous image above taken from the depresion era shows a mother in a Sepia state; two children try and receive some affections but she is care worn and indifferent toward them.

Chilly and are worse from cold.

Better from vigorous exercise or some sports activity. They are much less irritable after exercise.

Aggravation before menses or at menopause. <u>Prolapse, a pressure and bearing down as if everything will protrude from the pelvis.</u>

Nausea from the smell of food or when pregnant. Vaginitis (vaginal infection). Desire for vinegar. Lump sensation in the rectum. Psoriasis.

Dry cough, except in the morning where there is profuse expectoration.
Cases: 1. A women in her late 30's came to see me for irritability and psoriasis. The skin conditon covered most of her body.

About ten years previously she had lost interest in being married and lived alone ever since. She never wanted to have children.

The psoriasis started after a severe strep infection which had been treated with antibiotics. A day after taking Sepia 30c she got a fever and very sore throat. I asked her to wait rather than take the antibiotics again and within a week her infection was better, along with most of the psoriasis. Her vitality after that went very high, she became very social and later on had a boyfriend again. The psoriasis eventually completely disappeared.

This is another example of how suppression of an acute illness can lead to a chronic illness and for each person the susceptibility is differernt and therefore the next weakest link in the chain is different leading to different symptoms.

Case 2: In this case a women in her 40's had a prolapsed uterus.

She was very irritable especially before her periods at which time she could not tollerate anyone to touch her; even her husband and children. This had become much worse after taking birth control pills. She was always senstive to cold, craved vinegar and loved to exercise which made her feel physically better and put her in a much better mood. After Sepia 30c once a week she was better in all respects.

George Vithoulkas from his <u>Materia Medica Viva</u>: *Sepia will not express jealousy directly. What will it do? It will try to destroy things the other person loves. Whomever or whatever the other person loves. For example: a book. The partner reads a book and finds it fantastic. Suddenly the book disappears. It ended up in the fireplace. Or: "I love this song, this CD." Suddenly the CD is destroyed. Sepia doesn't say it directly. Instead, it tries to destroy beloved things. Or it says things it knows the other person is sensitive to. Sepia understands very quickly where someone has his weak points.* (Vithoulkas)

SILICA

(Elemental Silica – Glass)

MILD, DELICATE, REFINED, YIELDING, TIMID but stubborn.

Constipation and he perspires easily. Sweat on the head at night. Mild agreeable personality.

Silica can be used for very deep chronic illness. For ear infections that are often recurrent. The cervical glands are swollen. The middle ear fills up with pus. Impaired hearing from catarrh, or mucous and puss in the eustachian tube. The mastoid becomes infected. The tonsils are swollen and puss comes out of them. Bad breath from recurrent throat and tonsillar infections. Very slow recovery from ear infections or continuous ear infections. History of surgical tubes in the ear. Pale complexion.

LACK OF COURAGE, YIELDING, TIMID, Faint hearted AND REFINED, YET STUBBORN AND OBSTINATE.

They will say: "*I have my convictions* but I also have an aversion to argue them." *Too tired to argue and do not like to be in conflict with others.* Feels overwhelmed and pressured by other people. Fear of criticism. *Won't give up on what they believe.*

Thoughtful and will listen to reason. Insightful but timid.

Has the ability to do well, but doesn't have confidence in herself to accomplish it.

In newborn babies, the features are fine and delicate, the hair thin, and the head may be large with the top fontanelle staying open longer than normal.

Feels self conscious, so dwells on small details, to the point of being irresolute and wanting to give up. Performance anxiety, such as stage fright and exam phobia. Fear of making mistakes in general.

Worse from mental exertion, easily exhausted.

Constipation and *inactivity of the rectum*. There is great straining, the stool is partly expelled and then recedes again.

Perspiration of the hands, feet and axilla that is offensive and acrid. *Smelly feet at the end of the day. Headache b*etter from wrapping up the head warmly.

Repeated infections that go toward a suppurative process (infections that produce clear, yellow or green pus) such as felons (a painful swelling near the nail that is filled with puss), abscesses, boils, acne and ulcers.

Slow incomplete inflammations, such as a low fever that sticks around for days or months with no spike (which would resolve the infection in a more healthy person).

Tendency to swelling of the glands, indurations (hardening of the glands) and keloids (a hardened scar that is raised above the skin around it).

White spots on the finger nails, crippled nails (curved or distorted in some way). I*ngrown toe nails* (Nit-ac).

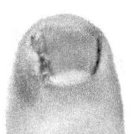

Chilliness and extreme sensitivity to cold and damp. Defects of the spine, such as scoliosis. Acne that leaves scars.

Silica has many similarities to Pulsatilla. They are both able to cure deep chronic tendencies. Both have a temperament that is *mild, yielding, timid,* lacking in self confidence. Silica is chilly while Pulsatilla is worse from heat.

Silica patients feel a *fear of failure*. Such as fear of an examination, or fear beginning new activities. Persons who need Silica are *refined*, feeling overly responsible about trifles, *sensitive, delicate, aesthic* and emotionally *closed.* It is not easy for them to express their emotions.
They prefer to hold in their emotions and work out their problems for themselves, or only speak to one very close confidant about their concerns and worries.

They have a great ability to be independent and listen to reason. Within the Silica constitution there is sometimes a type of over concern for details. It is a desire for precision, exactitude and perfection, combined with the need for things to be aesthetic. There is a desire to find a way to do things so that they avoid criticism. This can lead to everything being in order but sometimes lacking in new content.

They can be very responsible people from an early age. They have the ability to think deeply about complex issues but rather than try to change things they will tend to avoid conflicts. It is difficult for them to be assertive. They don't have the type of energy it takes to make changes, especially if it means convincing another person. This is partly because they are in a depleted state, and have to save their energy for the tasks that are the most necessary for survival. Those that can be accomplished

Study Guide

by the path of least resistance.

The person in a Silica state can be resisted and suppressed. They will go along with what the stronger person has told them to do. Yet at the same time have a strong enough identity to know what they believe. With Pulsatilla, the identity is often not as strong as that of Silica and they will believe the words of the stronger person. This is consistent with the idea that in those needing Pulsatilla there is the changeableness to a pathological degree. Yet in those needing Silica change does not occur so easily. They can be *obstinate* and *stubborn*, if they have enough confidence to stand up for themselves. This can even lead to a narrow-minded attitude, or to having fixed ideas about things.

Silica persons often care about how they look and the image they portray (Baryta even more so). Often they can be very devoted and serious toward what they believe in or to their profession. As the sense of responsibility develops, along with a desire for perfection, the end result can be overwork and mental exhaustion.

The fatigue of a Silica person can be so severe that it manifests as a type of chronic fatigue syndrome.

At least some of the following general and keynote symptoms of Silica have to be present in order for the remedy to be the simillimum:
- Sensitive to cold, to a draft, or cold and heat, but very rarely would they only have an aggravation from heat. They can be very sensitive to cold, with cold hands and feet
- Easy perspiration on the feet and the head
- Perspiration of the head during sleep (Calc-c). Hypersensitive to noise
- Constipation, hard stool. Most people that need Silica have some sort of constipation problem
- Nervous weakness
- Variable thirst
- Aggravation from milk
- Ingrown toe nails
- White spots on the nails of the fingers
- Poor assimilation of food

In the newborn

- Low birth weight
- <u>Premature birth</u>
- Weepy with frequent waking
- Eyes have a yellow discharge
- Aversion to mother's milk
- Diarrhea and vomiting from mother's milk
- Allergy to cow's milk
- Delays in development - gaining weight, muscle development emotional and mental developmental delays (Abrot)

Children in general
- Aggravation after vaccination
- <u>*Recurrent coryzas*</u> (runny nose)
- Obstruction of the nose (stuffy nose)
- Chronic tendency to colds
- *Sore throat*
- *Tonsillar infections*
- Otitis media
- Any chronic infection i.e. of the bones, pelvic organs, kidney, bladder, intestines, etc
- Slow learning to walk
- Delayed closure of the fontanelles (the bones of the head are open at birth. Generally, the back one is closed by two months and the top one is closed by 12 to 18 months)
- Diarrhea from dentition (new teeth pushing through the gums)
- Tendency for the teeth to decay
- Cervical adenopathy (swelling of the lymphatic glands)
- Curvature of the spine, known as scoliosis
- Asthma
- Bronchitis, rattling in the chest
- Pneumonia
- Loss of weight
- Stomach aches, worse to drink hot fluids as they cause sweating about the face, head and hot flushes
- Sweating on the head during sleep

Adolescence
- *Acne*
- Scoliosis
- Periodic headaches

Study Guide

- Warts on the soles of the feet
- Character slow to develop and assert itself
- Headaches aggravated by a draft
- Tears in the rectum from constipation
- Sleep walking

Adults
Many of the same symptoms as mentioned above only the ailments have progressed to a more severe degree.

There are many more symptoms that could be written concerning Silica such as "ringing in the ears" or "pains in the ankles" but for now, I believe this explanation is an adequate introduction to the remedy. It is best to use Silica when the physical symptoms, general, keynote and emotional symptoms all agree with the material that has been presented. If there are symptoms that totally contradict this information then study further for a better choice; perhaps Kali-silica, Natrum silica or one of the other Silica remedies would be a better choice. Recommendation: if Silica is indicated, give one 30c dose of the remedy every seven to ten days for six weeks, if there is not a general improvement in the persons health within the first two weeks; then search out a better remedy.

SPONGIA
(Sea Sponge)

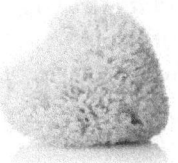

Dry cough won't stop. Wakes with a fright, can't breath.

Spongia is made from a roasted sea sponge. It is possible to use this to treat a variety of respiratory illnesses, including, croup, coughs and bronchitis.

<u>Dry hacking cough.</u> Dry croupy cough. Barking cough.

Materia Medica

The glands are often swollen and inflamed. The air passages are dry. There is a general aggravation from heat.

Dry tickle in the throat with a loud seal-like barking cough (croup). Throat feels constricted. Cough is better after eating or drinking.

Throat can be raw and sore. Hoarseness. Goitre (a swelling on the neck below the Adam's apple) with throat inflammation. Awakens suddenly after midnight wth pain and suffocation. Flushed, hot and frightened to death. Asthmatic cough. Cough worse before midnight. Weak sensation in the chest. Cough won't stop.

Nash: *The mental symptoms of Spongia show that it is a heart remedy. When a remedy produces the anxiety, fear, and dyspnoea found in Spongia, it will most likely turn out to be a cardiac remedy, unless these conditions are connected with irritation and inflammatory diseases of the brain. In this drug we find without any cerebral symptoms, marked anxiety, fear of death, and suffocation, associated with palpitation and uneasiness in the region of the heart. It is especially related to cases where there is pain and a sense of stuffiness and fulness in the cardiac region, in the chest, with dyspnoea, anxiety, fear of death, fear of the future, fear that something dreadful is going to happen. Wakens at night in great fear and it is some time before he can rationalize his surroundings (AESC.,LYC., SAMB., LACH., PHOS., and CARBO VEG.).*

The tendency to affect the glands is striking. As a matter of fact all the glands are affected; they gradually enlarge and become increasingly hard. Glands that have undergone inflammation and are increased in size become hard, or they take on hypertrophy.

Hypertrophy of the heart (KALMIA, SEPIA, NAJA). Spongia has cured endocarditis, cardiac croup and many other inflammatory diseases of the heart resulting from rheumatism. Hypertrophy of the thyroid, goitre, when the heart is affected and the eyes protruding.

Cervical glands enlarged; inveterate cases of enlarged testes; orchitis from a suppressed gonorrhoea, a cold or other causes; gradually increasing hardness.

The whole respiratory apparatus is acted upon; cardiac dyspnoea and the most severe forms of asthma. Dryness of the air passages with whistling and wheezing, seldom rattling, must sit up and bend forward; at times after great dyspnoea, white, tough mucus forms in the air passages, difficult to expectorate; it comes up and often has to be swallowed (ARN., CAUST., LACH., KALI C., KALI S., NUX MOS., SEP., STAPH.)

Dyspnoea worse lying down. The modality is common to its other complaints; violent, basilar headache forces him to sit up in bed and keep still. Holding the head in the upright position relieves the dull pressure in the occiput.

There are many headaches. In the occiput, in the forehead, congestive headaches, but most of them are associated with goitre, cardiac affections and asthma; they are due, probably, to sluggish circulation in the brain.

Face distressed in croup; anxious; livid; pale and bloated; blue, pale with sunken eyes; red with anxious expression; alternating red and pale; cold sweat. These symptoms are the natural effects of difficult breathing and are, therefore, not essential in the selection of a remedy. As primary symptoms, they would probably indicate ARS., but when due to cardiac difficulties, they are unimportant.

"Sore throat worse after eating sweet things. Thyroid gland swollen even with the chin; at night, suffocating spells, barking cough, with stinging in the throat and soreness in the abdomen." Enlargement of the tonsils. Difficult swallowing.

Spongia is the remedy when dyspnoea and cough are relieved by warm food; may be better from warm drinks.

Laryngeal troubles with great hoarseness, in individuals tending towards phthisis, with tubercular heredity, cachectic aspect, weak lungs, but no deposit of tubercle. But all at once hoarseness sets in.

There is a tendency for the larynx to become involved in phthisical patients that need Spongia. This patient takes an acute cold and it settles in the larynx with hoarseness.

Look out for that patient, for there is a tendency for tubercles to deposit where there is inflammation, and the infiltration instead of being fibrinous may become tubercular. Tendency for the larynx to be first involved in phthisical patients.

In Spongia do not look for the exudative, but the infiltrative form of croup. Hoarseness with loss of voice, great dryness of the larynx from a cold; coryza, sneezing, the whole chest rings, is as dry as a horn; voice hissing, croupy, nose dry.

There is very little accumulation of mucus, but at a late date ulceration begins and then there may be a copious expectoration of mucus. In proportion to the extent of rattling, this remedy is decreasingly indicated. HEPAR has the coarse rattling with much mucus.

At times an adult takes cold and rawness of the larynx and trachea is the result. On going to bed she is taken with a spasmodic constriction of the larynx. Laryngismus stridulus is commonly found in women. IGN., GELS., LAUROC. and Spongia. IGN. and GELS. will cure eight out of ten cases.

The larynx is sensitive to touch in croup, etc., like PHOS.

STAPHASAGRIA
(Delphinium Staphisagria)

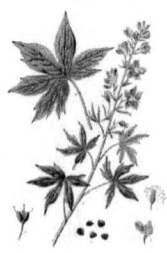

Indignation is the main idea for this remedy. They are offended by people who are rude to them or when they are not treated with enough respect.

Study Guide

They will often say: *"I can't believe I was treated that way, who would use such an awful tone of voice, who would not even show some manners"*. But instead of saying something back they stay silent and **suppress the anger.** This feeling of indignation is the defining feature of this remedy.

Case 1: patient in her 30's; she was planning on killing her x-husband, because when he came over to her house to look after their children he *'did not clean up after himself'*. This had gone on for years and she had never said anything about it (it was below her to bring it up). But it made her feel *extreme indignation ('he should know how to clean up and how to treat me with respect!!')*. I gave her some doses of Staphasagria and she was able to assurt herself so that she changed the locks on her house and had her x-husband take the children to his house. In effect she learned to use her voice and no longer was filled with bitter resentment and indignation.

These people are very sweet and mild when one has an interview of them. They talk softly and don't like to display anger. It is beneth their pride and dignity to get angry. Under the surface though is hurt and resentment.

Here is what Nash says about this remedy: *The mental symptoms are very important, and the impressions made upon the mind and thence upon the body guide to Staphisagria as a remedy. Excitable, easily aroused to anger, but seldom irascible, that is, easily disturbed and excited, but seldom manifests it. Suitable in cases where complaints come from pent up wrath, suppressed anger, suppressed feelings. The person becomes speechless from suppressed indignation, anger with indignation. Complaints brought on by these causes; irritable bladder with frequent urging to urinate, lasting many days after suppressed wrath, after insults. "Great indignation about things done by others or by himself; grieves about consequences."*

A gentleman comes in contact with one beneath his station and an altercation takes place, an argument which ends in insult, and the gentleman turns his back on the other. He goes home and suffers; he does not speak it out, but controls it and then suffers from it. He has sleepless nights and many days of fatigue, brain-fag; for days and weeks he cannot add nor subtract, makes mistakes in writing and speaking, has irritability of the bladder, colic, etc. Loss of memory with a sense of weight between the eyes; it is difficult to say whether this is a feeling in the head or an effort to describe a dullness of mind. Feels as if a ball of wood were in the forehead, or as if the whole cerebrum were made of wood; it feels numb. It is difficult to state whether it is a condition of the mind or head. Accompanying this sensation of a lump in the forehead is a feeling as if the whole back of the head were hollow; the patient may describe it as a feeling of numbness or a lack of sensation.

"Indifferent, low-spirited, dullness of mind after onanism." Staph. cures these conditions when they are the result of sexual excitement, masturbation, excesses in venery, allowing the mind to dwell too much on venereal subjects. Thinking on sexual relations. These patients are irritable, easily fatigued, most excitable, and when they have to control their emotions they suffer intensely. One who is in health can easily put aside a controversy, knowing that he has done what is right, but a Staph. patient when he has to control himself goes all to pieces, trembles from head to foot, loses his voice, his ability to work, cannot sleep and a headache follows.

Many a time a man has come into my office with blue lips, trembling hands, pains about the heart and all over, and he thinks he is going to die. He tells a story of an altercation and pent up wrath, and Staph. stops his trembling and quiets him. Without it he would have sleepless nights, brain-fag, prostration and headache. This state belongs especially to those who have indulged in sexual excesses. (Nash)

I have used this remedy to treat psoriasis, bladder infections and many other complaints.

Kent says: *The Staph. headache is a numb, dull pain in the occiput and forehead, especially in these nervous constitutions. "Sensation as of a round ball in the forehead, sitting firmly there even when shaking the head."*

Headaches from vexation and indignation. Crusty, squamous eruptions on the scalp.

"Painful sensitiveness of the scalp, skin peels off, with itching and smarting, worse in the evening and from getting warm."

The scales are lifted up by a watery exudate and the denuded surface is extremely sensitive to touch.

New growths about the lids and balls of the eyes, extremely painful to the touch. Meibomian tumors (Con., Thuja), in irritable children (Kreos).

Another feature in Staph, is its action on the glands; scrofulous glands; glands of the neck enlarge; enlarged and indurated ovaries and testes; stitching, tearing pains in the glands everywhere. Hardness and chronic induration.

Stitching, tearing pains along the course of the nerves; in the heart, and as in such a nervous patient the mind is likely to be on the heart, the stitching pains in the intercostals are supposed to be in the heart. Stitching pains directly through the chest to the back.

Swelling of the tonsils after the abuse of Mercury. Chronic tonsilitis, tonsils are not large but hard from previous attacks of acute tonsilitis; strumous diathesis; cross and irritable.
"Pains come on after eating."

The Staph. patient has much difficulty in the bowels. Subject to chronic diarrhoea and to constipation. Colic, twitching, tearing pains in the abdomen. Diarrhoea from cold water, from eating, from indignation, anger, with flatulence of a terribly offensive odor like spoiled eggs.

"Chronic diarrhoea or dysentery of weakly, sickly children after anger; after being punished, after emotions." (Coloc. and Cham.)
Staph. and Coloc. resemble each other. In both, eating and drinking cause griping and stool, both have colic as if stones were squeezing; Staph. in the intestines, head and testes; Coloc. in the intestines and ovaries; both are worse from anger. Caust., Coloc. and Staph. follow each other like Sulph., Calc. and Lyc.

It often happens that nervous women soon after marriage are attacked with frequent and painful urging to urinate which becomes extremely troublesome and may last many days. Staph. is very comforting to the young wife.

Urinary and Genitals: Great teasing and tearing all night long bloody urine; involuntary discharge of urine, acrid and corroding, with burning, worse from motion.

Profuse discharge of pale urine with burning and urging. Burning during and after urination.

Staph. has cured enlarged prostate with frequent urging to urinate, especially in old men; continued teasing with dribbling.

"Frequent urging to urinate, with a scanty discharge in thin stream or discharge of urine in drops; may be followed by a sensation as if the bladder were not fully emptied."

The most distressing symptom of the male genitals is excitability, but there is also impotence, great weakness of the sexual organs; the sexual desire is greatly increased but there is impotence.

Useful in the results of secret vice, long practiced.

"Seminal emissions followed by great chagrin and mortification, prostration, dyspnoea.

Effects of onanism or sexual excesses; loss of memory, hypochondriasis, taciturnity, face sunken, abashed look, nocturnal emissions, backache, weak legs, relaxed organs, deficiency of vital heat and tendency to take cold, deep sunken, red, and lusterless eyes, hair falls out; loss of prostatic fluid and impairment of sexual desire; dull and contusive pains in the testicles, voluptuous itching of the scrotum, atrophy of the testicles."

Think of the extremely nervous patient.

Dry, sensitive warts about the genitals, from sycosis or from the abuse of Mercury, which cause a tendency to warty growths. Moist red, offensive warts belong to Thuja.

The testes dwindle as well as become inflamed and swollen; genitals waste away.

Sensation as if there were worms crawling over him. Crawling, etc., in the female external genitals, Coff., Plat., Petrol., Apis, Tarent. hisp, the latter has. While outer parts feel as if insects were biting. and crawling, better from heat or cold.

In the female there is violent sexual excitement, nymphomania with extreme mental and physical impressions; mind has been dwelling too much on sexual subjects.

"Very sharp, shooting pains in the ovary, which is exquisitely sore to touch; pains extend along crural regions and thighs.

Menses irregular, late and profuse, sometimes wanting; first of pale blood, then dark and clotted.

Scorbutic diathesis, vegetations of the vagina; stinging, itching of the vulva."

Miscellaneous: Stitching in the region of the heart; trembling of the body with nervous excitement is an excellent indication for Staph.

Effects from loss of blood, shock, from surgical operations, injuries from sharp instruments, incised wounds. Stinging, etc., in surgical wounds, cuts; colic after lithotomy, urging to stool, qualmishness, worse from drinking.

Tetter on the hands, itches and burns in the evening after scratching; numbness in the tips of the fingers; arthritic nodosities on the fingers. I remember a patient suffering from gouty nodosities; he had lived a life of peculiar continence, dwelling on his vices, broken down in body. Staph. brought out an eruption on his legs as high up as the knees that looked like a pair of trousers.

One continuous coat of crusts which lasted a year before it dwindled, but he was greatly improved in his body and his enlarged joints gradually improved. The eruption was yellow, crusty, tough, leathery, and, when lifted up by the moisture beneath, it had to be cut off like a bandage; he was practically crippled; new crops came out on the parts clipped off. It was with difficulty that be walked, for the crusts cut him.

Bone troubles, exostoses, inflammation of the periosteum.

Acute articular rheumatism of fast or debilitated men, with shifting pains. Mercurial bone diseases. ulcers, caries, injuries caused by sharp, cutting instruments. Nightly bone pains. (Asa f., Merc., Sil.)

STRAMONIUM
(Thorn Apple)

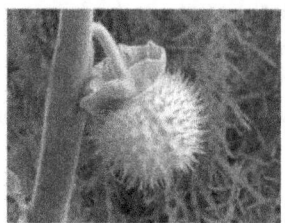

FEAR OF DARK. This symptom is present for almost every person who needs this remedy. *Terrified of the dark.*

After a fearful event the child has nightmares and can't sleep alone.

They feel they have been abandoned at night with the threat of being attacked by terrifying wild animals. There are many life experiences that can allow someone to feel alone and in danger but with Stramonium there is the idea that this is a terrifying experience such as a child that is left alone because they witnessed a parent being attacked or a parent taken from them in a violent manner.

Case 1: A child wakes up screaming from nightmares, she can't sleep alone or with the light out. A few months before she had been chased on Halloween.

Case 2: After being in the military he was afraid of every little sound and kept thinking he was still under attack.

Study Guide

Case 3: Seven year old boy: After his mother left to go look after her parents he developed convulsions and violent temper tantrums as he thought she had permanently abandoned him.

Case 4: After the car accident she was afraid of the dark, had panic attacks and could not be alone. Stramonium was the correct remedy in all of these cases.

Fear of dark tunnels of dogs, water and strangers.

Belladonna and Hyoscyamus are in the same family. These are similar remedies in many respects such as convulsions, spasms, violence and emotions out of control.

Boericke gives us a picture of the delirium during a fever: *Devout, earnest, beseeching and ceaseless talking. Loquacious, garrulous, laughing, singing, swearing, praying, rhyming. Sees ghosts, hears voices, talks with spirits. Rapid changes from joy to sadness. Violent and lewd. Delusions about his identity; thinks himself tall, double, a part missing. Religious mania. Cannot bear solitude or darkness; must have light and company. Sight of water or anything glittering brings on spasms. Delirium, with desire to escape (Bell; Bry; Rhus).*

From Nash: *Stram. is like an earthquake in its violence. The mind is in an uproar; cursing, tearing the clothes, violent speech, frenzy, erotomania, exposing of the person.*

These symptoms are found in continued fevers, insanity, cerebral congestion. It is useful in violent typhoids.

SULPHUR
(Elemental Sulphur)

RED LIPS – This symptoms is present in almost every patient who needs this remedy.

Materia Medica

EGOTISM, desire to be the center of attention. Sulphur people love compliments and affirmation.

ITCHING. Worse from heat. This is very typical for sulphur.
This remedy if the symptoms agree can treat almost any acute and chronic illness. It is the most common remedy in the repertory.

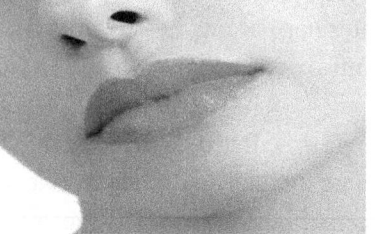

Craves attention from others. He or she desires COMPLIMENTS.

COLLECTS THINGS, MESSY; even rags seem beautiful. INVENTIVE MIND and CREATIVE. Can be the practical idealist or very philosophical with many theories. He sits in the book store all day reading about utopia; he thinks he is one of these ideal people. He tells his friends about what he knows and they wish he would stop as it is all in theory and he is boasting.

As we all know it is very tiring if people keep talking about themselves as if they have all the answers.

If the symptoms of the patients fit the overall symptom picture of Sulphur then one can rely on it thereafter to treat almost any acute illness for that patient. This may include: sore throat, ear ache, cough, flu, stomach ache or urinary tract infection.
What are the constitutional symptoms that can lead one to this remedy?
An irregular distribution of the circulation causing _burning pains_ or flushes of heat. Burning in the stomach.

THE SOLES OF THE FEET FEEL HOT WITH THE DESIRE TO UNCOVER THEM OR TO SEARCH FOR COLD SPOTS ON THE SHEETS. This is such a strong keynote that any remedy with Sulphur in it can have this symptoms such as: Aurum sulph, Lithium sulph, Natrum sulph, Kali-sulph, Mag-sulph, Sanicula etc. The same is true if your patient has red lips. Look to see which Sulphur remedy fits the best as any of them can have this keynote.

A constant sensation of heat in the head, chest, or feet. The lips, ears, nose, eyelids, and anus can become red and congested with blood. Bright red lips. *The skin is often red and itching,* allowing this remedy to treat

Study Guide

many types of skin eruptions. Scratching causes burning.

Tall and lean, stoop shouldered, untidy, too lazy to rouse himself, <u>worse from standing</u>, aversion to washing, and collects things, even rags, as they seem beautiful.

The practical idealist, the ragged philosopher, prideful, egotistical, haughty, imagines he is a great man, selfish and <u>*critical.*</u>

Anxiety about his family. Imagines something bad has happened to them if they are late returning home.

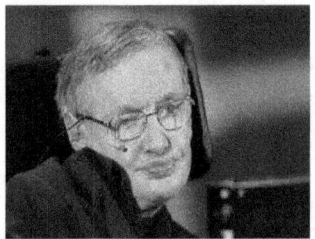

The scientist, the intellectual. The mind is stronger than the body.

Stephen Hawking, the famous scientist, writer, regarded as one of the most brilliant theoretical physicists since Einstein is most likely in need of Sulphur or one of the Sulphur remedies. Sulphur is listed for various types of paralysis.

Fear of heights.

Diarrhea that drives him out of bed early in the morning. The stool can be large and painful, the parts around the anus are red, itchy and excoriated (the skin is worn off).

Worse from being overheated. Hungry at 11 a.m. Has a desire for fats, spicy foods, and alcohol. Aversion to eggs. Feet sweat and give off an offensive odor. *Sleeping on the back is impossible or can cause nightmares. Skin that is aggravated by wool.*

Emotionally they may just like to get plenty of attention, but this can progress to a need for *constant compliments, egotism, overdeveloped pride, haughty nature or selfishness.* People who are full of themselves, they talk about their great accomplishments all the time i.e. "I am the greatest soccer player that ever lived."

The self centered teen: "I like to bang on the piano and won't stop because my song was not as long as the others. I like to be on stage and play the same music over and over because I, as we all know, I am the most important person, even though the music sonds terrible as they believe they don't have to practice." Teens who worry because they are not the most popular; find ways to be more popular. They have to form a click of loyal supporters. Dress up to get attention. Critical of others. Do things to get special attention from others.

From Nash: *Hering called the Sulphur patient "THE RAGGED PHILOSOPHER." The Sulphur scholar, the inventor, works day and night in threadbare clothes and battered hat; he has long, uncut hair and a dirty face; his study is uncleanly, it is untidy; books and leaves of books are piled up indiscriminately; there is no order. It seems that Sulphur produces this state of disorder, a state of untidiness, a state of uncleanliness, a state of "don't care how things go", and a state of selfishness.*

He becomes a FALSE PHILOSOPHER, and the more he goes on in this state the more he is disappointed because the world does not consider him the greatest man on earth. Old inventors work and work, and fail. The complaints that arise in this kind of case, even the acute complaints, will run to Sulphur. (Nash)

Carbon sulph is more balanced, less ego. Like to work hard. Stocky build.

SULPHUR IODATUM

Sulphur symptoms but hypoglycemic and more restlessness. So restless he can't learn. ADD children (Verat, Arsen-iod).

SULPHUROSUM ACID

Asthma and emphysema worse from smog, exhaust gases and smoke. Ulcerative inflammations of the mouth. Stomatitis.

TABACUM
(Tobacco)

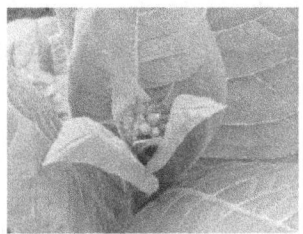

Nausea worse from being in a warm room, better standing in the cool air. Wants the ABDOMEN UNCOVERED with the nausea. MOTION SICKNESS *from riding in a car or boat.*

Boericke: *The symptomatology of Tabacum is exceedingly well marked. The nausea, giddiness, death-like pallor, vomiting, icy coldness, and sweat, with the intermittent pulse, are all most characteristic.*

Has marked antiseptic qualities, antidotal to cholera germs. Complete prostration of the entire muscular system.

Collapse. Gastralgia, enteralgia, seasickness, cholera infantum; cold, but wants abdomen uncovered.

Vigorous peristaltic activity diarrhœa. Produces high tension and arteriosclerosis of the coronary arteries.

Should prove the most homeopathic drug for angina pectoris, with coronaritis and high tension (Cartier). Constriction of throat, chest, bladder, rectum. Pallor, breathlessness, hard-cordlike pulse. (Boericke)

TARENTULA

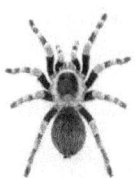

Strong sexual desire (Med, Hyos). Extremely restless. Loves music and to dance. Hyperactive children who love music and want to dance all the time.

Case 1: 26 year old women. On the weekends she goes out dancing; she tells herself not to have sex with strangers; but then every time brings home a different man for the night.

Case 2: 30 year old; he searches the Internet for casual sexual encounters when his wife is out of town. He tells me he can't go one day without sex.

Both of these patients loved music and to dance; they both did very well with this remedy as it helped their physical symptoms and the out of control sexuality (Anan, Calad, Bufo, Fl-ac, Hyos, Med, Orig, Sel).

Kent says about this remedy: *Desire to run about, to dance and jump up and down. Great fantastic dancing. Sometimes, music ameliorates all the symptoms and at other times it aggravates them. He becomes violently excited from music.*

Emaciation is so marked that it may be said sometimes that the flesh falls off from him. Creeping and crawling in the skin all over the body. Paralysis of any part of the body, or of all the limbs.

Study Guide

Trembling and jerking convulsions. It has an appearance very much like St. Vitus' Dance and hence has cured chorea when it was better from music. But it will also cure when worse from music.

The extreme restlessness of the limbs is like Ars., and it is a deep acting medicine like Ars., and it sometimes has cured where Ars. has failed, although it seemed well selected. Anxiety, restlessness, constant motion of the arms, legs, trunk and head. Restlessness of the limbs in the evening, in bed before going to sleep, like Ars. and Lyc.

It is full of pains in the body and limbs; pains in the bones; pains in the arms and in the joints. Periodicity is so well marked that it has been a marked curative remedy in intermittent fevers with restlessness of limbs, with aching of the bones, with stitching pains, with the anxiety, especially when these come in the evening and the fever lasts all night.

Chill in the evening followed by fever without sweat is a marked feature. Modalities: The patient himself is always sensitive to cold, so the pains in the limbs are worse in cold air and from becoming cold. (Kent) Compare to Medorrhinum and Hyos.

TAXUS BREVIFOLIA
(Yew Tree)

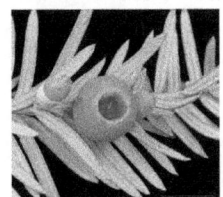

Memory loss …….. Sleepy in school ………. Timid……….

Taxol is severely toxic substance with many side effects one of which is the patient *looses their memory*.

In the proving we found the following symptom to be very prominent: ***'I forget what I set out to do, I forgot my purpose in life.' It also make the proves feel very sleepy.*** I have found this remedy useful for people who <u>can't learn to read.</u> *Sleepy in class or at church.* May be unable to speak. Forgetful. ***God fearing, mild and yielding, childlike.*** (Arbor Medica Vol II)

THUJA
(Northern White Cedar)

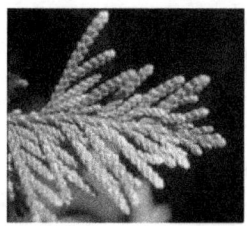

Can't accept themselves, hide the true self ….

The Thuja patient feels that if you really knew them you would reject them. This makes them try and hide their true identity.

They don't like who they really are or feel that there is something unacceptable about who they are, so they have to hide it.

Entrenched shame and mortification. No trust in themselves or in others.

They develop a survival strategy: a persona of what they feel others expect of them, this could be any persona. They loose their real identity so that when they get married or choose a career they find out that it was not based on what they really wanted or their true identity. At this point they can continue to try and connect with others through deception or can have a nervous breakdown as they feel that nothing they are doing is based on truth.

History of feeling that their parents could not or did not want to know them or accepted them for who they were. Therefore they try to change themselves so that the parent would connect and accept the false persona.

Very low confidence with a desire to please others or have a desire to have power over others.

They believe that others are like them so can't trust others. This can lead to manipulation of others to get power over them.

Tendency to warts and tumors. Ingrown toe nails. Aggravation from eating onions. Sensitive to cold and damp. Worse at 3 a.m.

Close remedies: Cypress family: Juniper, Redwood, Giant Sequoia. Tendency to lie: Salix alba, Opium, Morph.

Boericke: Its relation to the production of pathological vegetations condylomata, warty excrescences, spongy tumors is very important. Moist mucous tubercles. Bleeding fungus growths. Nevus. Excess of venosity.

The main action of Thuja is on the skin and genito-urinary organs, producing conditions that correspond with Hahnemann's sycotic dyscrasia, whose chief manifestation is the formation of wart-like excrescences upon mucous and cutaneous surfaces-fig-warts and condylomata. Has a specific antibacterial action, as in gonorrhea and vaccination. Suppressed gonorrhea, salpingitis. Ill-effects of vaccination. Sycotic pains, i.e, tearing in muscles and joints, worse at rest, better in dry weather, worse damp humid atmosphere; lameness. Hydrogenoid constitutions, whose blood is morbidly hydroscopic, so that damp air and water are inimical. Complaints from moonlight. Rapid exhaustion and emaciation. Left-sided and chilly medicine. Variola, aborts the pustule and prevents the suppurating fever. Vaccinosis, viz, inveterable skin troubles, neuralgia, etc.

Mind.--Fixed ideas, as if a strange person were at his side; as if soul and body were separated; as if something alive in abdomen (Croc). Emotional sensitiveness; music causes weeping and trembling.

Head.--Pain as if pierced by a nail (Coff; Ign). Neuralgia from tea (Selen). Left-sided headache. White, scaly dandruff; hair dry and falling out. Greasy skin of face.

Eyes.--Ciliary neuralgia; iritis. Eyelids agglutinated at night; dry, scaly. Styes and tarsal tumors (Staph). Acute and sub-acute inflammation of sclera. Sclera raised in patches, and looks bluish-red. Large, flat phlyctenules; indolent. Recurring episcleritis. Chronic scleritis. (Boericke)

From www. H-Pathy.com, Dr. Manisha Bhatia: *Thuja patients are very secretive; they will not permit themselves to be even looked at. They do not trust anybody easily and do not portray themselves truthfully. This will not happen suddenly; usually the patient suffers with low self-esteem and feelings of worthlessness. These inner doubts make the patient portray a pleasing and expected image to the world. This hiding of unpleasant aspects leads to a secretiveness. Patient learns to not display their real character anymore. You as a doctor always feel that some information is lacking or purposely withheld by the patient. Thuja patients are very reserved and suspicious. They do not allow any type of deep communication, as they are mistrustful and worry what might happen if they entered into deep communication. That is why they learn the art of manipulation.*

Thuja is a remedy which tends to alter the sycotic constitution, by changing the soil in which elements of the disease grow. There are three main precursors to the chronic conditions calling for Thuja: (1) Suppressed gonorrhea. (2) Suppressed warts. (3) Vaccination. If gonorrhea is checked by injection, by cold or by any other influence, constitutional symptoms may arise which call for Thuja. Thuja has a marked relationship to the smallpox vaccine, but has a lesser capacity to remove the untoward effects of other immunizations.

Regarding the nervous system, Thuja patient exhibits a manner which is hurried and impatient. Their movements are unnaturally active and hurried. There is a form of insanity or mania for which we find Thuja the only remedy, and that is one where there is a fixed idea in the patient's mind that he is made of some brittle substance, and he will be broken if touched. Or, he thinks that his body and soul are separated, or that a stranger is by his side. Another singular characteristic of Thuja is one that was first met with in an old maid. She experienced a sensation as though a living child were in her abdomen.

The action of the drug on the nervous system is further shown in various forms of neuralgia. Thus it is indicated in the form of headache in which the patient has a sensation as though a nail were being driven into the vertex, or into the frontal eminences.

Thuja is an excellent remedy for cases of gonorrhea where the discharge is thin and greenish, and there is scalding pain during urination. After urination there is a sensation as if a few drops of urine ran down the urethra.

Warts or condylomata appear on the genitals, at the anus, about the perineum and upon mucous surfaces. In the female organs, there are cauliflower like excrescences or fungus growths of venereal origin. There is thick green leucorrhoea. Thuja is of great use when articular rheumatism or prostatitis like complications result after the suppression of gonorrhea.

The hair is dry and split at the end; the scalp becomes scaly and covered with dry scurf. Also, Iritis with inflamed eyelids with a discharge that is thick and green.

Teeth decay at the edge of the gums, the crowns being apparently normal. Pyorrhea, ranula and varicose veins on tongue and mouth. These are some of the local complaints which occur in the sycotic soil and respond well to thuja.

Thuja patients are hard people. The hardness of their emotional expressions manifest even on the physical level, as hard tumors. Thuja has the singular property of softening hard tissue, even tissue naturally hard, as the nails. The warts may have a seedy look, or they may be of a cauliflower shape.

As regards physical generals, Thuja patients are chilly and worse from cold. There is general aggravation from damp weather.

Perspiration is oily and sweet smelling, or sometimes offensive. Patient shows specific intolerance to onions. There is craving and aversion to onions and garlic.

URTICA URENS
(Stinging nettle)

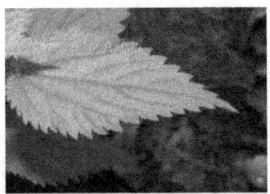

Sunburn ……. Any burn from heat or fire ……...

Other minor burns. urticaria, hives. Burning and itching of the skin.

Grief leading to hives (Grandgeorge). Sometimes this remedy is a better fit than Cantharis or Apis.

VERATRUM ALBUM
(Snow Rose)

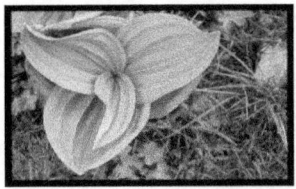

LACK OF VITAL HEAT, cold hands, feet and nose.

Feel as if they have fallen from a high social position (Elaps). *Worse from loosing their reputation. Worse after descrimination, after being shunned or blamed.*

Veratrum is a remedy that has saved many lives. It is used for infections that have progressed to a severe, and sometimes life threatening stage. These conditions would include: Pneumonia, gastroenteritis and mononucleosis. What are the symptoms that would lead one to giving this remedy?

The patient will be in bed, in a collapsed state. He will feel **very chilly,** having a blue and pale complexion. Vomiting with very low vitality.

In all cases that need Veratrum there is extreme coldness of the body. The patient will feel cold as death. Even though they try to stay warm, they will have cold hands, cold feet, cold head, cold nose, cold breath and cold perspiration.

VERY CHILLY, BUT WITH A DESIRE FOR COLD OR EVEN ICE DRINKS. This is a very peculiar symptom considering how chilly they feel.

The stomach or intestinal infections (gastroenteritis) can be diarrhea or vomiting or both together, *even at the same time.*

Severe retching, projectile vomiting. Cramping pains in the abdomen. This is a remedy you want to take with you when you are in a situation where the water is not clean.

The respiratory infections have the following symptoms:
- Hoarse weak voice
- Rattling in the chest
- Can't cough up the mucous
- Chronic bronchitis with the feeling they can't get enough air to breath
- Loud barking cough
- Blue or pale face
- Headache

<u>Desires sour things</u>, such as lemons or sour candy. Desires salt. Desires to chew on ice.

If the Veratrum symptoms become chronic then one may notice a tendency for the patient to reach for an ambitious goal and then through some life circumstance fall from this position. She or he will then feel angry and depressed from this reversal of fortune. They fail but then later the constitution turns to a sense of egotistical power with lots of talking or breathless preaching.

Religious mania. Restless with ideas so that he can not rest – feels on a mission to change the world. Delusions and mania.

Case 1: Mother of three, married, 34 years old. Calls me because she can't sleep. She thinks she is doing God's work and has 'grace.' She is excited but can't stop talking about it. 'I get so excited and feel God's power.' Some days though her mood goes the other way and she is very depressed; she thinks God will punish her for wanting to get credit for all the good things she does. 'I am a horrible sinner because I tried to be like God, people must look at me with pitty and distain. It is so selfish of me to do good things because when I do, I look down my nose at others.' (Verat: Mind, Egotism).

At these times she feels guilt, that I am so selfish and feel as though fallen from grace. When she comes in to my office she is talking rapidly, with great intensity as if something has to be done to help her right away. 'I want salvation; if I can't get it my family will leave me all alone, everyone will be in heaven except for me.' She is crying.

She has chronic diarrhea worse during her menses. (Verat). 'As I child I felt so alone, my father ditched me, why was I not good enough for him? he did not put me first, so I am so bitter and resentful - (fallen position). I tried to get attention from men by sleeping with them as a teenager. I slept with so many men but it did not help. Rather it made me feel bad about myself and I had a bad reputation. (falling again). I feel that I am in a prison, I can't feel good about myself, that is why only God can help me but I am doing Gods work for the wrong reasons; it is all for me and that is wrong!!, so I will be punished and end up alone. There is no way out. I feel hopeless. Craves ice cold drinks. Chill with the diarrhea.

Analysis: Veratrum is listed under *Religious Affections* and *Moods Alternating*. We see how the ego is undermined and tries to resurect itself. She has the perfect polarity for this remedy. Fallen reputation – her father left her and then further lost her reputation in her community. She feels God can help her but it does not work out. These are all themes for Veratrum album.

Two days after the Veratrum the diarrhea stops, she is able to sleep again. Two weeks later after a few doses of Veratrum album 30c she says: 'I don't feel so hopless now, I don't feel that I am falling from grace any longer, I am less tearful, I feel more confident and brave now, less nervous, I feel like I can get through all of this.' My stomach is half better. I am still very senstive to cold. It is May and I still need the heat on in the car. 'At night when I lie down now I feel at peace. The depression is 90% better. I am more patient with my children. Not so concerned about religion, she is more into playing baseball.

Analysis: She is still like a child growing up, she wants to play baseball all day. This is a very healthy step for her. Then she says: 'I am not taking so much offense at work and not feeling like they are going to fire me. Her body coldness sensitivity is much improved. She looks younger, happier and she is no longer having mania alternating with depression. It is now five months later and she has not relapsed. Able to accept her sexuality again and not feel guilt about it.

Here is what Kent says about the mental state of Veratrum: *Exalted state of religious frenzy, believes he is the risen Christ screams and screeches until he is blue in the face; head cold as ice, cold sweat, reaches out and exhorts to repentance. Exhorts to repent, preaches, howls, sings obscene songs, exposes the person. Fear and the effects of fear; fear of death and of being damned; imagines the world is on fire.*

Mania with desire to cut and tear everything, especially the clothes, with lewdness and lascivious talk.

Puerperal mania and convulsions, with violent cerebral congestion; bluish and bloated face; protruding eyes; wild shrieks, with disposition to bite and tear.

Loquacity, he talks rapidly.

She is inconsolable over a fancied misfortune; runs around the room howling and screaming or sits brooding, wailing and weeping."

Alternate states of brooding, screaming, and screeching. A few such remedies would empty our insane asylums, especially of recent cases. Insanity is curable if there are no incurable results of disease. Full of despair and hopelessness with approaching insanity.

"*Despair of his recovery, attempts suicide.*"
Insane people are not hopeless, those approaching insanity are but after

they become insane, they think that everybody is crazy except themselves. Those bowed down by great grief and despair are likely to go into a state of violent mania. Veratrum carries them through the state of despair.

"Melancholia, head hangs down, sits brooding in silence."
Young girls go on for years with menstrual difficulties, and preceding each menstrual nisus is a state of despair; never smiles, the world seems blue, everything is dark; these are preparing for a marked state of insanity.

Veratrum is a remedy that would keep many women out of the insane asylum, especially those with uterine troubles. Girls at puberty suffer with dysmenorrhoea, hysterical mental states, diarrhea, and vomiting. During the menses they become cold as death, lips blue, extremities cold and blue, dreadful pains, sensation of sinking, mania to kiss everybody, hysteria with coldness at the menstrual period, copious sweat, vomiting, and diarrhoea, etc.

Kent again adds to our understanding of the physical symptoms:
Coldness: *Hardly a group of symptoms will arise without this accompanying coldness. Coldness of discharges, coldness of the body. You would also wonder at the remarkable prostration attending the various groups of symptoms, complete relaxation and exhaustion, coldness. Profuse sweat, vomiting and diarrhea.*

Profuse watery discharges. These conditions occur without apparent provocation. In cholera or cholera morbus, it seems that the fluids run out of the body.

Lies in bed, relaxed prostrated, cold to the finger-tips, with corresponding blueness, fairly purple; lips cold and blue, countenance pinched and shrunken; great sensation of coldness as if the blood were ice-water; scalp cold; forehead covered with cold sweat; headache and exhaustion; coldness in spots over the body; extremities cold as death. Full of cramps; looks as if he would die.

This state comes out during the menses, during colic with nausea, with mania and violent delirium, with headache, with violent inflammations. Is it any wonder that Hahnemann predicted that Veratrum, Camphor, and

Cuprum would become remedies in the cure of cholera; he saw in their nature the ability to cure.

He saw the similitude. In cases of this sort which are characterized by superabundance of cramps, Cuprum is the simillimum. For those with coldness and blueness and scanty sweat, vomiting, and purging,

Camphor is the remedy. These are called "dry cholera;" they sink down and die without exhaustive discharges. In proportion as there are coldness, blueness and scanty discharges, Camphor is indicated.

In proportion as copiousness, blueness, and coldness are present, Veratrum is indicated. Secale has something of cholera in it. Podo. has exhaustive stools. Ars. anxious restlessness. (Kent)

VIOLA ODORATA
(Sweet Violet)

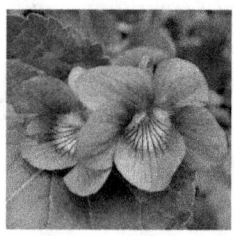

Sinusitis – one of the main remedies. Pains are worse from change in barometric pressure. Pain in mallar bones. Face pain pressing or pressure in maxillary sinuses.

Dull pain and congestion of the face from sinusitis. Worse from cold dry air. Worse to move the head. Ears feel full or bursting. Ear discharge. Lots of respiratory symptoms. Headache with visual disturbances. <u>Head pain from forehead over head to neck.</u> Feels better to be magnetized. Desire for activity, mood changeable.

Study Guide

Case 1: 33 y.o. (M.C) Female. Has had a cold for two weeks. Sore dry throat, tickling cough, yellow mucous. Sinusitis. Headache goes from forehead backward to cervical region. Worse from change of weather. Tries to be the perfect mother and hard on herself. Likes music. Plan: Viola-odorata 30c. Seven days later: Sinuses have drained. Overall 70% better. Cold symptoms all better. No more pain from ingrown toe nails. No more twitching. Mood better; less anxiety about her illness, less hard on herself. Asthma better (had this since a child). Headache all better. Less perspiration of neck at night.

Boericke: Head.--*Burning of the forehead. Vertigo; everything in head seems to whirl around. Heaviness of head, with sensation of weakness in muscles of nape of neck. Scalp tense; must knit the brows. Tendency to pain immediately above eyebrows. Throbbing under eye and temple. Headache across the forehead. Acts upon frontal sinuses. Hysterical attacks in tuberculous patients.*

Materia Medica

Supplemental Sections

APPENDIX ONE

CASE STUDIES

These cases give you a more realistic presentation of the case taking process along with what symptoms are collected, how to sort them out, how to apply the repertory and how to differentiate remedies.

Repertorize the following cases. This will give you practice in finding symptoms in the repertory and then look up and read the materia medica for the remedies that seem most likely to be needed.

Recommended Text for Materia Medica.

Materia Medica with Repertory. W. Boericke
Lectures on Homeopathic Materia Medica. J.T. Kent
Concordant Reference. Frans Vermeulen
Materia Medica Viva. G. Vithoulkas.
Leaders in Materia Medica. Nash
Allen's Keynotes With Nosodes. H. C. Allen

Case of Arnica Montana

Case 1: 27 Year old female native American. Main complaint: depression. Physical symptoms:

- Painful acne.
- Chronic pain in the lower back – diagnosed as a disc problem. At times I can't bend my lower back – very painful to bend forward. Many back spasms.
- Sore right shoulder – burning pain – pain with external pressure.

The shoulder pain is worse from exertion such as holding daughter or sports.

Emotional symptoms:

- I feel I will never succeed – so what is the point.
- Fear of failure.
- I often feel down on myself.
- I have trapped potential I can't move forward.
- Depression and anguish.
- Shy – difficult to express herself – difficult to be intimate with others and can't trust others.
- Fear of responsibility for other peoples feelings – it feels like a burden – I stew on it – I can't solve it so I feel inadequate.
- One time I had a boat accident – I nearly drowned – I had a fear to call for help as I felt no one would be there for me – I have a fear to be vulnerable.
- When I play music in front of others I fear I will die. Anxiety and stage fright.
- I have a fear of rejection.
- I don't like to feel alone and isolated and insecure but I do have those feelings at times.
- Grief from abandonment – my boyfriend left me – I felt betrayed.
- I find it difficult to trust again – fear to leave the house as I use to fear him and his mother would hurt me or take my child from me.
- I felt they put me down and made me feel not good enough – I felt disrespected.
- They made me feel not good enough – so I felt lost and without an identity – I was an alien – like there was a wall between me and others.
- So I worked hard on myself to get better.
- I feel I make mistakes and then feel inadequate.
- For a time I was bitter, angry and resentful at my x-boyfriend.
- So now I am very cautious.
- Fear to be alone to be physically attacked.
- I feel too vulnerable in public.

- Fear of rape and strangers.
- Fear of dark when outside.
- Fear of failure.
- Bites nails.

Discussion: Generally this patient has been beaten down emotionally, she feels emotionally bruised, vulnerable, inferior and small inside. She has become afraid and cautious as a result but wants to try again to succeed. Basically this is a case where the main limitation is TIMIDITY from being emotionally traumatized. Constantine Hering and James Kent both listed Arnica under timidity.

On repertorizaton Lycopodium was the first remedy according to RADAR.

This is understandable as she feels inadequate and fearful. We do not see any overcompensation or other strong keynotes for Lycopodium so I did not prescribe it.

In the rubric Cautious we find the following remedies: acon. alco. am-c. anac. arn. ars. aur-m-n. aur. bar-c. brom. cact. calc. carc. caust. chel. chin. cic. coff. Cupr. dros. graph. hyos. Ign.ip. kali-n. kali-s. lach. lact. LYC. m-arct. mang. nat-c. nat-m. nit-ac. nux-v. oci-sa. op. petr-ra. ph-ac. PULS. sil. spig. stram. sulph. tax. thuj. verat.

One could also consider Silica and Aurum from this list. To prescribe Silica we would like to see ingrown toe nails, extra perspiration and constipation – none of which she had. For Aurum we usually see a much heavier depression with the idea that "there is no way out and total hopelessness" although I think in a very severe Arnica case the patient may present this way. I think Arnica and Aurum share also the feeling that no matter how well they do something it is never good enough.

The other remedy I considered strongly was Lac caninum. It is listed under:

- Fear of failure
- Confidence, want of
- Timidity and ailments after being abused

Our patient though is not trying to please anyone in particular in order to feel included and safe and she did not have nightly salivation and so I rejected this remedy; these are two symptoms we usually see with Lac caninum.

The number two remedy in the repertorization was Carcinosin. This remedy is well known for people who have been beaten down, suppressed and struggle to regain an identity. My patient was not fastidious or overly sympathetic as these are two of the leading symptoms for Carcinosin.

Finally we come to the possibility of Arnica. In the repertorization it came up number three. It is listed under:

- Want of confidence
- Reproaching self
- Fear of injury
- Fear of coition, rape
- Fear of failure
- Suspicious
- Cautious
- Timidity
- Back injuries
- Shoulder injuries
- Fear of strangers

Painful acne

Based on this information I gave Arnica 200c one dose.

Her report back was: I feel more confident and worry less about my actions. The shoulder pain is much less. I feel more balanced overall. The first day after the remedy the acne was worse and then it improved. I feel less hesitation in my relationships with others as if I have more courage. I feel more expressive with others and less self conscious. I am less in doubt about my actions like I am in a more natural flow with life. My brain can focus better. I feel more confident when I play music. Less anger to the past and more forgiveness. Less fear to be outside at night – this is about 80 percent better. Much less low back pain. The shoulder feels 95 percent better. Much less nail biting.

We can think of Arnica for people who feel beaten down for one reason or another, emotionally black and blue from the trials of life. Financially beaten down, beaten down emotionally by a neglectful parent or suffering emotionally after a physical attack or beating. The human spirit is resilient it tries to stand up again, regain its confidence and make strides forward but this can be a fearful experience and not without suspicion of another attack. Arnica is the remedy for these cases and goes a long way to heal the original trauma and presenting symptoms.

Case 2:

Crateagus Oxycantha 12 year old boy.

October 2, 2012. For several years stomach aches every day which are progressively worse. Started as colic as a baby, then worse after a car accident at two years old. Accompanied by nausea. Sharp abdominal pains. Car sick easily. The nausea is worse when he has to go out to a place he does not want to go to. As we shall see he does not like to leave home because of his emotional anxiety.

The nausea is worse after eating and worse from oily food.

Chronic headaches almost every day.

Generally he feels anxiety in new places.

What else do you feel anxious about? I don't have enough time to do my homework and get everything done for school. I am also nervous around certain people, new people and people who I want to be friends with. I don't like people who have a strong personality, aggressive people.

I have high expectations to be perfect at things. I try to be neat and tidy. I don't want to try things that I am not good at. Sometimes I think to myself: I can't do it any better. If people knew that I made mistakes they would not be my friend, that is what I am worried about. I have a fear to be rejected. I fear if they are around me too much they would see my mistakes.

Remedies that we know are useful for fear of rejection are Carcinosin, Magnesiums, Natrums, Pinus contorta. For example Natrum carbonicum is very sensitive to the opinion of others.

In this patient I asked right away if he was tight in the jaw or cervical area and the answer was no. This information took me away from the idea of Pinus contorta.

He bites his nails a lot. He keeps his room very neat and clean like one would expect from Carcinosin. He wants to have it clean for his friends so that he won't be criticized. This is the exact symptom for Carcinosin.

What else bothers you? I worry for others (wow this is going to be an easy case of Carcinosin). If I see an injustice or see someone treated badly then I worry for them.

I wanted to rule out Phosphorus right away so I asked about his thirst which was below average. As we know in almost every case Phosphorus craves at least eight or ten large glasses of cold water a day.

(I went back to the idea of Carcinosin) Can you say no easily? I feel hurt so easily and feel obligated to say yes. I don't want to be reprimanded or get into trouble so that is why I am worried about my homework and how the teacher will react. This confirm the idea of Carcinosin, they feel guilt when they say 'no' and plus they feel sympathy for others so want to help them and are sensitive to criticism and so saying no is impossible for them. If you are thinking about giving Carcinosin and your patient can say 'no' easily such as: 'no I am tired I can't help you today' – then most likely

Carcinosin is not the remedy.

Do you like to help your mother? (this is another confirmation for Carcinosin.) No not especially he says. Some kids are a bit lazy we do not rule out this remedy because of this.

For eight years he has had to use Melatonin to help him get back to sleep. Without this medicine it takes him two or three hours to get to sleep. After a car accident at six months old he had night terrors for two years. In this accident his mother was injured. After this accident his mother said he wanted all his toys in a line.

His father had leukemia, depression and a drinking problem.

In Natrum cases we see a lot of resentment. It is not easy for them to forgive. So I asked him about this. I will forgive if they say they are sorry. With this one can move away from the Natrum idea.

I do though have anger and frustration which I keep inside. When I am upset I like some consolation and want a hug. For part of the interview he was holding his mothers hand. Again this is more like Carcinosin – they tend to suppress their anger but like close contact with others.

What fears do you have? I fear spiders and heights.

Tell me more about the stomach pain? It burns and aches.

I have good friends but I won't call them on the phone because I fear they will reject me. This is not like Carcinosin who feel with their friends secure, confident, look forward to the social interaction with them. During case taking one has to stay flexible and open to new ideas. For every remedy that seems obvious at some point in the interview there are four more that are very similar and may be a better match.

The father grew up in Utah in a place where there was nuclear testing. Perhaps this is not a true Carcinosin miasm?

Craves: spaghetti, pancakes, sour lemons, fruit, veggies.

He is very generous. (Car)

Colic as a baby. We see how strong this abdominal complaint is and so need to find a remedy that treats stomach ailments. Unfortunately almost every remedy treats stomach ailments and nausea is one of the most common symptoms besides pain.

How is your body reaction to temperature? I feel warm all the time (he is wearing shorts and apparently wears them all year round no matter how cold it gets). I want a fan on even in winter. This information is very upsetting to me because Carcinosin is not in this rubric and I have not seen a Carcinosin patient who could tolerate to be exposed to cold weather as in Washington State it is 0 to 10 degrees in the winter.

GENERALS - FANNED; being - desire to be: ant-t. apis ars. bapt. CARB-V. caust. chin. chlol. chlor. ferr. glon. hist. kali-n. lach. lyc. med. mim-p. nux-m. petr-ra. positr. puls. Sec. sulph. tab. zinc.

One has to now rethink the whole case from this new point of view. Each of these remedies needs to be seriously considered. For example for Apis we have: Low thirst, anxiety for others, warm blooded, loyal to parents, but the rest of the case does not fit. Causticum is sympathetic like this patient but Causticum is a lot more assertive. Pulsatilla is intolerant of heat, thirstless, Agravaion from fatty foods, sensitive to what others say, affectionate and likes consolation, fear of abandonment. This now becomes a real possibility.

He wants to only wear soft clothes. I have to be perfect at everything. Very indecisive.

Fear to start new things. His maternal grandfather had multiple myeloma.

Analysis: I felt this was a difficult choice between Carcinosin and Pulsatilla. Perhaps Magnesia Phosphoricum.

Plan: Carcinosin 30c one dose.

Ten Days Later. The stomach pains are no better; in fact they are worse. So much so, that seven days after the remedy the mother gave him coffee to antidote the remedy. After the coffee the sleepy feeling he was having all day with lower energy also got better and the stomach pains also were relieved. (Analysis: wrong remedy, more determination to find the correct remedy).

In what way do you worry for others? I want things fair for others; for example I feel bad if someone is left out. He does not like any conflict with others and would rather suffer than speak up for himself.

We usually can think of Magnesium for this type of sensitivity. The person who benefits from Magnesium remedy feels deeply disturbed when people argue around them – they can not tolerate it and will do anything to avoid conflict of this type. Luckily we have many Magnesium remedies to choose from. The rubric: Mind, quarreling aversion to and Mind, discords agg give us the remedies but one can choose from any Magnesium remedy if this symptom is clear.

The other remedy which one can consider here is Crataegus. In the proving the most obvious mental symptom was sensitiveness to unfairness and reprimand. One of the provers would not come to class as she felt that she had made a mistake with her homework. Another prover would not talk to her boyfriend as she thought he had been unfair with her by expecting her to pay for her meal at a restaurant. In the proving the work fairness came up over and over. IF THINGS ARE NOT FAIR I AM NOT GOING TO PARTICIPATE.

This is the idea of this remedy. There is tremendous fragility to betrayal, there has to be justice. There is an amazing sensitivity to criticism or doing things incorrectly.

This patient of ours has this exact sensitivity. I ask him more to be more certain.

Things have to be fair he says. If they are not fair I will stay home. That is why I can't invite other kids to my birthday party.

If one of them happened to be hurt or treated unfairly then it would be my fault. I can't guarantee this would not happen so I could not invite any of them over.

I have to be perfect for my teacher, I can't disappoint her, I can't upset her. I am awful, a bad person. I feel this when people are critical or when they won't be my friend. My one friend often cancels on me. Then I cry; and even God won't answer my prayers.

Here we see more detail about this remedy. A person who fears isolation, feels they are flawed and forsaken by God.

I eat then I am not full so I eat again.

I have been getting headaches and tension in my neck.

I don't like sun on me or too much heat. I sometimes have nausea with the headaches.

Mother and grandmother have high blood pressure.

Analysis: Crataegus fits the emotional picture exactly and the family history of blood pressure miasm helps to confirm this remedy.

Plan: Crataegus 30c one dose; then as needed.

Three Weeks Later

He has taken two doses so far. The headaches are almost totally gone. The nausea is 75% better. The anxiety is 75% better. I am looking forward to things now and can enjoy them.

His mother says he is louder now, more excited about things, silly and playful. He use to be so reserved, quiet, fearful and serious. He is acting like a normal twelve year old now.

He can not speak to his father about how he feels while in the past he would suppress all of his feelings as he was afraid he would disappoint his father.

He has stopped being afraid to drive in the car.

In the past the nausea was worse when the anxiety was worse. Now they are both better.

In the past I had a fear of the unknown and the unexpected – this is now better. Home was a secure and safe place.

I had a fear to look silly and wanted to control how others saw me as I did not want to be rejected. This is now better; I don't seem to care as much what others think.

Most of all I did not want to be left alone. So I would not contradict anyone especially my father.

With new people I would feel like an outcast. I had to be invited into the group. (Abies Canadensis).

I was so slow to make friends. The relationships would be

broken so easily as I had to pull away to protect myself. (Sensitive to betrayal: Pseudotsuga menziesii).

I would withdraw and sit in the corner silently. I would rather suffer than stand up for myself. I could not tolerate the guilt of feeling that I had disappointed my father.

If people really knew me they would not like me. (Thuja).

I had a core belief that there was something wrong with me. (Thuja). I still bite my nails. Still takes Melatonin.

As a child I would be angry if things were out of order.

I would get angry at myself if I did not live up to my high expectations; so I would hit my head on the door or hit myself in some way. I felt that I was stupid; but I don't think I am stupid any longer. I feel so much better about myself now.

I still want a fan to cool down.

I have a lot more energy and my mood is less changeable. I cry much less often now.

I still want to eat a lot.

Analysis: Correct remedy.

Plan: Crataegus 30c as needed which seems to be about one dose every two weeks.

Five Weeks Later

Over time he stopped using the fan. Less fussy about how he looks. He is still wearing shorts even though now it is December and very cold outside.

Eventually I gave him Crataegus 200c so that after this dose his stomach pains improved to 95% and finally to 100%.

Still bites his nails.

If he is treated unfairly now he can pull himself out of it and go on. It no longer affects him so deeply.

No longer feels anger or frustration.

Still has a fear of spiders and heights as before.

No bloating. (I was wondering if Carbo-veg could be used at some time?)

I no longer feel alone all the time as I use to.

Still has nausea from fats. Loves affection from his mother. Holds his mothers hand through the interview and in the car when she is driving.

About a week later he got a cold. A dose of Crataegus did not help. His mother called to say the cold was getting worse. Very stuffy in the sinuses with thick discharge. No thirst. Want mother to sit with him all day and read him stories.

Analysis: New layer. Wants consolation, no thirst, thick discharge, very warm blooded.

Plan: Pulsatilla 30c one dose.

Result: All better by the next day.

Two Months Later

No symptoms to speak of.

Mother says he is doing well in all aspects of his life and enjoying being a thirteen year old.

Materia Medica of Crataegus This remedy is indicated for people who seem to be even more sensitive to the opinion of others than Carcinosin. This leads them to suppress their emotions and thus we can see a connection to a reason for the high blood pressure.

They want others to treat them fairly and they also do their best to treat others fairly and not hurt others in any way. We see this same trait in Natrum muriaticum.

This is a remedy that can be used for headaches, stomach aches and nausea.

APPENDIX TWO

THE PERIODIC TABLE

This is supplemental information that can add to your knowledge of materia medica but there are many remedies here that are not necessary for the NPLEX exam.

If you learn the characteristic symptoms of each element you can learn to predict what a remedy will be like if one puts two elements together. As you know elements on the left of the table want to combine with elements on the right of the periodic table. Natrum phosphoricum is a good example. They are closed about who they are; like all Natrums, but want others to be open and friendly like we find in people who need phosphorus.

After plants the second most common source of our remedies is found on the periodic table.

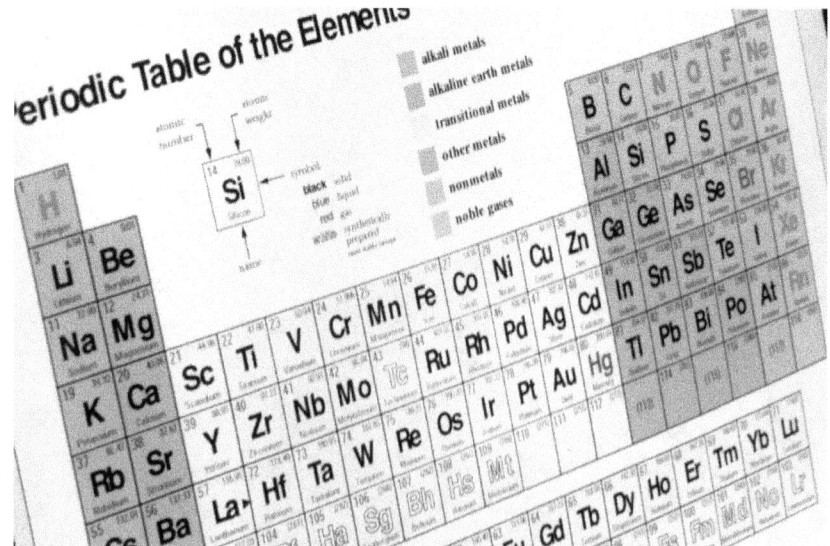

These are the basic elements from which our universe and all living things are made from. Most of the remedies from this list are either single elements such as Aurum metallicum – gold by itself or in combination with one other element such as Aurum muriaticum – gold chloride.

Hydrogen: The first element created in our universe. It is the element that has the closest experience to who made it and what was there just before it was created. Spiritual excitement followed by exhaustion or burn out. The heightened struggle for unity, to find a connection to what is our spiritual home. Yearning to transcend this material world, study incredibly hard to enter the spiritual world and finally accomplish this goal only to find they can't handle it and come apart. Believe they have contacted God, egotism, paranoid ideas. Absolute ideas. Acute spiritual mania. Followed by collapse and paranoia. (Proving by Jeremy Scherr)

Case 1: Man in early 40's, paranoid ideas, thinks he is going to be assassinated, delusion he is going to save the world, he wants to travel to meet up with others who have the same ideas. I meet with him and his family who wanted to avoid having him committed to a mental hospital. He tells me that he can teach me homeopathy because he just read my book (he opened the book and flipped through the pages). His ego is huge, he has grandiose ideas. He tells me he was meditating for months and finally met up with a supreme being. After a few doses of Hydrogen 30c and 200c he is much better. I see him a year later and he is still well; not paranoid and no more ideas about saving the world.

When hydrogen is added to other elements such as carbon, chloride and phosphorus it becomes an acid and the result is fatigue, indifference and collapse.

Picric acid: weakness of the mind.

Phosphoric acid: weak emotions.

Muriatic acid: physical weakness.

Helium: Dissociation. Difficult to take a full breath. Very little eye contact. Autism, won't speak or listen to parents. Only focus on his terms. Remain locked within themselves unapproachable and distant. Hypoesthesia, in the sense of skin anesthesia, insensitivity to cold, heat, even when pinching or scratching oneself on the face or on the body. Sensation of cardboard skin. Detached aversion to company. Anger if disturbed. Desire to laugh. Out of body experiences. History of abuse; life is too painful so leaves the body. Numbness to external world. (Salix-alba, Opium).

Lithium metallicum: Compressed or subdued emotions. Not allowed to express self as a child or feel they have to hide their real identity (Thuj). Suppressed emotions in order to conform. Try to conform but feel isolated and inhibited. May find it difficult to enjoy sex. *Arthritic nodules on the finger joints.* Exostosis. Osteoporosis. Stenosis - bone deposits on inside of spinal column leading to narrowing and pressure on the nerves). Osteoarthritis.

Lith-carb: Same as lithium metallicum but has easy weight gain, perspiration increased, more anxiety. A combination of Lithium and Graphite (Carbon) symptoms.

Lith-caust: A combination of Lithium and Causticum symptoms.

Case 1: 70 year old male. Stenosis of spine. Severe constant back pain extending into legs. Legs are restless. Arthritis in many joints. Helpful nature. After Lithium causticum arthritis much better, no more jumpy legs at night.

Lith-mur: Combination of Lithium and Natrum Muriaticum symptoms. Inhibited, timid, raw eczema and desire to do things perfectly.

Lith-phos: A combination of Lithium and Phosphorus symptoms. These people will be very tall, slender with thin bones. Inhibited, nervous, fear to be in new places but enjoy to watch life from a distance like reading novels or watching movies.

Lithium sulph: **Case 1:** Chronic sinusitis, hay fever and itchy scalp. Tall and slender, red lips. Suffers from bone spurs which are painful (Lithium). He likes order, works hard. Parents critical, feels inhibited, aversion to conflict. Closed emotions and tension. Difficult to laugh. After Lithium sulph sinus and hay fever markedly better; 80% in one week. More open, expressive, playful and relaxed. Sleep more refreshing. Calmer overall, more creative, feels happier. Tolerates salad better; less diarrhea from it. Four months on Lith-sulph 200c and his bone spurs at the base of the fingers have dissolved. Later on he developed back problems (rigid low back, sciatica, pain worse if sneeze) and this was resolved with Lithium sulph 1m in one week.

Beryllium:

Boron: Natrum biboracicum. Borax: Worse downward motion. Apthae. Oversensitivity and a weakness "on the surface of the nervous system."

This nausea is produced by the intense feelings that arise while engaged in serious thought. The patient wakes up in a terrible fright, as if his end had arrived. Similarly, hearing a sudden noise brings about this frightened reaction. The patient gives the impression of being absent minded at that moment and out of touch with the environment; this sudden noise brings him back to his body with a fright.
This reaction may be brought about by hearing a cry or an unexpected noise such as something dropping from a chair or a door closing unexpectedly. Hearing someone hawk or sneeze may provoke a fright, as may even very slight noises like the crumpling of paper, or the rustling of silk. Other fears to be found in Borax include fear of impending disease, fear of infection, and fear of falling. Another interesting point in these children is that they cry and shriek with pains before urinating or passing a stool. You may find cases of colics in babies, after suppressed aphthae. They suddenly scream and kick and equally suddenly turn quiet for 10 to 20 minutes, and then start again. They want to be carried about but the fits are not prevented. In cases of enteritis the child cries a great deal, its mouth is very sore, greenish stool passes every hour or two, a white coat covers the tongue and inside the cheeks, and a red eruption appears on the face. Excessively nervous, these children are especially affected by noise. A slight noise will wake them up. They are frightened on hearing a distant shot, and start in every limb on hearing an anxious cry. The three main keynotes on which Borax is usually prescribed are: 1. Aggravation from downward motion. - 2. Fretfulness, ill-humor, indolence and discontent before stool; but lively, contented, and cheerful after stool. - 3. Amelioration of mental and physical symptoms after 11p.m. Other keynotes: - Ingrowing of lashes, tangled hair that sticks together. -

Exhilaration after coition. - Mouth very hot in aphthae. - Greenish stool day and night. - Tip of nose shining red. Red noses of young women. - Waking as from fright. - Mother cannot nurse child due to thickened milk which tastes bad.

Carbon: Graphites: Overweight, stocky build, chilly. Down to earth, practical, family oriented, like to work. Mental confusion, forgetful. Aversion to salt and sweets. Diamond: Loss of identity, feel held back by others.

There many remedies with Carbon. Calc-carb, Natrum carb, Kali-carb, Baryta carb, Magnesia carb. Etc.

Carbon Sulph: No ego symptoms. More like graphites but with itching, worse from heat. Like to work. Responsible.

Nitrogen: This element expands functions (especially blood vessels) and releases emotions which then go to an excess. Loss of attachment and connection between different parts of the brain. Loss of moderation as the brain can't add layers of constraint upon the part that is excited.

N2, or liquid nitrogen is an extreme vasodilator. Throbbing and pulsating pains.

Nitrogen oxide gas: The syndrome called Nitrogen Narcosis *is a reversible alteration in consciousness that occurs while diving at depth.* The deeper the dive the stronger the symptoms. *The Greek word ναρκωσις (narcosis) is derived from narke, "temporary decline or loss of senses and movement, numbness", a term used by Homer and Hippocrates. Narcosis produces a state similar to drunkenness (alcohol intoxication), or nitrous oxide inhalation. It can occur during shallow dives, but does not usually become noticeable at depths less than 30 meters (100 ft).*

The most dangerous aspects of narcosis are the impairment of judgment, multi-tasking and coordination, and the loss of decision-making ability and focus. Other effects include vertigo and visual or auditory disturbances. The syndrome may cause exhilaration, giddiness, extreme anxiety, depression, or paranoia, depending on the individual diver and the diver's medical or personal history. When more serious, the diver may feel overconfident, disregarding normal safe diving practices. (Wikipedia) The brain is disconnected from consciousness as we see in Cannabis and Opium. It is a fearful experience to be disconnected in this way. On the other hand there is no inhibition thus leading to extreme confidence (Arg-nit), outgoing behaviour, fearlessness (Agar).

Glonoin - $C_3H_5N_3O_9$ - Vessels dilate. Throbbing headaches. Compressed anger which wants to explode. Congestion.

Amyl nitrosum: Throbbing headaces, fear something bad will happen.

Amyl nitrate.

With Nitric acid – HNO_3: we find no limits on anxiety. The connection with a protective and meaningful higher spirit-hydrogen is lost. The patient thus feels that there is no meaning in life, he is cynical and nihilistic. Hatred and unforgiveness are common symptoms for this remedy. Fear of death and suffering. Fear of death perhaps because there is nothing after as the connection to God is lost.

Arg-nit – expansive in a positive way but it goes to an extreme. Loves to perform, very social. Image: He is excited to climb the telephone pole but once he is up there he is afraid; this idea can be applied to a ten year old about to go on stage to give a recital. She is excited but once up there is frozen in fear and has diarrhea. On the other side he can be fearless as he thinks he can jump from a height or put his hand in a mouth of a shark. The rational part of the mind is inhibited and disconnected from the impulsive part of the mind. The fear then takes its turn and becomes exaggerated as not bridled by reality; fear to cross a bridge, fear of crowds, fear to look up at at tall building as it will fall on him. Argentum metallicum people are loquacious and friendly with enlarged knee joints but they do not go to extremes as we find in Argentum nitricum.

Kali – nitricum: One can predict this remedy is for extreme belief in rules, rigid belief systems and conformity. Rules are not connected to other values and norms of society. Believe or die!

Natrum – nitricum: One can predict this remedy could be for extreme grief, suicidal grief, grief that leads to extreme isolation.

Oxygen: I have not confirmed this information: Selfishness, feeling victimized and deprived of that which he feels he deserves. There is a quality of begging, pleading, and demanding to have his own way. He experiences the indignation of the loss of his self worth, which he blames on others and thereby feels victimized. Their sense of space is also disturbed: they can be so disorientated that it is not safe for them to drive a car. They make mistakes in speaking and writing or they don't know left from right anymore etc. Gloomy, depressed, empty, motionless. Aversion: sharp noises, as made by radios and televisions. Desired nothing, oranges.

Down's syndrome. Headache, in temples, amel. hot bath. Eyes dry, tired, -amel. closing them; heaviness and numbness of eyelids, as if they have been in chlorine. Hot face. Colds, much mucus, itching, blocked nose. Sore throat, scraping, amel. water and tea, rasping, as if something stuck in it. Low voice, deep voice. Respiration asthmatic, cough agg. morning. Wart on first joint of right index finger. Urticaria. Walking upright and gracefully. Locality: right. Weather: cold, as if freezing; or very hot. Time; agg. 5 pm, agg. 5 am. Desires: nothing, oranges. Aversion: cold drinks, bread. Sleep: yawning (2). Physical: agg. neon lights.

Natrum. Closed, alone. Serious, responsible, grief, hurt easily. Passive acceptance. Withdraw but hold onto ideas. Worse from sun. Very attached to the past. Desire for salt, worse or better from the sea.

Magnesium: Feels alone, forsaken. Mild. Worse from conflict. Sleep Unrefreshing. Cramps. Liver problems. Peace makers. Always want appeasement and for people to get along. Very disturbed by arguments.

Aluminum: Lack of identity. Impulses to be violent. Lost. Slow in mind, stasis. Constipation. Ailments appear slowly but very destructive. Dry skin. Itching with no eruption.

Silicon: Timid, yielding, thoughtful, mild, sensitive, obstinate. Ingrown toe nails. Extra perspiration on feet, hands or head. Chilly. Lean body type. Constipation.

Phosphorus: Desire to contact others, social. Empathy. Fears. Hemorrhages. Strong thirst for ice cold drinks. Fears and anxiety. Fear during a thunderstorm.

Sulfur: Strong ego, desire for recognition. Inventive. Strong imagination. Can be selfish, try to dominate others. Brag and or suffer from a loss in reputation. Lazy and procrastinate. Feel they need to gain the respect and appreciation from others. Often feel they are not appreciated by others. Heat or red in places. Red lips. Itchy skin.

Chlorum: Chlorine: Muriaticum: Grief, sentimental, strong attachments, hurt feelings easily. Worse from sun. Proper, polite. Stayed or controlled emotions. Suppressed emotions. Eczema, skin is raw and burns. Patient wants to be fanned like we see in Carbo-veg.

Potassium: Kali: Conscientious, strong sense of duty, practical. Strong principles. Rigid, rule and routine oriented. Difficult to be flexible, dogmatic. Control their emotions. Aversion to be tickled. Hard working, persevere. Worse 2 to 4 am. Can't sleep from 2 to 4 am. Stitching pains.

Swelling upper eyelid or lower lids. Wants things done a certain way. Place great importance on belonging to a group. Such as family. Insecurities relate to family and friends.

Argon: Content, lazy, self satisfied, not interested in bonding with others. No direction in life – does not want to get out of bed, go to school, or work or even look for work. Phlegmatic temperament (Sulph). Enjoy their own company to watch television or play video games. Only do the minimum amount of work. Very sensitive to hot and cold (Merc). If anyone puts pressure on them they get upset. Obstinate, want their own way. Aversion to conflict. Want to be beautiful and valued. Denial of things that are bothering then on a deeper level or that they need to take care of.

Case 1: 12 year old, fever and almost constant dry cough for three weeks. Tickling cough. Aversion to go to school, likes to be alone. Pale and low vitality. After Argon 30c energy returned next day, cough and fever better. Back at school and became very motivated about worldly events wanting to help others.

Calcium: Insecure, build a stable life. Fear of instability. Obstinate. Family oriented. Fear their confusion will be noticed. Fear of disapproval. Desire to be appreciated especially with Calc-sulph. Fear to be abnormal. Fear poverty, the future, disease. They like to feel protected. Worse from cold and damp. Myomas. Extra perspiration on hands, feet or head. Gain weight easily. Pale. Paper thin finger nails.

Scandium:

Titanium: Proving was done.

Vanadium: Exercise to look perfect. Insecure. Fasting.

Chromium: Chromium compounds are recommended for individuals that are hypersensitive and easily wounded. Because they are afraid of being hurt, they are particularly introverted and cautious in their behavior. (G.L.) Superficial perfectionism. The desire to have a good image Fear she is not beautiful. Feels her husband does not understand her or really love her, does not believe his sincerity. Reserved. Depression. Fear others will see he can't prove himself. Fear to fail, lack of courage. Embarrassed. Shame when things go wrong. Carry on regardless – strong determination. Small mistakes are felt like serious crimes. Fear to say the wrong thing and blunder. (Sch) Hypersensitive and easily wounded. Fear to be hurt. Introverted. Cautious. (G.L.)

Manganese: Manganum: Insecurity. Sensitive to music. Learning. Fine tuning. Fear of failure and criticism. <u>Sensitive to cold air in the ears.</u> The main characteristic of Manganum is their desire to help. They are very kind and love to please others. They also adapt easily to other people. This desire to help is more than a desire, it is a need that has to be fulfilled otherwise they get very restless. Desire for compliments. Sensitive people who like to please others and who hope they will be acknowledged for what they do.

They like others to notice how much they do and they like to be compliments on their efforts. Compliments put them at ease: they know they have done well and they can relax now. Criticism makes them feel very indignant (DD Staph, Colocynth). They may dream about reconciliation, because it will keep bothering them until it is solved. This shows in the frown on their forehead or the bitter expression on their face. It is a state of hurt and indignation that makes them want to avoid company altogether. Vrijlandt gives a typical example of a Manganum woman who has given a party and who won't rest until she gets a thank-you phone call from her guests the next day, saying they had a wonderful time. The same theme of pleasing others but wanting to be praised for her efforts. I can tolerate criticism as long as it is constructive'. This is the answer they will give you if you ask them how they react to criticism. If the criticism is purely destructive they get very bitter. They did so much and it still isn't enough. They tried so hard to please everybody and look what they get! This is the stage indicated by the rubric: 'Embittered mood, implacable, for a long time having a grudge against who offended him' (Allen), and 'Irreconcilable and long continued resentment against those who injure him' (Hering). They can be quite critical themselves too, although always in a mild form, because they mean it to be constructive.

Mang-acet: She tries to do her very best for each family and when the advice she gives isn't immediately accepted she feels she has done it wrong. Ear pain from cold air.

Iron - Ferrum: Long suffering, keep going through adversity, tough, obstinate. Never give up on a plan. Tenacity. Anemia. Sensitive to noise. Obesity. Red in the face.

Niccolum: Feel that they do not deserve to have many things. Can feel useless. Critical of self and others. Sensitive to injustice. Controlling, contrary, dictatorial. Rigid ideas. Guilt – as if a criminal. Also strives for congruency, as he wants to be simple, i.e. not part of a composite existence. Niccolum demands simplicity, because only thus can he be the only source and originator of his actions. Rejects being a part of a larger whole, because he cannot realize his projects fully in that way. He controls all things without mixing himself with them. It is this being the

Materia Medica

originator by virtue of God's simple unity that Niccolum envies. Niccolum makes of himself an isolated fragment of a larger social whole and can no longer procure anything. (Nees.)

Anger from contradiction. Disposition to contradict. Intolerant of contradiction. Asking for nothing. Aversion to change. Critical. Delusion accused. Delusion pursued, poisoned. Delusion policeman. Fastidious. Pride. Impulse to hurt others. Need to fight for others. Judgmental. More controlling than Kali remedies.

Cobalt: Overly sexual. Weakness in the lumbar area.

Copper: Cuprum: Cramps. Spasms, guilt. Bossy, want to be in charge. Controlling, forceful.

Zinc: Hyperactive, restless. Intelligent.

Gallium:

Germanium: Self conscious anxiety. Feel alone and inferior. Too sensitive.

Arsenic: Insecurity, feel the word is chaotic. Restless anxiety. Fastidious. Chilly. Selfish to have needs met. Fear of future.

Selenium: High sexuality. Hair falls out all over body.

Bromine: Guilt. Worse from dust and pollution. Kali-brom most restless guilt about being punished by God i.e. wringing hands, biting nails.

Krypton: Anxiety, the world is too chaotic. Anxiety mind is spinning out of control. Anxiety if leaves home. Tends toward perfectionism. Disconnect from family but wants them in the same room. Disconnect from reality, friends and co-workers. Feels in a dream, not in body, dissociative. Loneliness, alienated, loss of purpose. Difficult to be spontaneous. Can't accept change. Keeps the wall up to be separate. Hiccough and belching. Feels unworthy. Aversion to praise. Better when working. High standards but then feels he is a failure. Guilt and feels like a criminal. Out performs all others at work. Weakness, worse from the sun. Feels thick and can't move. Headaches worse from light. Wakes every tow hours. Very cold feet like ice. (Based on a cured case S.Olsen)

Rubidium:

Strontium: Insecure, desire for support from others. (J.R.U.)

Yttrium:

Zirconium:

Niobium: Suppression of creativity. (G.L.)

Molybdenum:

Technetium:

Ruthenium:

Rhodium:

Palladium:

Silver; Argentum: Creative, interactive, extroverted, quirky humor, love to entertain and be on stage but it frightens them. Excessive consistency. Need to follow a schedule. Punctual. Keep their word. Arg-nit: most social, creative, entertainers. Fear of heights and closed in spaces. Impulsive to do dangerous things. Stage fright, anticipation anxiety. Worse from sweets. Crave salt and sweets. Arg-met: loquacity, enlarged joints, cartilage hypertrophy.

Cadmium: Cancer remedies.

Cad-sulph. Repertory: Nausea from breathing deeply or from coughing. **Case 1:** Chronic sinusitis, very bad foot odor, emaciated, pain in teeth. Nausea from taking a deep breath. After Cad-sulph 30c better next day, vitality returned, able to eat again.

Indium:

Tin – Stannum: Weakness felt in the chest.

Antimony: Anger, feels reclusive, critical cold eyes. Anger when looked at. Ant-crud is sentimental and romantic but reclusive and can get into horrible moods with people so better to stay alone and write poetry. Ant-tart: anger and respiratory problems with sleepiness. Disdainful of others.

Iodine: In a hurry, restless. Worse from heat. Worse from fasting.

Tellurium:

Xenon: Case 1: Feels shunned. Others aren't good enough to be friends with (Platina). Talented, good grades, then gave up and did nothing. Checked out of life. Withdrawn. Scratch face and pimples till they get raw. Dejected. Won't show up for things. Cut off from fiancée, went on a trip instead. Won't go to work. Closed down. Dropped out of school. Wrapped up in self. Self-centered. Wants to be admired. Went to an ashram to find herself. Jerking of the shoulder. Can feel high like its a religious experience. Dropped uterus. Fear of failure. Not available to others. Body feels heavy. Feels spaced-out. Easy to get along with but can't connect or bond. Everything feels like a burden. Feels closed in and weak. Wants the best for her daughter for her to be brilliant. Diffuse, lack of structure.

Cesium:

Barium: Delusion inferior. Feel they have to be perfect. Self conscious anxiety about details. Irresolution, need support from others. Hiding away. Childlike. Need support from others.

Lanthanum:

Cerium:

Praseodymium:

Neodymium:

Promethium:

Samarium:

Europium:

Gadolinium:

Terbium:

Dysprosium:

Holmium:

Erbium:

Thulium:

Ytterbium:

Lutetium:

Hafnium:

Tantalum:

Tungsten:

Rhenium:

Osmium: – Delusion of being a criminal. Guilt, feel they have committed a crime.

Iridium:

Platinum: – Delusion better than others. Pride. Feels superior and looking down on others.

Aurum: Gold – Self reproach, work to achieve perfection. Feels worthless. Worse at night. Suicidal ideas. Must work toward his vision and success. Selfish motives. Desire to be the best at things. Can't fail. Must achieve and get to the top, to be the best and strive very hard for that. If achieve their goal will feel it is not enough and set a higher goal. Will work from morning till night. Fear to fail. Can't tolerate defeat.

Mercury: Suspicious. Hiding feelings. Closed emotions as don't trust anyone. Salivation at night. Many symptoms worse at night. Violent impulses. Worse hot and cold. Pale, decay, chronic infections. Offensive odors. Indented tongue.

Thallium: Pain in legs very intense. Paralysis.

Plumb: Lead: Stasis. Mind is slow. Contraction of tendons. Hard nodules on tendons in the palms of the hands.

Bismuth; Fear of being alone. Desire for company. Clinging. Intolerable pains in the abdomen, colic.

Polonium:

Astatine:

Radon: Cured case from Steve Olsen: Alone and isolated in the extreme. Hate mother and father. No friends, does not want to talk to anyone. Chronic nausea every day. Nausea and anemia. Severe depression. No meaning in life. She became very social, confident and involved with others in a positive way after this remedy. The anger and isolation also resolved.

Francium: No remedy yet made from this element. The information for the remedies below was obtained from a book by Patricia Le Roux. The Actinides.

Radium: Very dense metal. Luminescent blue. Extremely radioactive. Breaks down into Radon. Cancer.

Radon: Case 1: 17 y.o. Female. Won't leave her room. No ambition. Lack of confidence. Dresses up very beautiful. Jealous of sister. Hatred of mother (Pseudo-men) can't forgive (Nti-ac), critical. Isolated from family and friends. Anger at mother if mother asks her to do things. Depression, no meaning to life (Nit-ac), suicidal thoughts. Won't go to school. Sweet things like fruit taste to sweet. The slightest things other people do make the patient angry and so she needs to be alone. No sexual feelings. Ear pains from loud noise. Mouth ulcers, stomach ulcers. Ear pain from cold air. Chronic continuous nausea worse from the smell of perfumes. Anemia. Cracking of joints. Better from open air. Never hungry. Bleeding gums. Tension headaches worse from sun. Joint pains. During the interview she would either turn the chair around to face away from me or hide behind her long black hair with no eye contact, then shrug if I asked her a question. Sensitive to hot and cold. Wants to go and live on the street. Since grade one did not want to go to school. After Radon 30c she started to get better. Went back to school, took up music and performed in concerts. Make amends with her father and mother. Became a happy person, sexuality returned with abundance, lots of friends. Able to smile, appreciative of her accomplishments at school and became a beacon of positive vitality.

Rad-brom: Rheumatism, gout, acne, thrush, cancer, wounds that don't heal well, low blood pressure, burns slow to heal, pains with great weakness, feat to be alone in the dark, desire for company. Vertigo with occipital headache worse in bed. Occipital and vertex pain. Pain in eyes better from open air. Dry nasal cavities. Pain lower jaw, facial neuralgia. Mouth dry with metallic taste. Stomach empty feeling, nausea, aversion to sweets. Violent cramps in abdomen. Itching hemorrhoids. Nephritis, urinary tract symptoms. Itching vulvae. Irregular menses. Pain in right breast better from rubbing. Ache in back and neck worse from dropping head forward, better from standing or sitting erect. Lumbar or sacral backache, pains appear in the bones, better from continued motion. Backache between shoulders, better from walking. Pain in joints. They feel hard and brittle as if they would break on moving them. Arms feel heavy. Cracking in shoulder joint. Pains are worse at night. Dermatitis of fingers. Nails distorted. Restless sleep. Fever: feels cold internally, chattering of teeth until noon, followed by heat on the skin. Eruptions and dermatitis with burning and itching. Swelling and redness. Necrosis and ulceration. Itching all over the body. Burning of shin as if on fire. Skin cancer. Better open air, continued motion, hot bath, lying down, and pressure. Feeling of guilt, confusion. Insecure, observers. Disciplined. Critical. Shy. Passive. Feel rejected, withdrawn but angry.

Case 1: arthritis, wandering pains, rheumatic endocarditis, guilt that she can't meet expectations, few friends feels rejected, passive, fear of dark, irritable, rejects sympathy, fear of future, aversion to closed in spaces, isolated and feels rejected. Aversion to eggs, meat and fish. Sensation of burning between her shoulder blades.

Rad-iod: Allergies, hay fever, asthma. Lots of energy, restlessness. Worse from heat, hypoglycemia. Thin but excessive appetite. Feels undernourished. Loss of contact with culture.

Actinium: Cancer. Extremely radioactive.

Act-nit: Fever with shivering and marbled skin. Weakness, convulsions with the fever (107F, 41.7C). Pneumococcal septicemia. History of too much energy. Precocity, sarcastic. Retreats from others, self doubt. Withdrawn, controlled. Family history of cancer. Desires meat and fruit.

Protactinium: Cancer. Restless, difficult to concentrate, partial failure in school. Trouble maker, expelled from school. Social, open and likes sports. Obstinate, won't study things he doesn't like. Too much energy. Likes meat and fruit. History of ear infections.

Thorium: Cancer. Chronic catarrh. Wrinkles in the brow. Severe trauma – feel life is falling apart. Fear of new things. Can't keep up at school. Fear to take the first step. Not aware of her strength. Craves eggs and fruit.

Thor-oxy: Low self esteem, selfish, demanding. Tormenting itching at night. Can't face any challenge, won't even try, given up. No interest in anything. Sexually abused, feels like a victim, dependent upon others for everything. Likes to wear dirty clothes, unkempt. Communicates better with adults. Withdrawn socially, constant irritable mood.

Thor-nit: Self doubt, depression, can't study. Trauma – life falls apart, then testicular cancer. Withdrawn. No energy, feels as if breaking apart, craves carbonated drinks.

Thor-mur: Loss of a parent. Talented at art. Arthritic pains, swelling of joints. Autoimmune diseases. Desire for fruit, aversion to eggs and vegetables.

Neptunium: Cancer. Suppression of serious illness.

Nep-nit: Eczema, betrayal, isolation, depression. Too much vitality then later total exhaustion. Creative parents. Judo champion. Methodical. Pretends to have lots of friends. Very anxious to do a test or have an examination. Dyslexia and mistakes in spelling. Quick to evaluate situations and clairvoyant. Over mature for his age. Respected by others. Worry about the future. Strong sense of duty. Fastidious.

Nep-mur: Recurrent ear infections. Plump, jovial. Loss of a parent. Wakes howling with pain in the ear. Feels destroyed my circumstances of life.

Uranium: It is found frequently in nature; it is found in sea water. The half life is 4.5 to 700 million years. 92 protons and from 125 to 150 neutrons depending on the isotope. Cancer. Generous mood, sympathetic, sad, loneliness. Slender. Edema around the eyes. Inflamed eye lids. Ear inflammation. Acne, boils on the face. Ulcers of the stomach and duodenum – pain better from eating. Bleeding from stomach. Sudden and persistent vomiting causing dehydration. Inflamed peritoneum, enteritis. Inflamed bladder and or kidneys. Fishy odor to urine. Bronchitis and pneumonia.

Uran-met: Episodic vomiting with violent abdominal pains. Can't sleep since house was robbed and burned down. Accident prone. Self confident and rarely afraid. Attention to detail, worldly and responsible. Calm; reassures her mother. Strong sense of duty. Independent and responsible. Restless sleep. Craves fish. Acid reflux.

Uran-acet:

Uran-ars: Cancer. Anxiety about health.

Uran-mur: Failing school. Mother alcoholic. Gifted child but under performs. Well behaved, perfect child. Mild mannered. Strong sense of duty, control, responsible. Grief. Craves fruit. Aversion to eggs and vegetables.

Uran-nit: Eczema and leukemia. Complains from overwork. Strong sense of Duty. Introverted. Craving for salt.

Uran-oxy: Indignant from being abused. Stubborn insomnia. Mature for his age. Loves red meat. Selfish, demanding. Abused victim. Low self worth. Lazy, neglected, vagrant.

Americium: Does not exist in nature. Cancer.

Amer-nit: Proving by Sherr: (not yet published) Depression and anxiety. Sleep disorders. Hives. Organized and methodical. Cynical and sarcastic. Aversion to milk, desire for meat.

Amer-mur: Slender, full of energy. Loss of mother or father. Fits of anger, nightmares. Depressed, won't play. Resentment, sensitive, grief.

Plutonium: Cancer. Desire for order or will feel threatened. Sensation of heaviness. Feel their own center is being oppressed. Feel they have to express their feelings immediately. Changeable moods. Pressure in the forehead, heaviness. Pressure at the vertex like an explosion. Burning pain in the eyes. Dry throat. Cutting pain the abdomen worse from bending forward. Distended abdomen. Vomiting and diarrhea. Pulmonary fibrosis and lung cancer. Sensation of heaviness in the breasts. Paralysis of the sacral region; pain extends to the back of the thigh and hollow of the knee. Pains as if bones are fractured. Can't walk, worse from walking. Better from heat, hard pressure, short sleep and massage. Sensation of heaviness in limbs. Pains in the heels. Can't sleep as feels too hot. Paralytic fatigue, has to lie down. Chilly and shivering, but heat in the face and head. Aggression or deeply religious.

Plut-nit: Viral illness, fatigue, can't breathe at night. Throws anger fits like an animal. Allergic and asthmatic. Precise, fastidious, systematic and organized. Responsible. Overly sensitive, isolated. People seem to reject her. Craving for meat and raw meat.

Plut-mur: Singer; lost voice. Loss of a parent at a young age. Betrayal, resentment. Becomes devoted to something. Loves to dance wildly. Wakeful and too excited. Too much energy or falling apart with grief.

Curium: Cancer. History of suppression of ...

Cur-nit: Refined in the arts. Isolated but enjoys to study. Isolated. Swollen lymph nodes and enlarged spleen with very low vitality. Feels near death, no meaning left in life. Likes meat and delicacies. Nightmares.

Cur-mur: Tall for age. Brilliant at one thing. Suppression of eczema. Life threatening asthma.

History of parental alienation. Resentment. Likes salt. Aversion to onions. Very dry skin.

Berkelium: No remedy made from this element.

Californium: Cancer. History of suppression of …..

Calif –nit: Near death, collapsed state, deep wrinkles on forehead, curled up into a ball, no ambition, anxiety about health, no connection to God. Unforgiveness. History of deep depression.

Calif-mur: Near death, deep wrinkles around mouth, overly sensitive, history of grief and disappointment. Sentimental, refined, and withdrawn into self, worse from sun. Gives up eventually. Suicidal thoughts.

Einsteinium: Atomic number 99. No remedy made yet from this element. Too unstable and too radioactive as are all of the elements from this point onward.

Fermium: No remedy made from this element. Half life up to 200 days.

Mendelevium: No remedy made from this element. Made artificially; only a few atoms ever made, which lasted for less than a second.

Nobelium: No remedy made from this element. Radioactive metal not found in nature i.e. only artificially made.

Rutherfordium: No remedy made from this element.

Lawrencium: No remedy made from this element. Half life only a few seconds to 3.6 hours.

APPENDIX THREE

Wound Healing

Study the local symptoms of the infection and what has changed since the infection began. These will be the best symptoms to finding the correct remedy. If you can

ARNICA MONTANA – To stop the bleeding, and bruising of a wound.

FICUS RELIGOSA – If Arnica will not stop the hemorrhage then often this remedy will. After a severe injury or car accident.

MILLEFOLIUM - Can also be used for hemorrhages. Bright red blood. Bruised soreness.

BELLIS PERENNIS – Injury to internal organs. Sprains and bruises. After excessive physical exercise; sore all over, severe strain.

CALENDULA – This is the most important remedy for infections from wounds.

CINNAMON – Hemorrhage after childbirth.

IPECAC – Hemorrhage with nausea.

Study Guide

Systemic Infections

ECHINACEA

Links 4/98, pg. 204-206, Keith Avedissian

- Blood poisoning from infected wounds with marked debility in thinking and feeling very tired.

- Two case examples centered around a wound that became infected, the condition didn't resolve with antibiotics, and there was a gradual debilitation of the patient, both mental and physical. The patients did not have the energy to do anything, had to force themselves to do what was required. Great difficulty focusing the mind. There was a feeling of exhaustion with a great desire to go to sleep.

- Rubrics: Generalities, Wounds, dissecting.

  Generalities, Wounds, suppurating.

  Confusion of mind with sleepiness.

  Stupefaction as if intoxicated.

  Thinking, aversion to.

  Work, aversion to mental.

- Useful in conditions with suppuration of wounds, infections where there is blood poisoning with foul discharged, marked debility, sleepiness, difficulty in concentration and slowness both physically and mentally.

- Vermuelen: Patients feel weak and tired, aching in the muscles, slowness in every action, speaks slowly, replies slowly, walks slowly.

- Mentally they feel confused, depressed, can't exert the mind. Doesn't wish to think or study. Drowsy, could not read, senses seemed to be numbed, difficulty to apply the mind.

- DD: Baptisia (infections and septic states, prostration, persistent drowsiness, sensation of soreness all over, bruised, tired all over, heaviness, parts lain on feel sore and bruised and bed feels too hard, discharges are foul – but they feel scattered all over the bed), Gelsemium (weakness, debility, aching, soreness – but they want to lie and do nothing and their condition doesn't usually arise from a septic state), Arnica (aching, soreness, septic conditions, restlessness, feeling as if the bed is too hard, drowsiness, loss of strength – but the attitude is that they feel OK and they try to keep going), Pyrogenium (septicemia with fever, foul discharges, putrid, aching, bruised feeling, prostration, soreness of muscles, bed feels too hard, restlessness, sense of duality – but pulse can be abnormally quick or out of proportion to their temperature), Anthracinum (affected parts burn as if on fire)

BUFO RANA
(Toad)

Lymphangitis; after a cut the infection spreads up the lymph vessels. Blood poisoning.

· Important in treatment of convulsions, mental retardation, delayed development. (RM)

· Appearance: coarse-looking, stupid-looking, lazy or sleepy look, thick lips (not always).

· Frequently protruded tongue, or lapping motion of tongue (GV, AG).

· Typical patient is mentally slow and unrefined, basic and instinctive (not always).

· Can be normal or even gifted in specific mental capacities or skills (A. Geukens).

· Easily angered when misunderstood (A. Geukens) - Difficulty expressing themselves, and easily angered when misunderstood (DG).

- In most cases there is a strong focus on sexuality. Strong desire for masturbation and a great preoccupation with pornographic material. (RM)

- Desire to be alone to pursue solitary pleasures, such as masturbation – can't postpone pleasure.

- Love of music (A. Geukens), may be gifted at playing musical instruments (DG).

- Bites nails (A. Geukens)

- Childish and immature mind, speech, behavior (Baryta carbonica) with cunning deceitfulness (Tarentula) (Sankaran)

- Convulsions, epileptic seizures – often from excitement or anger or connected with sexual excitement (A. Geukens)

-- Headache after an attack

-- Rolling head, shaking head (A. Geukens)

-- Tongue lapping before or during attack

-- Mouth wide open before an attack

-- Eyes turned upwards during convulsions

-- With unintelligible speech

-- Biting tongue

- Autism, lack of emotionality (A. Geukens)

- Want of moral feeling (2)

- Cure for lymphangitis: from a cut on the arm – inflamed lymph with a blue streak running up arm to lymph node.

- Infections and inflammations – not just lymphangitis

- Infections around nails, hangnails (David Mundy)

Links 1987-90, Notes from Geukens Seminar

Case 1: A man whose only interest was mathematics and computers, to the exclusion of his family. When disturbed he would fly into a rage. His first presenting symptom was an inflammation of the tibia. Wife described him as a dictatorial man who had sex with no emotional attachment, his only interest was computers.

- Comment: This case shows the more intelligent type of Bufo. Bufo arouses the lowest passions, e.g. sex and rage, but we may often observe that one part of the brain is highly developed, e.g. a great gift for music, an extremely developed sense of equilibrium as seen in circus people, or the highly specialized academic.

- Inflammations: Important in this remedy, and not limited just to the arm.

Links 3/93, pg. 18-19, Rajesh Shah

- For respiratory disorders – bronchial asthma, allergic laryngitis, chronic bronchitis

- Based on 18 cases, two cured case examples given in the article

Indications:

1. Tickling in larynx which excites cough

2. Aggravation 1-4 a.m.; 3 a.m. ... Bufo wakes between 1-4 a.m. with tickling sensation in throat leading to cough and dyspnea; this is specific to Bufo. Hering writes: "Cough provoked towards 3 to 4 a.m. by a tickling in the larynx which he feels only at this hour." This resembles Kali-carb (dryness in larynx at 3 a.m.) but Bufo has been used successfully where Kali-carb had failed with such a time modality.

3. Other sensations – stitching, sticking, stinging, burning – which excite the cough, often experienced at 3 a.m. or in the evening hours.

4. Paroxysmal or violent cough, or deep hacking cough, or hollow cough.

Study Guide

5. Dyspnoea

Rubrics:

- Cough, night, 1 to 4 a.m.
- Cough, night, 3 a.m.
- Cough, night 3 to 4 a.m.
- Tickling in the larynx from cough
- Tickling in the larynx from cough, 3 to 4 a.m.
- Sticking in the larynx from cough, 1 to 4 a.m.
- Stinging or burning in the larynx from cough
- Stitching in the larynx from cough, evening
- Hacking, violent, hollow, hoarse, deep, dry
- Ag: eating, motion, excitement, getting feet cold
- Amel: diarrhea, frequent stool
- Dyspnea
- Agg: midnight, after 3 a.m.
- Agg: lying down, impossible
- Agg: ascending
- Amel: sitting bent forward

Links 3/93, pg. 24-25, Alfons Geukens, Bufo and Epilepsy, Down's Syndrome

- Most children with Down's syndrome are Bufo children – you will never cure these children but you can treat their physical symptoms and change their character so much that they can make contact with the outside world or don't get attacks of anger anymore.

- Feeble-minded children with neurological problems, especially epileptic attacks, and also acne.

Symptoms: Epileptic attacks – primary generality of Bufo, one of the most important remedies.

Gait, staggering

> Extremities, awkwardness.
>
> Extremities, in-coordination.
>
> Limited mental development, difficulties understanding.
>
> Childish appearance.
>
> Stupid, foolish appearance.

Impatience – never sits still, cannot wait, has to be be busy all the time

> Anger from being misunderstood.
>
> Eyes turn upwards – an expression of autism.
>
> Children start masturbating early.
>
> Memory about certain things may be remarkable – card games, dates, numbers, etc. Acne – Bufo is an important remedy in acne, like Bovista.

Guiding symptoms

Patients most sensitive to Bufo are usually intellectually **retarded** and have a child-like mind. They laugh and cry for no apparent reason. These patients are often depraved and **obsessed with sex.** May be talented in one area. Lazy, sleepy look or look stupid. Pornographers.

Modalities

Worse in warm room and on awakening.

Better from bathing or cold air or from putting feet in hot water.

Study Guide

Main Areas of Pathology

Lymphangitis –After a cut or bite an infection with red/blue k up the arm. Pain runs in streaks up the arm or leg. **Prominent lines of lymphangitis**.

Backwardness at school – A **progressive deterioration of the intellectual faculties** ranging from confusion and loss of memory to complete imbecility with **sexual obsessions**.

Epilepsy – people having seizures assume a toad-like aspect

Comparisons - Person reasons like a child, talks like a child, whimpers like a child, cries like a child, wants to be petted like a child just as with Baryta carbonica

Case 1: - The New England Journal of Homeopathy
Fall/Winter 1998, Vol.7 No.2, Frank Gruber MD

Mary is a 42 year old mildly retarded woman who came to my office with her sister in April of 1997 with a chief complaint of epileptic seizures. She was taking Tegretol 400 mg. each morning and had been on that medication for about 3 years. Prior to that she had been on 4-5 different seizure medications in an attempt to control her seizures. The medications, including the Tegretol, did not control the seizures.

Earlier in her life Mary had grand mal seizures. Currently they are focal seizures which consist of twitching starting in the left hand, moving up the left arm and continuing upwards to the face, especially around the mouth and eye. They are usually on the right side of the face. She usually does not have twitching in the legs and does not lose consciousness during these types of seizures. She does still occasionally have grand mal seizures during which she does lose consciousness. The seizures last for a minute or so and leave her with no adverse affects afterwards.

The seizures started at age 14 right after menarche. While they can occur at any time of the month, they continue to be aggravated by the menses. They worsen mainly before the menses but can also be somewhat worse right after. They are not so prevalent *during* the menses. They are worse during stress. The menses are not regular but never occur more than once a month.

Mary also has scoliosis and has a Harrington rod to support her spine. She has a history of very mild osteoarthritis of the left hand and both ankles.

Mary is a very affable, pleasant woman who seems eager to please. I meet her in the waiting room where she is sitting reading a paperback book. I ask her what she's reading and she mentions that it's a romance novel. She responds easily to my questions, volunteers information to the point of being quite chatty and talks loudly in an animated way.

It seems that Mary was premature and that she almost died at birth, although neither she nor her sister know the details. They just know that Mary "didn't get enough oxygen in the womb." She was slow learning to walk and talk and was always in special education classes in school.

Mary lives with her mother, who has been ill for a long time. She essentially waits on her mom hand and foot. Mary is normally easy going but can get very stubborn or even have tantrums if she doesn't want to do something. She can be sensitive and easily offended. She watches children's TV shows.

Mostly Mary reads romance novels. She has 3 bookcases full of paperback romance novels. I note that while I am putting symptoms into the computer and shift attention from her for a minute or two, she opens her romance novel and begins to read. She describes the novels as "very racy" and smiles. She denies masturbating.

Mary has difficulty with spelling but her memory is good. All of her senses seem slightly off to her, especially her hearing and vision. Her balance is also slightly off. Sometimes she has a tendency to fall slightly to the left while walking or standing.

David Mundy Seminar, June 14/99, Vancouver

Study Guide

Video case – male, age 21, interviewed in front of a class, mostly women. Speech is indistinct, mumbling. Chronic ear infection with hearing loss. Cheesy smelling discharges. Tonsillitis as a child. Keeps repeating the word 'infection'. Pretended he couldn't hear in university – cunning, deceitful. Asked about what he thinks caused his ear problems – "I'm not too sure" followed by a long pause – means he is sure, but isn't saying – he's hiding something. Says he chose to work in the family business, wasn't pushed into it – actually the opposite is true. Married his girlfriend when she got pregnant – said he'd already chosen to marry her, wasn't pushed into it – actually the opposite is true. Recently became a Christian, realized things in his family weren't normal. His father is key to the case – he talks a lot about how he was 'brought up' and about 'breaking away' from his father's influence. Unusual situation between sister and his father – father took photos of sister in various stages of undress. Father gave him pornographic material when he was 8. That's when his ear infections began. Was fascinated with pornography – only gave it up 2 months ago although he'd been a Christian for a year by that point. Father is a Buddhist – doesn't support his Christianity. Thinks of sex as separate from love – something you do alone. Masturbates 3 times a day. Wife is his first sexual relationship, but he's confused by sex and love. He says he's "gone off" his girlfriend since she got pregnant. Sexual desire gone since he got married. Feels under pressure to perform but would rather masturbate. "I'm not ashamed of my body or anything like that" but "I have to urinate in a private cubicle". Mistakes about his sexual orientation – "I'm not attracted to men or anything like that." Talks about not having had girlfriends or boyfriends. "I'm not attracted to the other sex" (i.e. this indicates the female sex). High IQ, seems intelligent.

- Confirming keynote: he has infections around his nails, hangnails.

- Analysis: He was revealing as well as secretive – shameless. He wants instant sexual gratification in private. Sexual depravity. Frequent masturbation. Like an animal – separates sex from love. Infections also indicate Bufo Rana. Very childlike in the things he says. Sexually and emotionally immature. Shameless.

- Remedy: Bufo Rana 200c one dose.

- Results: Major improvements physically and emotionally. His whole attitude towards sex changed – more interested in sex with his wife now. "I'm like a rabbit now." Watching videos on love and sexual intimacy. Left his father's business – broke from his father's influence. Became quite charming after the remedy - kiss a frog and become Prince Charming! Voice is no longer indistinct, much clearer.

- Comments: Bufo Rana does not have to be mentally slow or retarded (stereotype is of low intellect, retardation). They can be normal intelligent people, or very talented in one particular area (i.e. musicians), but sexually or emotionally retarded.

- Phatak: "depravity due to bad inheritance" – i.e. the way he was brought up

BAPTISIA TINCTORIA
(Wild indigo)

- Acute illnesses like severe influenza, malaria, typhoid, serious infections, septicemia, etc.

- Great exhaustion, restlessness, and chilliness.

- Great drowsiness, may fall asleep while talking.

- May seem to be in a stupor, as if drugged or comatose.

- May have the feeling that they are "scattered in bits", children describe it as "all in bits", as though legs and arms are not connected to body, as if body parts are fragmented.

- Thoughts may also be scattered, confused, hard to pull them together.

- Muscles feel sore and aching, stiff and heavy.

- Bed feels to hard and body feels bruised.

- Moves about restlessly, trying to get comfortable – or too weak to move at all.

- Unable to sleep because can't get thoughts together, feels too fragmented.
- May become delirious, incoherent ramblings.
- May have problems breathing with feeling of suffocation.
- Great thirst, but can only take small amounts.
- Offensive discharges – breath, sweat, stools, urine.
- Mouth tastes foul and may be bleeding from mouth, black blood.
- May be needed after typhus vaccinations.

Constitutionally: (SO)

- People who have been shattered, fragmented, cut off
- Confusion of identity.
- Loss of thoughts.

Constitutional Themes from IFH Case Proceedings 1993, p. 281

- Fragmentation, of being in pieces, divided, scattered, of trying to put the pieces back together but not being able to do so.
- Despair that the pieces will never come together and that the center will never be found.
- Sense of separation or disconnection from himself, from reality, from other people, from the outside world – may be a sense of being outside himself, or there being another self outside himself.
- Inability to sleep because of scattered feeling in his mind. Kent says: "He cannot sleep because he cannot get the pieces together. If he could get matters together, he could go to sleep, and these parts that are talking to each other keep him awake."

- Stupor – mind is gone, confusion, in constant argument with all his parts.

- Downward motion, moving down into the mud, descending into a pit, a sewer, a cess-pool, into the mud, etc. Kent talks about "in a mine, in a swamp, down in the mud, in the sewers, foul gases."

- Brain feels toxic, congested. Blood feels poisoned. Kent talks about confusion and blood accumulation in the brain with a toxic feeling.

- Restlessness, movement.

- History of pneumonia in some patients.

- Very offensive discharges in acute illnesses – breath, stool, urine, sweat.

- Soreness and heaviness and aching of muscles (fibromyalgia).

- Bleeding from the mouth, black blood.

- Heaviness of the head – feels too large, heavy, numb.

Case 1: – Schizophrenia – Theme of fragmentation, of scattering: "Parts of my body are awake, but parts are asleep. Reality gets too fragmented. Everything was falling apart; trying to keep it all together. I can't get them together. They don't come together. They don't stick together. I couldn't understand what people were saying to me, like parts of me were just shut down. Different parts are battling; different pieces of the puzzle. Sometimes I try to gather them together to appear like I'm normal. Most of me is scattered all over the place, like one leg here and the other over there. A state of fragments. So many levels disconnected from each other, most often warring with each other. I can't put it all together. I try to pull the different aspects together. I feel a sense of losing all the parts of me. There is no core – just components. I feel scattered all over the place. No connection. No way to pull together. Crazy feelings in my head and a sense of disconnection with all the other parts. To sleep I try to focus – there are so many things racing around. I try to focus everything together, to pull all the pieces together. One part behaves like this, and the other part says behave like that. And there are many parts saying this and that. I don't know who I am. I am so many different parts. I don't know how to gather the portions together. So fragmented. I shatter into tiny, tiny pieces. I am unable to connect the pieces. Parts of me are everywhere in the room. I once went to a House of Mirrors – it was the closest expression of how I experience myself – my head in one mirror, and one arm here, another arm in a different place, all separate." Theme of separation from self, from reality, disconnection from others: "Everything can become unreal, nothing makes sense. She kissed my face, not really me." Feeling separate from family, disconnected from everyone. Also had: bleeding mouth, blood oozing from the mouth, bleeding is black with a foul smell. Also describes a toxic feeling in his brain, a feeling of congestion in the brain, a sewer in his head, a toxic polluted feeling. "The blood is stuck in my brain." Also, theme of being in a pit or in mud is strong. He describes his room as being like a pit, down in the basement, with a foul smell, putrid, toxic, decaying, feels like a dark muddy hole, going into the sewer at night. Rearranging things compulsively as a way of making order.

Case 2: – chronic fatigue, fibromyalgia, food allergies, chronic inability to sleep. "I think I am covering all parts of me – but I am sure there are parts I am missing. It feels that way anyway. I get completely scattered with any type of upset. Now things are scattered all over the place. I don't know where I am. I feel I am spinning apart, things are splitting off all over the place. I can't sleep, anxious, like some part of me is wanting to sleep, and the parts of my body are just restless and can't get in sync somehow. I just watched myself falling to pieces. Felt like I was dissolving all over the place. Too easily shattered. Feeling of disconnection from myself, as if my body parts were not connected. I feel all over the place. All dispersed. No center. Desperately trying to gather things together. I'm afraid of losing control. I feel I have lost control and all the pieces are scattered about. I feel I am desperately trying to collect all the pieces and pull myself into a whole again, to integrate it all. I felt so separate from everything. It feels like my brain isn't working. I feel confused all the time. Thoughts disappear. My intellectual abilities dissolved." Describes childhood sexual abuse: "I really was a mess. Shattered. I really didn't know who I was or what I was. I felt so disconnected and scattered. Sleepless, trying to find some continuity, something that would pull all the pieces together." Heaviness of the head. Describes her family: "a lot of dark, deep, low, cess-pool type secrets, like an infectious mass of toxins in our family." After remedy: "I feel like I might be pulling out of the mud."

Case 3: – Acute case of flu and tonsillitis. "I can't collect myself. I feel so dispersed. I feel really shattered. Suddenly I am down again; tired and wading through the mud. Incredible confusion. Who am I? Am I someone else. Mind in a stupor. A feeling of being all over the place – part of me wanting this and the other part not wanting it. I feel weird. All over the place – part here and part there. No continuity. I'm falling to pieces."

- Mainly seen in **acute serious infections**, but it may occur in less serious infections as well. The key is **rapid onset** of these septic states.

- **Stupor, falls asleep while being spoken to or in mid sentence**

- **Confused as if drunk.**

- **Illusion that the body is double**

- limbs separated and conversing with each other, can't sleep because body seems scattered about and cannot collect pieces.

Pathology:

Typhoid fever, epidemic influenza, Mumps, Pharyngitis, Sepsis, Tonsilitis, Dysentery, threatened Abortion, Apoplexy., Appendicitis., Biliousness., Brain softening., Cancer., Consumption., Diphtheria., Enteric fever., Eye, affections of., Gall-bladder, affections of., Gastric fever., Headache, bilious., Hectic fever., Hysteria, Influenza., Stricture of Esophagus., Plague., Relapsing fever., Sewer gas-poisoning., Shivering., Stomatitis., Tabes mesenterica., Tinea capitis, Tongue ulcerated., Typhus., Variola., Worms.

Psychology

- This remedy works in acute illnesses when indicated.

- A state of mental confusion where the person is in a constant argument with his/her body parts. The person feels that there is two of him/her and will talk about the other person in bed with them. In this state of delirium, the patient is trying to put him/herself back together again.

- Schizophrenia.

Generals:

> All exhalations and discharges fetid. The odor is cadaverous, pungent, and penetrating

> In whatever position the patient lies, the parts rested upon feel sore and bruised

> Ulceration of mucosal membranes

Head:

- Stupid, besotted expression to the face
- Red, dusky congestion of the face

Throat:

> Painless sore throat; tonsils – dusky red inflammation or ulcer of the throat

Stomach:

> Esophagus feels constricted down to stomach, can only swallow liquids

> Distended abdomen, with tenderness

> Eyes:

1. Congestion; Redness; Pains in eyes and back of eyes

Modalities

< On waking, walking, open air, cold wind, autumn or hot weather.

PYROGENIUM

Infected wounds with fever.

- Puerperal septicemia – severe blood infection after childbirth – almost a specific for this condition.

- When the pulse rate is too fast for a moderate fever - can hear his own heart – or too slow for a high fever (i.e. disparity between the pulse rate and the temperature).

- Aching through the whole body; sore, bruised feeling.

- Bronchitis, pneumonia.

- High fevers – reportedly curative in delirium with symptoms similar to Baptisia (RM).

- Great restlessness during fever.

- Offensiveness of bodily discharges.

BED FEELS TOO HARD. (B),nash).

Loquacious .

Consciousness of heart, palpitations.

> motion (changing position), heat, hot bath, pressure.

Pathology

Abscess, cellulitis, influenza, lymphangitis, puerperal fever or endometriosis, sepsis, skin ulcers.

Comparisons: Bapt, Rhus-t, Ars, Sulph, Ail

MYRISTICA

Infections after physical trauma.

Infections around the nails. Fellons. (Silica, Hepar,)

Suppuration of the middle ear.

Anal fistula.

Case 1: 72 year old female. Cracked tooth. Hard swelling on gum about the size of a walnut. Patient says: "It feels numb. Had a fever of 100 for a day. Not sensitive to cold or heat. Impatient with her illness: "I have work to do."

Plan: I gave her **Myristica** 30c two doses a day. In three days the swelling is 95% better, infection all better in four days. Never needed antibiotics.

All the snake remedies can treat systemic infections: Bothrops, Cench, Crot-cas Crot-h, Elaps, Lach, Naja, Vip. Some authors like Farokh Master have expanded on this list.

APPENDIX FOUR

SNAKE REMEDIES

All of the snake remedies are extremely useful. I use at least one of them a week. It is worth learning all of them. They often suffer from excessive attachment which brings them great suffering. To learn more: <u>Snakes and Simillimum</u> by Farokh Master. Also: <u>Insight into the Consciousness of Snake Remedies</u> by Sadhana Thakkar. Also reference Kent, Clark, Nash and Boericke.

Cenchris Contortrix
Copperhead

Suspicious, fear of rape, feels persecuted. Worse from tight clothing about the neck. Salivation during sleep. Chilliness. Right sided symptoms. Feels abandoned, not supported. Has to feels secure and safe at home. Needs a relationship to feel safe. May look like Pulsatilla.

Anger from being rejected. Intolerant of tight clothing.

Here is Sadhana Thakkar's <u>Insight into the Consciousness of Snake Remedies</u> summary of this remedy: *Insecurity, fears to be abandoned, feels forsaken, rejected, sad, neglected, alone, insignificant, not good enough, worthless, a failure, hurt and punished. Crave a relationship and affection (Puls, Lac-can). Act polite, makes apologies. Lump sensation in the throat.*

React to this feeling by competing for attention or with jealous rage.

Wants to be noticed as a special hero, wants to act out to prove they are better than others, on guard to do battle, very quick to anger to attack back. Anger if see abuse or injustice. Wants to prove they are important. Anger at insults wants to attack back but will try to suppress the anger as he does not want to be rejected.

Able to kill animals. Fear she may hurt others as her anger is so strong.

Fear others will try to attack them, kill them, chase them, rape them.

May be a case of sexual abuse, feels alone, not good enough, wants to kill the perpetrator.

Ailments from injustice tries to prove self and redeem reputation.

So much anxiety can't sleep with palpitations.

Worse cold damp weather. Worse hot damp weather.

Dreams of robbers, dangerous places, being attacked, rape, burned, sexual dreams. Wake with a start or in a trance.

Wakes 3 to 5 am. Desires raw meet, cold beer, wine, spices.

No sense of smell or taste. Hives, urticaria. Epistaxis. Clotted menses.

PNS: Weepy, breasts tender, lymph glands tender, night sweats.

Allergy to metals. Hypoglycemic. Better from physical activity. (Thakkar)

Coma, presentment of death. Delusions she will be sent to the asylum, feels someone is behind him. Feels persecuted. Fear to go to sleep. Forsaken, jealous. Throat choking on going to sleep. Respiration arrested on going to sleep.

Right ovary affected. Difficult empty swallowing and swallowing of solids, swallowing of liquids is easy. Throat pain is better from warm drinks. Symptoms come on at once from lying down. Aggravated from 3 p.m. To 8 p.m., gradually better toward midnight.

Worse from tight clothing like other snake remedies. General distrust, suspicious and fear especially of rape. Sensitive to cold but desires cold drinks. Right sided.

Farokh Master from his book: <u>Snakes to Simillimum</u>: (highly recommended text): Conflict with sexuality after rape or from strict parental or religious upbringing. Feel strong sexual feelings but then withdraw due to fears and suspicion.

Suppressed anger. (Staph) Curious about different topics. Like to read. Anxiety with chattering of the teeth and trembling.

Extremely selfish, envious and jealous from being unloved.

Not able to give, uncharitable.

Sexual attraction and eroticism – they put a lot of energy into attracting a partner but then they have a fear to be raped. Really into sexual gratification.

Suspicious. Believe others are plotting against them. Feel they can't trust their family. Feel betrayed by family and friends.

Frequent sighing. Procrastination. Chilly, better from warm coverings.

Periodicity. Worse in spring. Tends to faint easily. Worse on waking like diarrhea, headache, palpitations.

Salivation at night during sleep. Metallic taste in mouth. Besotted expression (Lach, Bapt, Gels).

Craves salted bacon. Nausea better from ice. Feels whole body is enlarged.

Swelling and edema. Cellulites.
Worse at 3 pm. (Ang, Apis, Bell, Chin-sul, Thuj), esp fever, chill, cough, heart symptoms, urinary symptoms.

Periodicity marked, complaints at same time every day.

Worse in the Spring (Lach).

Tendency to faint. Worse on waking: diarrhea, cough, headache, palpitations etc.
Hypertensive headaches, sinusitis headaches. Pain in occiput, root of nose, forehead during menses, above the eyes during menses, left frontal

eminence extending to the right side and teeth.

Lacrimation with cough (Squill). Twitching of left eye-lid. Swelling of eye lids like a bag of water.

Allergic rhinitis and sinusitis. Swollen turbinates. Bloated face, eyes dull, heavy look.

Chapped and cracked lips.
Mottled face (Crot-c, Bapt, Lach). Expression besotted. Swelling of upper lip.

Can swallow only liquids, solid food causes gagging.

Gagging from cough (Agar, Cina, Ip). Cough from exertion.
Throat pain worse from empty swallowing and better from warm drinks.

Chronic pharyngitis, from hose dust, coloring agents. Choking on clearing the throat, from clothing, on going to sleep, better from bowing the head. Tries to hawk up mucous, constant swallowing. Albumen mucous, bloody, gelatinous, tenacious, defficult to detach, draws from post nares.

Craves salty bacon (Calc-p, Mez, Sanic, Tub.) Extreme thirst for cold water, small quantities. Nausea better from ice.

Vomits undigested food and white mucous. Abdomen sensitiveness to clothing tight (Bov, Calc, Nux-v). Diaphragm is sensitive to touch. Abdomen is very distended after eating. Sensation of a band around the abdomen.

Sensation abdomen is full of water. Colon tender to touch. Hard on left side. Chronic mucous colitis. IBS. Ulcerative colitis. Diarrhea on waking, driving out of bed.

Involuntary stool on passing flatus and during sleep.

Prolapse of rectum. Frequent urination after mental exertion. Involuntary urination with cough. Pain left kidney, better drawing up legs.

Copious menses. Ovarian neuralgia worse before menses. Herpes labia.

Palpitations when lying of right side. All cardiac symptoms are worse on lying. Anxiety on going to sleep. Fear of death with heart symptoms. Fear to go to sleep.

Restless in bed, moves about a lot. Sensation heart is falling into an abdomen. Anxiety about heart and patient says: "I shall die" over and over.

Worse lying on left side, better to lie on right side.
Arrested respiration on going to sleep. Stops breathing on going to sleep unless he sits up and bends forward (Kali-bi, Spong).
In sleep feels suffocated and choking.

Nates cold at night in bed.
Wants to cross feet or feet up when sitting.

Sour perspiration. Abscesses.
(Farokh Master)

Guiding Symptoms
Marked alteration of moods. Restlessness due to SUSPICION of constant threats towards oneself.

VIVID DREAMS - horrible & lascivious.

Increased sexual desire. Cardiorespiratory complaints (dyspnea, angina pectoris, palpitations).

Excessive swelling. Anxiety about the heart, when lying in bed.
Modalities & Generals

Mental and physical restlessness. Right sided symptoms. Intolerant of tight clothing. Whole body seems enlarged to bursting.

Allergies in spring. Forgetful, absent-minded, alternating moods.

Desire: Cold drinks; in evening with dry mouth & for small quantities, salt, bacon, to wander.

Aversion: breakfast, food.
Worse: Pressure, lying down, afternoon and night, being disturbed.

Psychology
Constant threat from the surroundings and to ones own chastity.
Extremely SUSPICIOUS and mistrustful about the people who are around her.

Anger from interruption; averse to being disturbed - time passes too slowly.

Delusions people are behind or beside him or that he is being persecuted.

Dreams of being pursued and bitten by wild animals/snakes, of frightful nakedness, rape, being pursued for the purpose of threats, of indecent behavior between man and woman, of animals copulating.

Censorious. Forebodings; presentiment of sudden death. Anxiety in evening in bed while lying.

Fear of being bitten by snake. Aversion to domestic duties. Desire to wander, restless. Forgetful, absent-minded, alternating moods.

JEALOUSLY.

Pathology
Extreme realization of the Heart - feels DISTENDED, fills whole chest, as if it fell down in abdomen, fluttering under left scapula.
Anxiety about the heart with palpitations, fluttering sensation, pulse rate increased and feeble.

Sudden, SHARP STITCHING pain in the heart followed by a dull pain.

Diarrhea consistency of bran porridge, gray color, gushing, frequent, watery, with a dark sediment at first without pain then great pain before stool < PM.

Sputtering flatus with bloating of abdomen after the smallest amount of food.

Dyspnea as if dying from, anxiety, during sleep (Sleep apnea).

Suffocating feeling after lying down in the evening.

Must lie with the head drawn back or will choke and suffocate.

Frequent sighing. Dry, hacking cough, coming on at 3PM, continues throughout the evening.

Cough < walking fast, upstairs, at night, after retiring, causes watering of left eye.

Comparison
Arsenic: dyspnea, mental & physical restlessness, thirst for small quantities of water. Anxiety, blue in the face, better to bend foreward. Septicemia.

Lach: necessity for loose clothing, jealousy, suspicious, more loquacious.
Ignatia: fear of something deadly happening, mood changes.

Croc-sat: Alternating moods.
Crotalus: Lost sense of position and direction.
Puls: Forsaken, desire for relationship.

Case One:
Male, age 29, recurrent colds and coryza. Also dyspnea every summer. Likes to spend money freely, doesn't worry about tomorrow. His passion is watching horror movies – "I like the suddenness – a hand coming out of the grave, somebody stabbing someone suddenly" Absent-minded, forgetful – when driving a car he doesn't know how he got where he was – has had several accidents because his mind wanders while driving. Dislikes doing things with his family. Likes blue movies, fantasizes about it. Loves traveling – fascinated by greenery and animals. Fear of water. Dreams of snakes in the water. Dreams of being attacked by a snake and then drowning. Dreams of being chased, pursued. Dreams of naked women. Mistrustful of his family and friends. Envious and suspicious about his young brother. Rubrics: Fear of death (i.e. from his dreams), Dreams of naked people, Dreams of snakes, Forgetful as to where she is going, Absentminded, Envy, Suspicious, mistrustful, Domestic duty, aversion to; Indifference, duties to; Wander, desire to; Clothing, intolerance of. Remedy: Cenchris 30c. Result: Aggravation of dyspnea, a sensation of choking at the collar. Mood was better. Sinus problems improved gradually. Remedy repeated twice in next year with good results. (Links 1/96, pg. 25-26, Sudhir Baldota)
Master, F.J. <u>Snakes in Homeopathic Grass</u> . Jain Publishing Co., New Delhi, India 1994:
Inability to respond or act when necessary.

Characteristic Particulars
- causes generalized swelling especially of upper eyelids (D/D Kali-c).
- causes paralysis.
- with swelling of the whole body feels it is enlarged as if it would burst.
- hate tight clothing – feels unbearable
- restlessness, nervousness, thirst for small quantities of water (D/D Ars).
(F. Master)

Crotalus cascavella

Large area of urticaria or hives all over the body. Sensation of coldness in stomach after eating (Elaps). Can't tolerate tight clothing on throat and abdomen. Delusions or fear of ghosts/voice/someone beside or behind them. Keynote: Burning hives over large areas or parts of the body is characteristic. Cardiac symptoms, hypertension. Passive hemorrhage of dark blood. Dreams of Spiders. Right sided paralysis. Weakness from pleasure. Feels isolated, unloved and forsaken. Feels persecuted. (Chin, Cocaine, Dros, Kali-br, Lac-leo, Vesp, Zinc). Suppressed anger leading to deeds of rage. (Anac, Bell, China, Con Hyos, Nux, Stram). Cruelty, desire to cut. Destructive. Feels cheated or let down by others close to him. i.e. stabbed in the back. Lots of grudges and feels vengeful but feel they don't have the power to retaliate. Destructive but also fear to be harmed. Duty bound and so suffers from pangs of guilt. Egotistical and haughty like Platina. Abusive and ambitious. Amorous, censorious, jealous, malicious. Feels forsaken and neglected. Delusion of being a great person, superior and tall. (F. Master)

Crotalus horridus
Rattlesnake

Associated to low septic states and a general disorganization of the blood caused by septic toxaemia or zymotic diseases (low grade infectious diseases).
A hemorrhagic or cancerous constitution in diseases that are of a putrid type coming on with great rapidity and reaching putridity very quickly.

Marked Features
- *Periodicity*– every spring as the warm weather comes on their. Symptoms get worse from:
- *Sleep*– tend to sleep into aggravations. Pains that come on after sleep.
- *Trembling*– of the limbs, tremulous. Weakness. Protruding the tongue it quivers. Muscles that twitch.

Hemorrhages
- cases that come on with great rapidity, breaking down the blood, relaxation of the blood vessels, bleeding from all the orifices of the body and rapidly increasing unconsciousness. Stroke. Septic hemorrhage.
-a thin, dark fluid decomposed blood that is difficult to coagulate, hence clots are not usually detected in the hemorrhage. Hemorrhage of the retina and eccymotic spots in different parts of the body.
- gastric hemorrhage in which large quantities of almost black, water, sanguinous blood is brought up
- bleeding from the anus that is black, thin coffee-ground stools.

Offensiveness
- bleeding with putridity,
- diphtheria,
- Ebola (also give 30c three doses a day for three days to prevent this illness).
- typhoid with bleeding and putridity,
- evacuations and discharges are offensive,
- breath offensive,
- stomach cancer, vomiting large quantities of bile mixed with blood,
- stomach ulcers with dark hemorrhage that does not coagulate(Salix alba),
- after hemorrhage the body looks like wax, anemic, pale yellow. The body appears mottled black and blue mixed with yellow. Yellow color of the eyes,

Constriction
- sensation of constriction of the throat, only able to swallow liquid food,
- tends to be more sensitive on the skin on the right side of the body,
- can not bear clothes around the stomach,
-produces profound nervous shock and prostration (expect to see if

bitten),
- marked trembling,
- disorganization of fluids and tissue – start to break down,
- right sided symptoms,
- malignant septic states,
- Yellow Fever, Cholera.

Mentals
- snappy + irritable (Nux-v).
- furious at slightest annoyance (Nux-vom)
- fear of death, thoughts constantly dwelling on death.
- fear of evil/danger.
- desire to travel – due to fear of evil/danger.
- suspicious of friends.
- feels surrounded by enemies.
- antipathy to his family (nasty).
- loquacious.
- stumbles over words.
- when down and debilitated appear intoxicated.
- mild delirium, stupor, drowsiness.
- aversion to certain persons/members of family
- death thoughts of.
- delusions surrounded by enemies.
- suspicious, escape attempts to.

Aversion to family members, sensitive to certain persons. **Desire for company**, craves attention, **LOUD.** Dreams of an enormous hairy spider which tried to climb on him. *Mental exertion aggravates*; indolence, aversion to mental work, sensitive to reading (ADD), mistakes in reading and writing. **Loquacious but muttering**, talking to himself. Fury at trifles, Snappish and **irritable.** Vivaciousness.

Image: *Fat, robust, besotted, hungry drunkard, purple face, delirium tremors.*

Generalities: Very sensitive to changes in temperature. <BEGINNING OF SLEEP, sleeps into aggravation. < RIGHT SIDE.

Food and drinks: PORK and ALCOHOL, craves intoxicating drinks, cannot resist.

Pathology: Hemorrhagic tendencies, from any orifice. Passive, dark, unclotted blood. Hemorrhagic fevers.

MALIGNANT conditions, SEPSIS, boils, carbuncles and eruptions.

Case: 17 y old female, jeans black hair, overweight. Has **ADD,** can't learn anything. The most important thing is her social life. She was adopted when she was 2y old. Her mother was 14y old when she gave birth and had abortions prior to that. Angry *with her step parents. Yells at them and hits her mother.* Loves junk food. Likes swimming and animals. Very impulsive. She'll do anything to please other people especially her friends (she would steel money from parents and than give it to her friends). Low self esteem. She is **LOUD,** talks a lot, *can't stop talking (Loquacious)*, acts like clown in class b/**c she wants attention and recognition.** Compliment very important to her. *Three inch chocolate brown area on her chest.* **NOSEBLEEDS** since she was toddler, **Right sided.** Very closed, does not open up easily even to closest friends. *She's warm but when it is warm outside she's really cold.* Angry from contradiction, short tempered, get mad over dumbest stuff. Likes SNAKES, hates *spiders*(Arachnophobia)can't stand holding a toy spider.

Naja

Similar to Lachesis however, the hemorrhagic and septic tendencies are notably absent and the valvular and cardiac symptoms are prominent.

Exaggerates problems; obsession, dwells on unimportant or minor problems.

Case 1: Main complaint is heart palpitations, irregular heart beat and anger. She hated her husband and therefore got divorced from him. But now since he got married to someone else she hates him even more and has become obsessed with him. She feels that he is doing her wrong, that is; he is causing her suffering by getting married again. In the repertory we see the symptoms: Mind, will contradiction of: Naja and Mind, antagonism with self: Naja. This described her well, if she hates him so much why can't she let go of him? After Naja 30c once a week for two months she is much better, peaceful, able to let go of her husband, no more anger, heart is feeling well with no more palpitations. This brings up a good point. The most common thing a patient will say after you give them the simillimum is that they feel peaceful.

Constriction of the throat, intolerant of collars. Sensation of suffocation at night, wakes up gasping. Aggravation from lying on left side.

Aggravation at night. Valvular lesions or disorders – the tendency for valvular lesions is so strong that it is almost a specific in valvular lesions in children.

Cardiac problems (angina, arrhythmia, endocarditis, congestive heart failure). Violent palpitations, < exertion, < talking, < lying on left side. Asthma or cardiac asthma, < night. Left ovarian cysts and pains.

David Mundy, June 14/99, Seminar in Vancouver

Case: Female, car accident, blow on back of head, whiplash, back pain. Wouldn't talk much in the interview, said very little. Fear of high places. Feelings of bitterness towards mother after a bitter, confrontational divorce. Religious – feels well when at peace with her creator. Tried Mag-mur, which can be very reserved, but didn't work. Next interview – extremely strong sense of duty to mother in spite of her feelings of bitterness towards her.

The most dutiful snake is Naja – the highest sense of duty to the family – compelled to do their duty even if the person is treating them dreadfully.

Although snake people are usually loquacious, they can also be very quiet, even silent. Naja is one that can be quiet, still, noble. Naja can be quite subdued – DD: Pulsatilla.

Believe they are someone of note. Delusion – she has suffered wrong; Delusion – injured by surroundings (or other people); Delusion – that she is neglected, that she deserves better.

Delusion – wrong, everything is, but can't be rectified.

Antagonism of self – this means a conflict of the self, a battle going on inside the self, an internal battle (e.g. Shall I be good or bad?) Anac, Sepia, Aurum ……… note that this is similar to Will, contradiction of – which is an external action opposed to internal will …… so in this case she has an internal conflict, she can't stand her mother but her strong sense of duty requires her to help her mother (Note: Radar lists Naja under Will, Contradiction of … not under Antagonism of Will)

Fear or fascination with snakes. Dreams of being chased, dreams of flying; Dreams of fire, fascination with fire. Predisposition to back and neck injuries. Sensation of being struck at the back of the head. Chilly. Affects the heart. Less septic, pushy, offensive, malignant than Crot-h.

Vipera berus

Lower limbs feel they will burst when they are allowed to hand down.

Blood and Blood Vessels
 - Inflammation of blood vessels.
 - Hemorrhages.
 - Paralysis especially of lower extremities: paralysis moves upwards.
 - Affects kidney:haematuria.
 - Affects liver: enlargement sever pain extends to Right shoulder + hip). Cirrhosis of liver with black spots on the abdomen.

Keynotes
 - Pain in extremities so part must be elevated.
 - Pain is unbearable as if it would burst.
 - Inflammation of veins in legs, acute phlebitis).
 - Boils or carbuncles, septic ulcers of legs).
 - Edema of legs with tendency to ulcerate in diabetes and heart disease.

Mental
- Irrational talking, wild sexual excitement, adultery, everything that is prohibited becomes a temptation. Hatred and revenge, rage and fury. Jealousy. Competitive, increased ambition but when not achieved he becomes gloomy and discontented. Forsaken feeling leading to despair, discouragement, dullness, irritability and sadness. Indifference. Egotism can't bear any contradiction. Lingering guilt about past sins, feels pursued. Fear will be poisoned.
- Delirium raving. Speech inarticulate, incoherent.

Mental confusion, delirium, dullness, muttering. Torpor. Premonition of death. Arrested development in children mentally (Bart.c, Calc.c, Tub,Calc.p). < cold. < touch. Worse from clothing, tears it off. **Varicose veins. Thrombosis (formation of clots).**

Acute or chronic phlebitis (inflammation of vein).

Aggravation from leg hanging down, needs to elevate it.

Swelling, bursting sensation, or tremendous pain when the leg is hanging down. Lymph edema especially the right side with bloody vomiting and diarrhea.

IFH Case Proceedings 1993, Jeff Baker, pg. 45

Patient's left tibia was crushed in a car accident in Mexico, developed a local and systemic infection. Wound site became gangrenous. Refused amputation. On antibiotics for 3 years. Multiple surgeries. Six years later, his main symptom is swelling when standing (3). "It feels puffy, like it's filling up." Tremendous need to elevate his leg. Even sits on the floor while waiting in line in supermarket. Used to have drug addictions. Frequently cleared his throat. Twitch around the eyes.

Drug addiction especially by injection. Wet gangrene. Pains extend upward. Face ⁓ Excessively swollen. Lips and tongue swollen, livid, protruding. Tongue dry, brown, black. Speech difficult. Liver ⁓ VIOLENT PAIN IN ENLARGED LIVER, with jaundice and fever;

extends to shoulder and hip. Extremities ⊼ When they are allowed to hang down, it seems as if they would BURST, and the pain is unbearable. Varicose veins and acute phlebitis. Severe cramps in lower extremities. Skin ⊼ livid. Skin peels in larges plates. Lymphangioma, boils, carbuncles, with BURSTING sensation, relieved by elevating parts. Ailments of menopause. Edema of glottis. Poly-neuritis, polio-myelitis – causes a temporary increase in reflexes, a paraplegia of the lower extremities extending upwards. Kidneys ⊼ induces hematuria. Cardiac dropsy. Functions of heart, lungs and bladder suddenly cease. Surgical wounds won't heal and open up again. Wounds become gangrenous, bleed, oozing out black offensive sanguinous discharge. Wounds become septic. Pain and weakness of the jaws. Periodicity, symptoms recur annually for years. Sleepiness from pains. Apoplexy and thrombosis. Edema parts become red, hot, hard and tender. Finally become numb. Poliomelitis, motor neuron disease, muscular atrophy, ALS. The paralysis with weakness that extends upwards. Deep tendon reflexes exaggerated. Polyneuritis. Angiosarcoma. Headache with nausea, vomiting. Worse from changes of weather. Paralysis of lids. Vision dim and lost in right eye. Drooping of eye lids. Diabetic retinopathy. Epistaxis with vertigo. Biting of tongue, grinding of teeth. Salivation during stools. Swelling of tongue, fills the whole mouth. Clenched jaw.

Case 1: Leonard (M. A., xxvi. 103) gave Vipera acontica carinata to a lady suffering from climacteric hemorrhage; flow red with dark clots; excessive to prostration and faintness. After diarrhea, greenish and bloody, most violent pain in the enlarged liver, with jaundice and fever, pain extending from liver to shoulder and down to hip; Vipera immediately removed the pain and reduced the liver to its normal size.

Case 2: A kid had smashed his hand with a hammer. It was all swollen up and painful. All these acute remedies passed through my mind. But he was holding his hand up in the air. I asked him to put it down, and he didn't like that one bit. The longer it was down, the worse pain he was in. So I gave him *Vipera.* First. And in less that 24 hours I saw him again and there was no swelling and he had no pain. This was after his getting progressively worse for three days. (JC)

APPENDIX FIVE

On-Line Resources

Pharmacies:

Boiron USA: http://www.boironusa.com/

1-800-blu-tube

Boiron Canada: 1-800-461-2066

Stock of the most common remedies.

http://boiron.ca/en/

Hahnemann Laboratories (California)
www.hahnemannlabs.com

Ainsworths (England)
   www.ainsworths.com

Helios Homeopathic Pharmacy: England. A reliable source for almost every remedy. They can also make up new remedies for provings.

http://www.helios.co.uk/

Remedia Homeopathic Pharmacy – Austria

Caries many of the new remedies that are difficult to find.

http://www.remedia.at/homeopathy/index.html

Books, Courses, Software, Journals.

Nature Reveals

Most new and old homeopathic books available to buy within Canada.

http://www.nature-reveals.com/

Homeopathic Educational Services

Most new and old books.

http://www.homeopathic.com/

Books, Online Courses, Radar Software

http://wholehealthnow.com/

www.vithoulkas.com

Repertory Software

Radar Opus :
http://www.archibel.com/homeopathic_software.html

Complete Repertory – available for download online.

http://www.completedynamics.com/

Vithoulkas Compass – available to use online.

http://www.vithoulkascompass.com/

www.wholehealthnow.com

MacRepertory

http://www.kenthomeopathic.com/macrepertory.html

On Line Materia Medica

http://homeoint.org/books3/kentmm/index.htm

ABC homeopathy: https://abchomeopathy.com/

Hpathy.com:

http://hpathy.com/

Video Teaching, Courses

http://www.vithoulkas.com/

Journals

The Homeopathic Academy of Naturopathic Physicians

http://www.hanp.net/simillimum/about

American Journal

http://www.homeopathyusa.org/journal

Spectrum of Homeopathy

http://www.narayana-publishers.com/index.php

Europe

http://www.homeopathyeurope.org/links/homeopathic-links/journals-1/free-journals

Australian Journal:
http://www.njhonline.com/abstract/australian_journal.shtml

Research Updates

Audesapeare collects research articles and posts the papers online.

http://www.audesapere.in/

New Provings

http://www.provings.info/en/einleitung-proving.html

Materia Medica

http://abchomeopathy.com/

http://homeoint.org/books3/kentmm/index.htm

There are countless sites that provide materia medica and toxicology information about individual remedies.

Naturopathic websites:

Homeopathic Academy of Naturopathic Physicians
    www.hanp.net

Homeopathic organizations with websites:

National Center for Homeopathy (USA)
    www.homeopathic.org

Homeopathic websites, local and international:

Homeopathic Internet Resources
www.holisticmed.com/www/homeopathy.html

Homéopathe International (free English books)
http://homeoint.org/english/index.htm
    http://hpathy.com/

End.

ABOUT THE AUTHOR

Steven Olsen ND, DHNAP is a teacher at the Boucher Institute of Naturopathic Medicine. He has been in full-time practice since January of 1988. He is the author of several provings which are included in his books Homeopathy - Nature's Way to Better Health and Arbor Medica.

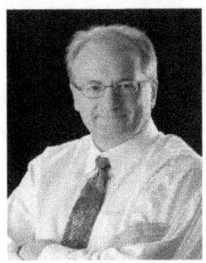

Works Published:

A Case of Hysteria: Simillimum, The Journal of the Homeopathic Academy of Naturopathic Physicians, Winter 1999. Vol, XII, Issue 4.

Trees and Plants That Heal 1997 Proving of five new remedies.

Winning Strategies of Case Analysis: A short course for RADAR and the Vithoulkas Expert System. Co-authored by George Vithoulkas.

A Case of Paranoid Schizophrenia. Proceedings of the IFH 1994 Professional Case Conference.

The Breakdown State of Baryta Carbonica. Proceedings of the IFH 1993 Professional Case Conference.

Anxiety and Costochrondritis. Simillimum, The Journal of the Homeopathic Academy of Naturopathic Physicians, Spring 1993.

A Case of Chronic Tendonitis. Proceedings of the IFH 1992 Professional Case Conference.

Psuedotsuga menziesii, Proving with Cured Cases. IFH Professional Case Conference: 1997, Seattle. WA.

Arbor Medica – vol. One and Two. New provings of tree remedies with cases.

www.ingramcontent.com/pod-product-compliance
Lightning Source LLC
Chambersburg PA
CBHW051758170526
45167CB00005B/1794